Advance Praise

"With great mastery, Peter Fraenkel pulls back the curtain to reveal the inner workings of his three-decade-long practice with the most precarious couples. *Last Chance Couple Therapy* is a curious and illuminating read for therapists, coaches, and clinicians."
—**Esther Perel,** psychotherapist, author, and host of *Where Should We Begin?*

"All couple therapists need to read this amazing book that opens the door to a very important, but overlooked group of couples: those on the brink of divorce or worse, a loveless life together. These couples deserve to see a therapist who uses a research- and theory-based therapy approach to help them restore hope and happiness. Now all couple therapists can reach and help these couples by following the program Dr. Fraenkel presents in this new and exciting book. He is also one of the best writers you will read in the plethora of books on couple therapy, so not only will you learn this exciting new approach, but you will really enjoy reading the book."
—**Howard Markman,** PhD, founder of the PREP approach, and coauthor of *Fighting for Your Marriage*

"This remarkable book, based on more than three decades of clinical work and richly illustrated with many detailed case vignettes, is a must-read for any couple therapist—and not only for those working with seemingly hopeless couples presenting with a long history of failed therapies. Fraenkel's 'open-hearted surgery' approach demonstrates convincingly that by continuously generating a vast range of different creative contexts, even the most entrenched couples get a chance to change their interactions and improve their lives. Amazing!"
—**Prof. Dr. Eia Asen,** Anna Freud Centre and University College London

"Peter Fraenkel's brilliant new book focuses on a crucial, special group of clients in couple therapy, those for whom the therapy really is the last chance. Anchored in his Therapeutic Palette approach that draws from a wide range of therapies, Fraenkel offers a keen understanding of these couples as well as the complex integrative therapy that can help them resolve this life crisis. Filled with poignant clinical vignettes and workable guidance for practice and drawing from Fraenkel's highly innovative toolkit for intervention that includes music and art,

this clearly is the definitive book on this subject and the book that couple therapists should read this year."
—**Jay L. Lebow,** PhD, ABPP, senior scholar and clinical professor, the Family Institute at Northwestern and Northwestern University, Evanston, Illinois

"Couples on the brink of divorce challenge even experienced therapists. *Last Chance Couple Therapy* offers courage for both therapist and couple to 'experiment in possibility' while commitment to their bond is precarious. Grounded in clinical wisdom and research, Peter Fraenkel helps readers feel their intense pain, hurt, and anger, while offering a creative and integrative palette of clinical interventions that promote relational movement toward change."
—**Carmen Knudson-Martin,** PhD, professor emerita, Lewis & Clark College, and coauthor of *Socioculturally Attuned Family Therapy: Guidelines for Equitable Theory and Practice*

"This is a very practical book for therapists who are working with last chance couples. I think the ideas shared in the case discussions are highly illuminating and can be applied can be applied to couples throughout the world. I highly recommend it!"
—**Wai-Yung Lee,** PhD, founding president and clinical director of Asian Academy of Family Therapy

"Feeling stumped by a couple? Dreading the next session with people who've been bonded in misery for decades? Frightened of a case where abuse and violence lurk? Peter Fraenkel's new book on 'last chance' couple therapy should steady your nerves. Masterful and encyclopedic, but also sociable and practical, Fraenkel offers a road map for getting through the session, and getting results over time. He has done the hard work for us. Reading the research and clinical literature deeply, he proffers a clinical method (the 'Therapeutic Palette') that is empirically validated, creative and flexible, and most important, battle-tested with clinical examples from his own practice over many years. Experienced therapists and early career clinicians should keep this book at the ready—we are all in his debt."
—**Virginia Goldner,** PhD, adjunct clinical professor, NYU Postdoctoral Program in Psychoanalysis and Psychotherapy, and Faculty Emeritus, Ackerman Institute for the Family

"An extraordinary long time overview experience on difficult couple conflicts. Dr. Fraenkel goes through evidence from research and clinical practices based on psychoeducational to neurobiological aspects, without getting away from recent systemic theoretical perspectives. Many clinical vignettes are included that show his gift as a drummer, taking account time sequences on couples' rhythms, and his light sense of collaboration that includes Buddhism as well as art and craft into last chance couple therapy."

—**Javier Vicencio**, MD, MRCPsych, MscFT, Crisol Postgraduate Center on Family Therapy, Mexico

"Love this book! I am sure any couple therapist will devour it in in a few hours. There is so much to learn here, and foremost, this is a book written well, not like what often happens with clinical literature—maybe because this is a book written with understanding as much as with love and passion for the psychotherapeutic craft. Peter Fraenkel has written extensively about couple and family therapy, without any arrogance, but with tremendous assertiveness. As in a successful jam session, he is not afraid to break with orthodoxy, while also integrating traditional research and wisely grounding it in the real clinical world. Like a good jazz player, Fraenkel embraces flexibility while honoring all what we know about couple therapy. The therapy stories are fascinating, the instructions are clear, he knows well who he cites. Fraenkel does not evade reflecting about the most daunting difficulties with couples that are in pain and testing any simple intervention. One of the big lessons in this book is that we need to think about fostering experimentation and action. Reflection will then emerge as a gift. If that happens, the couple will renew their trust in you as a potential help, and thus make it possible to move forward as a couple. Working with couples, Peter Fraenkel doesn't seem to miss a beat and the book doesn't either, from its first to last page. It is packed with good ideas, a Therapeutic Palette that we can integrate into our own toolbox. I was able to give a name to so many of the things we do with couples when we bring the best of ourselves, without making us the center of the work."

—**Gonzalo Bacigalupe**, EdD, MPH, professor, Department of Counseling and School Psychology, College of Education and Human Development, University of Massachusetts

LAST CHANCE
COUPLE THERAPY

Bringing Relationships Back
From the Brink

PETER FRAENKEL

Norton Professional Books

An Imprint of W. W. Norton & Company
Celebrating a Century of Independent Publishing

This book is intended as a general information resource for professionals practicing in the field of psychotherapy and mental health. It is not a substitute for appropriate training or clinical supervision. Standards of clinical practice and protocol change over time. No technique or recommendation is guaranteed to be safe or effective in all circumstances, and neither the publisher nor the author(s) can guarantee the complete accuracy, efficacy, or appropriateness of any particular recommendation in every respect.

The names and identifying details of patients described in this book have been changed. Any URLs displayed in this book link or refer to websites that existed as of press time. The publisher is not responsible for, and should not be deemed to endorse or recommend, any website, app, or other content that it did not create. The author, also, is not responsible for any third-party material.

For information about permission to reproduce selections from this book, write to Permissions, W. W. Norton & Company, Inc., 500 Fifth Avenue, New York, NY 10110

For information about special discounts for bulk purchases, please contact W. W. Norton Special Sales at specialsales@wwnorton.com or 800-233-4830

Manufacturing by Versa Press
Production manager: Gwen Cullen

Library of Congress Cataloging-in-Publication Data

Names: Fraenkel, Peter, author.
Title: Last chance couple therapy : bringing relationships back from the brink / Peter Fraenkel.
Description: First edition. | New York : W.W. Norton & Company, Inc., [2023] | Includes bibliographical references. | Summary: "This book will draw upon a prominent multi-perspectival integrative approach to couple therapy, known as the Therapeutic Palette (TP), to describe how to work effectively with last chance couples"—Provided by publisher.
Identifiers: LCCN 2022007578 | ISBN 9781324016250 (cloth) | ISBN 9781324016267 (epub)
Subjects: LCSH: Couples therapy.
Classification: LCC RC488.5 .F684 2023 | DDC 616.89/1562—dc23/eng/20220716
LC record available at https://lccn.loc.gov/2022007578

W. W. Norton & Company, Inc., 500 Fifth Avenue, New York, NY 10110
www.wwnorton.com

W. W. Norton & Company Ltd., 15 Carlisle Street, London W1D 3BS

1 2 3 4 5 6 7 8 9 0

I dedicate this book to all the colleagues, students, and couples from whom I've learned, and to the couples who will put their trust in me, my colleagues, and students from this moment on.

CONTENTS

ACKNOWLEDGMENTS

First and foremost, I want to thank all the couples I've worked with over decades for inviting me into their lives and struggles, and for placing their hope in me. I've learned so much more from this work than can ever be communicated in professional publications, and I hope this book reflects some of the nuance and specificity required in assisting couples to figure out their preferred path.

I am deeply grateful to my many colleagues in couple and family therapy, and in the field of psychotherapy and research more generally, from whom I have learned so much and been inspired in my thinking and work as a therapist and teacher. Many of their contributions to my work are indicated in this book, and I hope that I have done sufficient justice in referencing their ideas, therapeutic practices, and research findings. Some I've had to privilege of studying with directly, and others I consider "mentors from afar."

I am also grateful to the colleagues, organizations, and institutions that have invited me to teach about working with last-chance couples, or about components of this work, which allowed me the opportunity to refine and extend my thinking over time. In particular, I wish to thank my original professional home base, the Ackerman Institute for the Family, where I presented my first workshop on this work in 1999; the American Family Therapy Academy; the Psychotherapy Networker Symposium; the "Treating Couples" conference of Harvard Medical School and the Cambridge Health Alliance; Therapy Training Boston; the American Psychological Association's Division 43; Society for the Exploration of Psychotherapy Integration; the International Family Therapy Association; National Council on Family Relations; Council on Contemporary Families; Chicago Center for Family Health; Tulane School of Social Work, New Orleans; Department of Child Psychiatry, New York University Medical Center, New York; Derner Institute for Advanced Psychological Studies, Garden City, New York; Department of Psychiatry, Beth Israel Medical Center, New York; the Mel and Phyllis Zachter Institute for Advanced Professional Education at OHEL Children's Home and Family Services, Brooklyn, New York; Department of Family Practice Medicine, Wyckoff Heights Medical Center, Brooklyn, New York; Penn Council for Relationships, Philadelphia; Family Services of Morris County, Morristown, New Jersey; Department of Psychiatry, Elizabeth General Medical Center, Elizabeth, New Jersey; Jewish Family Services, Providence, Rhode Island; Conference of the Coalition for Marriage, Family, and Couples Education, Washington, DC; Department of Family Relations and Applied Nutrition, University of Guelph, Guelph, Canada; Dalhousie University School of Social Work, Halifax, Nova Scotia; George Hull Centre for Children and Families, Toronto; the Association of Family Therapy, Institute for Family Therapy, RELATE, and Marlborough Family Service, London; Department of Psychiatry, University of Crete, Iraklion, Crete, Greece; Aiglé, Buenos Aires; Instituto Chileno de Terapia Familiar, Santiago, Chile; Crisol Centro de Postgrado en Terapia Familiar, Mexico City; Centro de Terapia Familiar y de Pareja, Cholula, Mexico; Institut für Systemische Therapie, Vienna; Department of Social Medicine, University of Heidelberg, and the Helm Sterlin Institut, Heidelberg, Germany; Munich Institute for Systemic and Integrative Therapy and the Munich College of Family Therapy, Munich; Ausbildungsinstitute Meilen für Systemische Therapie und Beratung, Zurich; Department of Psychology, Boğaziçi University, and Bilgi University, Istanbul; Nibbana Counseling and Psychotherapy Centre, Chennai, India; Hong Kong Institute of Education, Hong Kong; and the Amani Counseling Centre, Nairobi, Kenya. Presenting my ideas and practices in working with couples both nationally and internationally honed my multicultural sensitivity and developed my understanding that theories and techniques developed in one cultural context may not apply so well to couples in other cultures, and must be adapted to fit the diverse ways in which couples' intimacy and beliefs about power between partners are construed.

I also want to thank my editor at Norton, Deborah Malmud, for her enthusiasm for this project, and the Norton editorial and production teams.

On the personal side, I want to thank my son Noah, with whom I had engaging weekly conversations about politics, music, and cooking, providing a welcome diversion from writing this book. And I want to thank my daughter Lena, for all the laughs and stories about her life, and for applying her great organizational skills to collating all the references from each chapter into one coherent list. If this book ever gets translated into German, it will be Lena who does the translating—she's the best!

Last Chance Couple Therapy

AN OVERVIEW OF WORKING WITH LAST CHANCE COUPLES

IT WAS 1995 WHEN I encountered my first last chance couple. Just a few years into my private practice in New York City, I'd had excellent training in couple and family therapy at the New York University Medical Center's Family Studies Unit, and a year of additional training with one of the founders of the field, Dr. Salvador Minuchin. Yet I was not prepared for the special challenges that this couple presented. Richard, a tall, handsome, and rather imposing man, was a well-established organizational consultant in his early 40s, and Jennifer was an attractive, successful head of marketing for a major media company in her mid-30s. They paused at the threshold of my office. With a slight sneer mixed with a touch of resignation, Richard looked down at me and announced, "We're the couple from hell. We've seen three other couple therapists, with no success. You're our last chance!" I smiled and replied, "Well, welcome to purgatory!" They laughed as I welcomed them through the doorway. Little did I know then that I had spontaneously created in that moment an important framework for working with all last chance couples: to establish a liminal or temporary space of neither being committed to staying together nor fully deciding to end the marriage, so as to engage in what I later came to call "experiments in possibility."

Together for five years, the couple described persistent high-conflict arguments on all manner of topics: how to spend their weekends, decisions about purchases, how to handle the every-other-week visits with Richard's son by a previous marriage, whether to have a child together, and more. Initially drawn to one another physically and intellectually, their sex life had plummeted, and they rarely engaged in their previously pleasurable conversations about art and politics. Whereas they initially explored the wide world of New York City fine dining, they now rarely went out, and meals were inevitably poisoned by conflicts about their home life.

I suggested we might start with me teaching them some research-supported communication and problem-solving skills to help them communicate better about their various challenges and to give them some concrete evidence that their relationship could possibly improve. I suggested that only with such evidence would they be able to determine whether to stay together. With more than a touch of arrogant self-assurance, Richard noted, "You know, I'm a very experienced consultant—I think I'm a good listener." Jennifer grimaced slightly, raised her eyebrows, and tilted her head as if saying, "Hmm, I'm not so sure about that!" At the time I was directing PREP at NYU's Millhauser Laboratories and later at the NYU Child Study Center. PREP stands for Prevention and Relationship Enhancement Program, a distress- and divorce-prevention program based at the University of Denver's Center for Family and Marital Studies. It is based on some of the most rigorous empirical study of what distinguishes happy from unhappy couples over time, and includes communication skills shown to greatly decrease conflict and promote successful problem solving.

As I did in countless couple workshops, I reviewed the four major patterns of problematic communication (and some subflavors of one pattern, escalation) and taught them the Speaker-Listener Technique, a form of structured reflective listening. Jennifer took the role of Speaker first, speaking only for 15 seconds, and, to his obvious befuddlement, Richard had difficulty repeating back her words. After three tries, he finally showed that he'd heard her. The mask of arrogant self-confidence fell from his face, and he said quietly, "Well, maybe I'm not as good a listener as I thought I was." Jumping in to reassure him a bit, I said it was common to have much more difficulty paying attention to one's intimate partner than to people in other relationships, and that he likely was a fine listener as a consultant. The couple went on to learn these skills and left the session saying that for the first time in years, they had some hope that they could work things out. And after a few more sessions to address their specific issues, some exploration of the emotional trigger points from their families of origin, and a few exercises to restart their pleasurable connection, they decided to stay together. One year later, they let me know they'd had a child, and they remained happy.

In our first session, wishing not to be their fourth failed attempt at therapy, I'd asked the couple about their previous therapies. They reported that all three therapists had engaged them in several weeks of discussions about the history of their problems, then explored their families of origin and the problems in their previous relationships. These therapies seemed to count on a common belief that insight and understanding would automatically lead to change, but this never occurred for Jennifer and Richard. The therapists never taught them any communication skills, but rather would interrupt their escalating conflicts and have each partner speak to the therapist while the other listened, with the therapist sometimes pronouncing a solution to the issue at hand. But these solutions never worked out, because the underlying issues of dysfunctional communication, and the power struggles that ensued whenever Richard and Jennifer argued, were not addressed with concrete suggestions about how to interact differently.

Furthermore, none of the therapists overtly addressed that the couple was at a choice point about their future together. Jennifer and Richard were not confident that the relationship was viable and were hoping therapy might help them develop new ways of being together. They needed observable evidence that it was worth continuing to try. They weren't even sure they wanted to continue coming to sessions, but the therapists simply proceeded as if Jennifer and Richard were still committed to the relationship and to the therapy. The couple felt that the therapists didn't recognize the precariousness of their bond and, in frustration, they quit.

THERAPY WITH COUPLES ON THE BRINK OF DIVORCE: A LARGE YET UNDERTHEORIZED GROUP

A large number of couples seek couple therapy when they are already close to separation, divorce, or dissolution in the case of those that never married. Doss and colleagues (2004) conducted a survey with couples seeking marital therapy and found that almost half—46%—did so due to "divorce/separation concerns" (p. 610). This is not surprising, in that couples seek therapy on average six years after experiencing serious problems (Notarius & Buongiorno, 1992). Just one-fourth of couples seek therapy prior to initiating divorce (Albrecht et al., 1983; Johnson et al., 2001), and many last chance couples are represented in this group of severely distressed couples. Couples who sought therapy to "clarify the relationship" (in other words, the relationship's viability and partners' degree of commitment to sustaining it) were much more likely to separate following a course of therapy than those couples whose intentions prior to therapy were to "improve the relationship" (Owen et al., 2012, p. 179). In their study of "mixed-agenda couples" (in which one partner wishes to maintain the relationship and the other is considering dissolving it), Doherty and colleagues (2015) found them highly distressed: "The average marital adjustment score was 6.98, compared to the marital distress cutoff score of 13 for the brief version of the Dyadic Adjustment Scale" (p. 251). In half of the sample, couples had consulted with a divorce attorney prior to seeking counseling.

Given the long-established highly negative impact on mental and physical health of marital distress on adult partners (Amato, 2000) as well as on children (Amato, 2000; Cummings & Davies, 1994; Davies & Cummings, 2006; Repetti et al., 2002), it might be expected that couples would seek therapy much sooner. Couples give a range of reasons for not doing so: a spouse who is reluctant to do therapy, one partner thinking that there were no problems serious enough to address in therapy, or a concern about violating their privacy (Wolcott, 1986). In cisgender heterosexual couples, wives are much more likely than husbands to initiate the search for couple therapy (Doss et al., 2003). Yet my clinical experience suggests that it is often wives who also initiate the couple's conversation about possible separation, meaning that male partners who may have been reluctant earlier on to address emerging issues are suddenly thrust into the role of seeking therapy and trying to convince their female partner to work on the relationship. As is discussed in Chapter 1, this creates special challenges in forming a solid therapeutic alliance with both partners so that they will continue in treatment, because the female partner may feel that his efforts are "too little and too late." She may feel extremely hopeless and even suspicious about his true willingness and commitment to change, given that she's tried for years to get him to address the problems and go to therapy.

Many books on couple therapy provide case vignettes of couples on the brink of divorce, but there are few studies on the particular challenges these couples present in therapy, and even fewer well-articulated models for working with them (see review by Doherty et al., 2015). Doherty and colleagues' "discernment counseling" is a major, important exception (Doherty et al., 2015; Doherty & Harris, 2017). Discernment counseling involves a series of individual meetings with each partner to determine whether they are willing to commit to a course of marital therapy; if so, couples are asked to make a six-month commitment to a series of sessions. Discernment counseling has been found somewhat effective, resulting in almost half of couples (47%) deciding to pursue counseling toward improving the relationship, with 41% deciding to pursue divorce, and another 12% deciding to stay together but without therapy, suggesting that these couples may have decided to endure their unhappiness. However, even in those that pursued therapy, only 36% had reconciled by the end of treatment, meaning that only approximately one-sixth of mixed-agenda couples who sought discernment counseling were happier together (although at the time of their follow-up, another 6% were still attempting to reconcile, and 13% were "on hold" [Doherty et al., 2015, p. 252]).

The present approach differs from discernment counseling in several important ways. First, rather than conducting a series of individual sessions with each partner to determine whether they will make a commitment to therapy, sessions are largely conjoint. If the couple remains in therapy beyond a few initial sessions, each partner is seen for at least one individual session, to provide each with an opportunity to discuss issues confidentially, although at the end of each individual meeting, the therapist asks the partner what material can be brought back to the conjoint sessions, and most partners agree to share almost everything discussed individually in the next conjoint meeting. My experience is that the partner who is considering leaving wants to witness observable change in the other and in the interactional quality of the relationship before even committing to a second session. When I have suggested a series of individual meetings with partners à la discernment counseling, the ambivalent partner has flatly rejected the idea, saying that they do not need individual meetings but, rather, clear evidence that the other partner is willing to make long-requested changes, or apologize for violating their safety, trust, or other values (through an affair, alcohol or substance abuse, or aggression). This rejection of the slower, more discussion-oriented assessment approach that characterizes discernment counseling in favor of a more action-oriented "show me the proof that you will change" approach may also be a regional difference between couples seen in New York City, where life is fast paced (and where people drawn to New York may be more oriented to fast results and immediate gratification), versus couples seen in the Midwest (Minnesota, specifically), where Doherty and colleagues developed discernment counseling.

Two short vignettes will give a picture of the type of impatient, challenging, results-oriented couples I often see here in the Big Apple.

Although I've never lived in the Midwest, I think this type of couple is probably rarer there than here. Teresa, 46, and Mark, 53, both white, were both high-powered finance professionals. Both were multimillionaires in their own right (Mark was one of the most successful people ever in his field). Mark was divorced with a teenaged child by a previous marriage; Teresa was divorced with two teenaged children of her own; and they had a 10-year-old daughter together. Married for 11 years, they were on the brink of divorce, largely due to Mark's heavy drinking and cocaine use, and his abusive behavior when drunk.

For our first session, Teresa was dressed in Wall Street attire; Mark in a sleek, silvery golfing outfit and brand-new-looking high-end sneakers. The couple sat down, and with a provocative smirk on his face, Mark said, "You should know straight away that I think therapy is a bunch of bullshit." Teresa, who had dragged him to this session and who had told me in our initial phone call that Mark would be "resistant," looked at me with a mix of "Told you so" and "Please try to engage him!" I smiled back and said, "To tell you the truth, I often think therapy is bullshit myself, and I've been doing it for 30 years. So for me, each session is a test of whether therapy is bullshit or not." Mark registered a look of surprise at my comeback but maintained his stiff, somewhat pulled-back posture as I began asking them about the challenges they were facing, as well as about how they met and what they enjoyed about being together. After Teresa raised the issue of Mark's behavior when he was drunk or high, and he minimized it, I countered with a comment that "alcohol, being a liquid, and coke, a dust, have a way of spreading into a relationship in ways that we don't intend when we're using them, and with all due respect, Mark, it sounds like your use has gotten a bit out of control—or at least, that you get a bit out of control when you use them, and I can see that you're a guy who likes to be in charge." Mark smiled and sort of agreed. As the session ended, he smiled at me, this time in an appreciative albeit still teasing way, and, using a finance term for a positive development, said, "I'm impressed with you, 'on the upside.'" Teresa looked relieved. The therapy was launched.

At a different place on the socioeconomic spectrum, Bill, a 50-year-old white Irish American electrician who had dropped out of school at 15 due to an undiagnosed learning disability, and Laura, a 46-year-old white Italian American high school graduate and high-level administrative assistant, both with kids from previous marriages, were on the brink of breaking up (they had not formally married, but had been together for six years, and had recently bought a home together in Queens). Constant fighting and conflict between Laura and one of

Bill's young adult daughters, and between Bill and Laura's two similarly aged children from her prior marriage who lived with them, led Laura to contact me to see if they could learn to communicate ("without fucking bashing each other's heads in, with words I mean, there's been no hitting or nothin' like that"). In the first session, Laura immediately launched into an angry, expletive-filled description of Bill's behavior, and Bill countered with, "You see, Doc, this is what I'm dealin' with. She's got a mouth on her, this one." Laura responded, "Oh yeah, me?? What about you, you stupid fuck!" Both were considering breaking up, and while Laura said I came highly recommended, she had not had a good experience with a previous individual therapist and was doubtful that therapy could help: "All she ever did was ask me how I was feeling and about my childhood, when I had real problems now with this one," meaning Bill. Bill had never been in therapy. ("That's for crazy people, and I ain't crazy. . . . She is [nodding his head sideways in Laura's direction], but I'm not.") Bill also explained that he was Irish Catholic and that "we Irish don't talk about our feelings. It's just not what we do."

The heat was on me to show them that I could help them make a difference, and I had to produce in this session, or I was sure I would not see them again. As I did with Richard and Jennifer, I told them about what research had shown about patterns of problematic communication and taught them the Speaker-Listener Technique. Both came from families filled with the same sort of high-conflict interactions they engaged in, and this communication technique was a revelation for them. (Chapter 4 provides a detailed description of how to teach high-conflict couples these skills.) Encouraged by this simple demonstration of how quickly things could change, they decided to continue for several months and made remarkable changes, resolving their issues around each other's kids and increasing their pleasurable activities, with each being able to express the vulnerable feelings under their anger, and with Bill agreeing to shoulder some of the housework. The therapy ended in one of the cutest sessions I've ever experienced, with them frequently hugging and smiling, and Bill thanking me for "changing us."

These two vignettes and many others in this book speak to a major difference in the present approach and that of discernment counseling in terms of forming the therapeutic contract and building motivation to engage in treatment. In the present approach, couples have immediate opportunities to observe changes in their interactions that then result in positive changes in their beliefs and emotions. These changes provide motivation to continue. In discernment counseling, careful individual assessment of partners' level of motivation results in a decision about whether or not to pursue therapy, but the partners have not had opportunities to witness positive "enactments" (Minuchin et al., 2014) or demonstrations of change. Although the present approach has not been subjected to careful empirical study of outcomes, I can report that I have a much higher rate of success than the approximately one-sixth of couples Doherty and colleagues report ending in reconciliation.

Another difference between Doherty and colleagues' (Doherty et al., 2015; Doherty & Harris, 2017) approach and the one you will learn in this book is that last chance couples include both those with mixed agendas and those in which both partners are considering ending the relationship. When both partners are viewing the exit door, it is even more challenging to develop a working alliance and get them on board to experiment with change.

THE BASICS OF WORKING WITH LAST CHANCE COUPLES

Let's take a look at the basic principles and practices of working with last chance couples and how these are different from working with couples committed to a future together. Along the way, I'll point out common mistakes therapists make with last chance couples, based on what I've heard from couples themselves about their previous attempts at therapy. All these points are discussed in detail in subsequent chapters.

Need for a Tentative Therapeutic Contract

The failures of these previous therapies, and the success of my first seat-of-the-pants attempt with a last chance couple, taught me some critical truths about how to work with such couples. Most couple therapies and the books that provide guidance for this work tacitly begin with the assumption that partners are committed to staying in the relationship. At the end of one session, the therapist summarizes what's been said and understood in that hour, assigns some form of intersession activity meant to move things forward in the assumed project of staying together, and pulls out their phone or paper appointment book to schedule the next session.

Not so with last chance couples. The last chance couple is defined by at least one, if not both, partners entering therapy with serious thoughts about ending the relationship and, in the case of married couples, serious thoughts about initiating separation and divorce. In many instances, one partner has already moved out and may have engaged a lawyer to begin divorce proceedings. Failed prior attempts at conjoint and individual therapy have littered the couple's history with the debris of broken dreams and hopelessness. At this juncture, the therapist cannot assume blithely that the partners want to stay together—or even return for a next session. Different techniques are needed in formulating the therapeutic contract, and in engaging couples to try one more time. It's the eleventh if not the twelfth hour of their lives together, and they want immediate observable evidence that things might actually change for the better. Chapter 1 provides a detailed guide to establishing a viable, flexible therapeutic alliance and contract.

Need to Validate and Make Space for the Ambivalent Partner's Desire to Leave the Relationship

As I will describe in step-by-step detail, the therapist needs to validate in the first session the ambivalent partner's (or both ambivalent partners') at-best mixed feelings about continuing in the relationship and about doing therapy at all. Commonly used cheerful reframes such as, "The fact that you made it to this first session despite your struggles shows some commitment to each other and trying to work things out!" or another common desperate attempt to shine a positive light—"The fact that you are so angry at each other shows you really care!"—will at best result in bemused, bitter half smiles meant to soothe the well-meaning nice therapist's naive feelings and at worst may lead one or both partners to conclude, "This therapist doesn't get us." After all, one or both partners may be attending the first session mostly with the intention of getting help dissolving the relationship without incurring further distress and animosity. Or, somewhat more cynically, they've shown up because the lawyer they consulted suggested they do so to demonstrate that they tried, so as to obtain a better divorce or custody settlement (even though they had no intention of working on things).

Rather than settling into an unstated multisession course of therapy, the contract for working together needs to be constructed on a session-by-session basis. At the beginning of each session, the therapist should ask, "What would be one thing we could achieve today that might make you feel this therapy is worth it?" And at the end of each hour, the therapist must ask the couple to evaluate whether the session was helpful enough for them to want to return for a next session—or whether they want to think about it over the week and decide whether to return.

An Initial Focus on the Present and Near Future Rather Than the Past

Rather than extensively exploring their history of pain over many weeks, hoping that venting their feelings and understanding each other's perspectives will somehow relieve their suffering, the therapist needs to help the couple experiment with possibilities in and after the first session by offering them tools and techniques that can lead to observable change for reducing conflict and promoting pleasurable connection. One sad advantage to working with many last chance couples is that they have refined their problematic patterns into a "lean, mean fighting machine." These patterns are well described in almost 50 years of research on distressed couples. In this book you will learn how to quickly detect the presence of these patterns, which travel across and underlie the various issues couples struggle with—money, sex, in-laws, child-rearing, housework, leisure time, and more. The skillful couple therapist must focus more on the process of couple interaction and not become bamboozled by the extensive menu of specific topics or contents about which couples conflict. Premier couple researcher John Gottman (2011) found years ago that he could predict with 93% accuracy the future of a relationship from observing just six minutes of videotaped interaction. Although this finding might seem astonishing, it's not surprising at all when you watch how distressed partners often treat one another in second-by-second exchanges of criticism, contempt, defensiveness, withdrawal and stonewalling, invalidation, and negative interpretations or attributions about each other's intentions and feelings. Add those sample seconds up to minutes, hours, days, weeks, months, and years, and that reliable six-minute sample of their lives together holds one key to transforming their reality—the need to alter destructive interactional patterns. Letting couples engage in such interactions for more than a few minutes in your sessions is not only not productive (apologies for the double negative)—it's downright destructive. Don't be surprised if, at some point, the fighting couple turns their wrath upon you, saying, "Why are we paying YOU?! We can do this at home for free!" And they're right.

Of course, the therapist needs to provide opportunities for each partner to describe their suffering and must empathize with each of them, no matter how wildly different their accounts of their shared history might be. This stance of "multipartiality" begins to model a way for each partner to realize that their fix on reality might be quite different than the partner's, but both are largely true—if not always in observable fact, then in felt experience—and can be heard with compassion. As I discuss in Chapter 1, the emotional, empathic bond between the therapist and each partner is critical to engaging them in therapy and helping them feel supported enough to try new things. However, just as the beautiful ghosts that appear in a scene of the classic film *Raiders of the Lost Ark* eventually turn into frightening skeletal images, continuing to invite the story of suffering turns sour rather quickly and further embeds the partners in the painful past.

Although much accumulated therapy theory suggests that talking about painful feelings is necessary for moving on from the past, when couples have been interacting in problematic ways for months to years, in some sense, they have no actual past—it is one long, continuous, and unchanging present that may stretch back decades. To create an experiential past, the therapist must invite couples to experiment with new, preferred patterns that help them bifurcate time into the problematic past and the more hopeful and pleasurable "present-toward-the-future." Contemporary research and clinical work with trauma support this focus on engaging clients to start reconstructing their lives through positive action rather than endless revisiting of their traumatic memories (van der Kolk, 2014). As the great Vietnamese Buddhist leader Thich Nhat Hanh wrote, "We want to take care of the future. But the future will be made of only one substance: the present moment. The best way to take care of the future is to do our best to take care of the present moment" (Nhat Hanh, 2006, p. 233). And the only way to put the past truly in its place is first to distinguish that past from a different present.

Once some notable changes have occurred in couples' present interactions, therapy is in a better place to explore in depth the experiences, attitudes, beliefs, and emotions from each partner's family and culture of origin, although these themes often get raised and addressed somewhat even as the couple is learning new ways of interacting. Chapter 2 introduces my Therapeutic Palette integrative approach to couple therapy, which provides a flexible, client-driven guide to when to focus on the present, past, and future; when to address behaviors, emotions, thoughts, and physiological arousal; and when to be more or less directive.

Avoid Initial Focus on Strengths and Positive Narratives

Another popular approach to working with couples mired in their painful past is to invite them to share what narrative therapists call "unique outcomes" (Freedman & Combs, 1996) and solution-focused therapists call "exceptions" (de Shazer, 1985; Hoyt, 2015)—times, however rare, when the couple communicated well, solved problems, and enjoyed each other. Although this is a fine approach for less distressed couples, when one or both partners arrive at a first session determined to convince the therapist, the partner, and perhaps themselves once again that their relationship is hopeless, attempts to elicit such positive memories often fall flat and may lead the couple to believe that the therapist does not take their extreme distress seriously. Asking the partners how they first met and what it was that attracted one to the other is useful and can provide the therapist a sense of the degree of positive, pleasurable connection that once characterized their relationship. When partners share a genesis story of intellectual and sexual passion, shared values, common dreams of the future, and enjoyable adventures small and large, this often bodes well for the future of a relationship that may have been contaminated by lack of communication skills, numerous stressors and disappointments, and plain old neglect and failure to water the flower of their *we*. Conversely, a story of early connection with little passion—in which partners paired mostly because "it seemed the right thing to do at the time"—suggests the therapeutic road ahead may be treacherous at best.

Hearing the story of initial attraction also often provides important clues about the qualities of each partner that have now become the end points of a polarized continuum on which many conflicts occur: "I loved his slow pace and relaxed vibe" has now become "He's a slug. I can't get him off the couch on the weekend." And "She was so energetic and exciting. She livened me up" has now become "She's always pushing me and rushing around, trying to do a million things. It's killing me!" (Working with these sorts of polarized differences is discussed in detail in Chapters 3 and 5.) However, when a therapist with good intentions continues to attempt to excavate the couple's hidden resources and strengths and shine light on the "subordinated preferred narrative" when the couple repeatedly insists, "It's been a long time since we felt that way for each other, and no, we never communicated well about problems, nor did our parents, grandparents, great-grandparents, or anyone that we know of in our respective genetic lineage," this well-meaning focus on submerged strengths will backfire, with couples becoming irritated once again that the therapist doesn't "get us and where we're at now."

Need to Restart Pleasure While Working on Reducing Pain

Another common mistake in working with couples generally and especially with last chance couples is to focus entirely on reducing their conflict while neglecting their fading sources of pleasure. Even with these couples who are at the extreme end of unhappiness, the therapist needs to help them experiment, not only with more productive and effective forms of communicating, regulating negative emotion, reconciling (if possible) their differing visions of their future, and overcoming hurtful events such as violence or affairs. At the same time and from the beginning of therapy, the couple needs guidance and encouragement to experiment with restarting the Bunsen burner of pleasure and passion. After all, partners do not pair up solely or mostly based on their premonition that the other will be a great person with whom to solve the inevitable problems and snafus of life. Partners are attracted physically, intellectually, spiritually—they enjoy being around each other, and even "get a kick out of each other" (Fraenkel, 2001b). They love the quirky way the other tells a story or a joke, their sleepy but sensual face in the morning light. They glow with pride while their partner describes to friends an interesting idea or project at work; their hearts brim with love and compassion when their partner tells of a perceived defeat, a loss of confidence, and they want to hold them and make it all better. They love the other's touch, they love each other's smell. Without a sense that those pleasures can be restored and expanded, few couples will want to venture into a future together, and therapy becomes just hard work, one more chore in a long to-do list. They resonate sadly to Tina Turner's classic tune, "What's Love Got to Do With It?," and may resolve to trudge on for the sake of stability, appearances, or the kids. But they won't emerge from a solely problem-focused therapy with much more inspiration to keep on truckin'. For what? In the words of another classic tune by Peggy Lee, they may wonder, "Is That All There Is?" We therapists can help couples become much more than lean, mean competent problem-solving machines. Chapters 4 and 8 provide a cornucopia of couple pleasure-boosting practices.

Therapist Self-Awareness and Self-Care

Let's be real: Working with couples in crisis, on the brink of divorce or unmarried dissolution, can be negatively arousing and exhausting. I often think of this work as "open-hearted surgery": We are working with couples whose distress and dysfunctionality is on the extreme end of the spectrum, uncovering relational traumas, and witnessing levels of hatred and acts of hurtfulness and destruction that resemble the worst international or interethnic conflicts—but between two people who share a life, a home, often children, a social network—and who started out with the intention of forming a supportive, loving life. As one of my most valued and wisest colleagues, Virginia Goldner (2014), writes:

> Couples in crisis may present in many different ways, content issues and personality styles run the gamut—but whether theatrically voiced or floating in the ether, something is always the same—the shock, the fear of collapse, the profound confusion over what is going on—a situation that incites extreme reactivity, paranoia, hypersensitivity, the feeling of "carrying my guts in a bag," as one man said. . . . When the one you love keeps hurting you, when the one who hurts you doesn't try to make it better, when the one you need abandons or frightens you, when the one you know becomes impenetrable or unknown to you, when the one who knows you no longer recognizes you—these are the ubiquitous traumas of love lost. (p. 403)

To fully grasp the pain and complex entangled roots in the vernal pool of their conflict, we must be open-hearted—willing to feel their pain, imagine their experiences, and attempt to sympathize with each partner, including partners who've done outrageously destructive things to the other. The effects on us therapists can be profoundly upsetting. Not only is their behavior objectively disturbing; their stories can evoke memories of our own relational failures or those we witnessed growing up, and the associated feelings of hurt, anger, shame, and guilt. Goldner (2014) writes:

> Any couple therapist knows the drill. Two partners who politely introduce themselves, tolerating the necessary small talk and business details with appropriate compliance, but clearly itching for the moment when, having now placed themselves in your esteemed professional hands, they can finally let loose and leave

the mess to you. Of course it's too early to be forced into the position of containing the extreme states and dangerous ways of people you don't know from Adam. But whether too early in the treatment, or too late in your day, these people will have their way with you. (p. 402)

In the afterword of this book, I address how to prepare and sustain yourself for this demanding work. It is essential to have a good grasp of one's own relational history so as to use it productively as a resonating chamber but, at the same time, not fall into trying to save your parents' marriage (or your own) through the work with the couple in front of you. And it is essential to engage in self-care, both during sessions and at the end of a long day and week, lest you become too reactive and burn out.

THE FOUR TYPES OF LAST CHANCE COUPLE SCENARIOS

Over 30 years of experience working with a variety of couples who announce that this therapy is their last chance, I've discerned four basic types of concerns that have propelled these couples to question their future together. A couple may present with one or more of these scenarios; thus, these are not types of last chance couples but rather types of last chance scenarios. Chapters 4 through 9 present the specific techniques needed to address these different scenarios, along with illustrative cases of couples where the therapy led them to stay together, and a few where the therapy resulted in them deciding to separate, but with more peace and mutual understanding.

High Conflict

High-conflict couples engage in patterns well documented by the research of Gottman, Markman and Stanley, Bradbury and Fincham, and others as risk factors for distress and divorce: escalation, withdrawal (and its extreme version, stonewalling), invalidation, and negative interpretations, and the expressed emotions of criticism, contempt, and defensiveness. Numerous authors have described useful methods for working with such couples, whether last chance or not (Baucom et al., 2015; Fishbane, 2013; Fraenkel, 2011; Fruzetti, 2006; Gottman & Gottman, 2015a, 2015b; Nielsen, 2016b; Scheinkman & Fishbane, 2004; Wachtel, 2019; and many others). My approach incorporates several theoretical perspectives and their associated techniques to help couples learn new, productive ways of communicating and solving problems; how to identify and express the more gentle feelings and attachment insecurities underneath explosive anger (Johnson, 2019); how to use mindfulness activities to self-soothe and regulate or modulate (Jurist, 2018) high levels of negative arousal that tend to hijack the higher cortical functioning of the brain (Fishbane, 2013); how to soothe the partner through compassionate listening; how to identify and address broader themes of power and control, closeness and caring, respect and recognition, personal integrity and safety, commitment, trust, and acceptance that erupt into specific issues and arguments (Markman, Stanley, et al., 2010); how to identify each partner's emotional triggers or vulnerabilities based on family- and culture-of-origin upbringing; and how to separate from the often-unproductive maps of relationship learned in those contexts (Scheinkman & Fishbane, 2004). Chapter 4 focuses on action-oriented techniques for working with high conflict, and Chapter 5 discusses incorporating more insight-oriented approaches and blending those with action-oriented techniques.

Value and Safety Violations

These are couples in which one or both partners have engaged in behaviors that violate values such as monogamy, trust, and honesty, or that jeopardize the emotional, financial, or physical safety of the other—alcohol or drug overuse, gambling or other egregious financial misbehavior, affairs, and behaviors on the continuum of intimidation, abuse, and violence. My approach to these issues, detailed in Chapters 6 (infidelity) and 7 (violence and substance overuse), again draws and expands upon a range of theories and practices including those already named, as well as the work of Perel (2017) and Spring (2020) on infidelity; the integrative feminist, systemic, psychodynamic approach to interpersonal violence pioneered by Goldner and colleagues (Goldner, 1998; Goldner et al., 1990); and the cognitive–behavioral approach to couples with a partner who overuses alcohol or other substances (McCrady & Epstein, 2015).

Mismatched Projected Life Chronologies

Couples mismatched in their "projected life chronologies"—hopes and plans for what they want to achieve and have in their lives, like financial security, home ownership, children, retirement—may not experience high conflict, but nevertheless find themselves in a log-jam that threatens the relationship's future. When they first met and fell in love, these partners assumed (often without discussing it) that they shared the same goals, dreams, and path through life, but lo and behold, their images of their futures now diverge markedly. In many cases, partners agree on what they want to have happen in their lives, but drastically differ about when they want to attain these things. I address these issues in Chapter 8.

Low Passion and Pleasure: Emotional and Sexual Disengagement

The fire is out, the engine is cold, the attraction and pleasure have evaporated, and it's not clear that they have enough mutual attraction to sustain a life together. These are the most difficult couples to treat, as there's little glue (attachment) and spark (passion) left to drive change efforts. The fibers of connection are frayed, making it difficult to confront the problems they must resolve. They may at one point have been high-conflict couples, and the flames of discord have burned them out. Or they may have been conflict avoidant from the start. They fear reconnecting lest that result in fighting, and, along with learning safer ways to communicate, they need suggestions and much encouragement to experiment with small but significant steps toward reigniting pleasure. Chapter 9 presents an approach to working with low- and no-passion couples.

Underlying Themes: Time and Emotion Modulation

Two interrelated themes underlie many couple problems in each of these last chance scenarios: How partners become polarized and "dys-synchronous" around the temporal or "time side" of life and behavior, and how they become polarized around emotional experience, expression, and emotion regulation or modulation. Temporal polarization occurs through differences in pace, punctuality, time perspective (emphasis on the present versus the past versus the future), time orientation (degree of adherence to clock and calendar), daily and weekly rhythms, and preferences for how to allocate time, as well as the aforementioned personal life chronologies. Differences in emotion modulation appear as one partner being quite expressive and the other less so; one partner being excitement oriented while the other seeks calmness and an emotional steady state; one partner focusing mostly on positive experiences while the other focuses more on the negatives and problems; and other differences in emotional style. In Chapter 3 I propose a theory that links these two broad aspects of human life, and an approach to bringing these often-unconscious themes into the light and reducing these polarizations. I draw largely on my extensive clinical studies of couples that are dyssynchronous in all matters related to time (Fraenkel, 1994, 2001c, 2011, 2018; Fraenkel & Wilson, 2000).

SUMMARY

Last chance couples come in two basic forms: mixed-agenda couples in which one partner is considering relationship dissolution and the other wishes to maintain the relationship, and those in which both partners are considering a breakup. They present with one or more scenarios: high conflict, value and safety violations, mismatched projected life chronologies, or low levels of passion. The therapeutic approach described in this book privileges action-oriented techniques initially, allowing couples an opportunity to witness actual change and disconfirm their long-held negative beliefs about one another and the relationship's potential, thereby gaining hope that therapy can be effective. Exploration of family- and culture-of-origin issues may occur briefly in initial sessions, but often must wait until each partner is convinced that change is possible in the present toward the future. Work on increasing pleasure and connection occurs concurrently with work on reducing conflictual interactions, invoking apologies, addressing external stressors, finding consensus and compromise, and other work to reduce risk factors and polarizations. The therapy is cast as a set of experiments in possibility, and the therapeutic contract is constructed on a session-by-session basis, fully acknowledging the strong desires of one or both partners to leave the marriage. A great deal of attention is paid to the therapist's "micromoves" that sustain a positive, empathic connection with each partner. We turn now to these micromoves, as without a strong therapeutic alliance the specific techniques described throughout the book will be ineffective.

A NOTE ON HOW THIS BOOK IS ORGANIZED

The initial chapters on the therapeutic alliance (Chapter 1), an integrative approach to working with couples (Chapter 2), and the broad themes of temporal/time-related differences, the unconscious ways in which partners regulate or modulate one another's emotions, and how these temporal and emotion-based patterns are often intertwined and become polarized (Chapter 3) provide general themes upon which I draw in discussing work with high-conflict couples (Chapters 4 and 5), couples in which one partner has violated the values and safety of the other through an affair (Chapter 6) or intimidation/violence or over-use of alcohol or other substances (Chapter 7), couples mismatched in their projected life chronologies or desires for certain things to happen by certain points in time (Chapter 8), and low- or no-passion couples (Chapter 9). As a result, at times I repeat points made in the first three chapters to illustrate how to use these ideas and techniques with couples in the four types of last chance scenarios. I do this also because I'm aware that readers sometimes skip to chapters on issues about which they are most interested and therefore cannot assume they've read the first three chapters thoroughly. Likewise, at times I discuss a particular couple to illustrate one point (for instance, how to sustain the therapeutic alliance when pointing out problematic non-verbal behavior by one partner) and then return to that couple to illustrate further points. This approach fits with the overall integrative perspective, in which any particular couple's issues can be viewed through multiple theoretical lenses. I hope that this provides a sense of continuity in how to work in a multitheoretical manner. I also want to note that the vignettes are based on actual couples with whom I worked. Because issues of partners' social locations in terms of race, ethnicity, social class, gender and gender identity, and other aspects of identity are important in working with them, I have retained those locational descriptors. However, I have taken appropriate care as required by the American Psychological Association to remove other identifying details.

CHAPTER 1

FORMING AND MAINTAINING THE THERAPEUTIC ALLIANCE

The Therapist as a Collaborative Expert

T HE RELATIONSHIP BETWEEN THE THERAPIST and the couple—
the therapeutic alliance—is the cornerstone of effective therapy.
Unless the partners each feel heard, understood, and cared for by the
therapist, they will not feel emotionally safe and willing to hear the
therapist's comments about their contributions to the problems in the
back-and-forth of couple conflict. Nor will they be willing to experiment with the therapist's suggestions for change. This chapter reviews
the emerging research on what leads to a strong therapeutic alliance
and what interferes with building and maintaining that crucial relationship. Short vignettes illustrate the often-delicate dance therapists
must engage in to affirm each partner's different points of view on
the problem and their respective needs for therapy and in the couple's
relationship.

THE ROLE OF COURAGE IN CHANGE: AN UNDEREXPLORED COMMON FACTOR

Before embarking on a review of what research has shown contributes to a strong therapeutic alliance, I want to address a term that
has been absent from most discussions of the therapy process: *courage*, and its correlative change-support act, *encouragement*. Central to

the alliance is the therapist encouraging couples to try new ways of interacting and new ways of viewing one another. The definition of *encourage* speaks to four key activities of the therapist:

1a: to inspire with courage, spirit, or hope: HEARTEN
1b: to attempt to persuade: URGE
2:   to spur on: STIMULATE
3:   to give help or patronage to: FOSTER (Merriam-Webster, n.d.b)

Whichever techniques we use in working with couples, a common factor in all therapy is to provide reasons to hope, so as to "respirit" and reenergize clients, to urge couples to try new things, to stimulate their existing, underutilized resources, and to foster or support them as they struggle to experiment with possibilities. The term *courage* comes from the Old French (12th century) term *corage*, meaning "the heart, as the seat of emotions." With last chance couples, in which partners' hearts have been broken or hardened, encouragement is therefore a central aspect of what we do.

Surprisingly, the role of courage in helping clients instigate change in their lives has not been discussed much in the psychotherapy literature, and not emphasized in publications on couple therapy. Existential psychologist Rollo May (1975) wrote that courage is needed "to relate to other human beings. . . . [Social courage is] the capacity to risk one's self in the hope of achieving meaningful intimacy. It is the courage to invest one's self over a period of time in a relationship that will demand increasing openness" (p. 17). He explains further:

> Intimacy requires courage because risk is inescapable. We cannot know at the outset how the relationship will affect us. Like a chemical mixture, if one of us is changed, both of us will be. Will we grow in self-actualization, or will it destroy us? The one thing we can be certain of is that if we let ourselves fully into the relationship for good or evil, we will not come out unaffected. (p. 17)

Although establishing a strong therapeutic alliance with any couple can be challenging, it is much harder with a last chance couple. These couples have tried to love each other and live together; things went wrong, and they now feel damaged and regret their choice. Partners often feel destroyed by each other, and hopeless, especially if they've already tried a round of couple therapy with little to no success. Without a sense of confidence that the therapist knows what to do, and without the therapist's emotional support and encouragement, last chance couples will not muster the courage needed to "take a chance on love"—to try new, initially awkward ways of communicating, solving problems, affirming and validating each other's feelings and points of view, making love in mutually pleasurable ways, and all the other new behaviors and ways of thinking and feeling that couples need to establish in order to move from unhappy to truly fulfilled.

Moreover, the qualities of an effective therapist at the core of the therapeutic alliance—the so-called common factors of warmth, genuineness, being relatable, and being knowledgeable about how to structure the change process—are therapeutic in their own right (Davis et al., 2012; Sprenkle et al., 2009). Common factors are viewed as aspects of therapy that cut across different models. Couple partners absorb these qualities and feel soothed in ways that they may never have experienced in their families growing up. The therapist models compassion and creativity in bridging differences and resolving problems, which the partners learn to apply to one another. I propose that fostering courage is yet another common factor essential to all approaches to therapy, and certainly to work with last chance couples.

WHAT ARE THE ELEMENTS OF THE THERAPEUTIC ALLIANCE? HOW DOES IT AFFECT THERAPY OUTCOMES?

The term *therapeutic alliance* as applied to couple therapy refers to the quality of the relationship between the therapist, the couple, and each partner, and the degree to which couples are engaged together in the therapy process. The therapeutic alliance has three components, as described by Bordin (1979) and as measured by a frequently used scale (the Working Alliance Inventory; Tracey & Kokotovic, 1989): degree of agreement between therapist and client on the goals of therapy, agreement on the tasks of therapy (what the client needs to do and what the client can expect the therapist to do), and the quality of the bond between therapist and client. Another alliance scale, the Couple Therapeutic Alliance Scale (CTAS-R; Pinsof, 1994) is based on the same tripartite definition of the alliance, but examines the alliance in all the relationships that occur in couple therapy: self–therapist (each partner's sense of the alliance between themselves and the therapist), partner–therapist (each partner's sense of the alliance between their partner and the therapist), couple–therapist (each partner's sense of the alliance between the therapist and the couple as a unit), and self–partner or partner to partner (each partner's sense of the degree of the alliance with their partner about the therapy's goals, tasks, and feelings about the therapist). Although there is an enormous research literature on factors that affect the therapeutic alliance in individual psychotherapy (see, e.g., Eubanks et al., 2018; Horvath & Bedi, 2002; Martin et al., 2000), research on the TA in couple therapy is relatively new. However, several important findings have already emerged, with great significance for working with last chance couples.

In one large archival study of partners who had at least one session of couple therapy (Moore et al., 2013), it was found that people who felt "very pressured" to attend therapy rated their level of motivation as significantly lower than those who were no more than "somewhat pressured" (on a scale from "not at all pressured" to "very pressured"). The authors based their study on the well-known "stages of change" model of Prochaska and DiClemente (1992), developed in work with clients who overused alcohol and substances, in which they categorize clients as being at one of five stages of readiness to change: precontemplation (not very interested in changing and tending to attribute their problems to others); contemplation (thinking about possibly changing but so far having taken no action to do so); preparation (clients planning to engage in change efforts soon); action (engaging in observable, behavioral change efforts); and maintenance (engaging in regular behavior to prevent relapse and sustain gains). The literature on motivation and engagement of clients who are mandated for treatment has produced mixed findings—some studies showing lower motivation and more resistance to treatment, whereas others show increased motivation. However, Moore et al. (2013) examined not only legally mandated clients but those whom they described as "soft mandated"—receiving pressure from family (including the other partner) but not facing legal consequences for nonattendance. They found that partners who felt "very pressured" to go to therapy were significantly less motivated to change than those who experienced lower levels of pressure.

Knobloch-Fedders et al. (2007) conducted one of the first prospective studies specifically on the therapeutic alliance in couple therapy. They assessed couple partners' alliance after the first and the eighth sessions. Several important findings emerged. First, there was little change in the therapeutic alliance from the first to the eighth session. The authors note that this suggests "alliance building may be one of the most important therapeutic tasks of the first conjoint session" (p. 254). Second, there were some interesting gender differences in their sample of cisgender heterosexual couples: Women's perception of their male partner's degree of strong alliance to the therapist was associated with better outcomes in therapy, whereas men's ratings of their female partner's alliance to the therapist were unrelated to change in therapy. Additionally, women's ratings of the alliance with their male partner about the treatment were significantly associated with positive change: Men's ratings of their alliance with their female partners about the therapy were not related to change.

This makes sense—in my experience, and I'll bet in yours, with heterosexual couples, it is usually the woman who finds me through talking with a friend or colleague who's a former satisfied client of mine, or online through my website, or from her individual therapist; and it's the woman who makes the initial call and often expresses concerns about her male partner not believing in therapy, not really wanting to come to therapy, or not seeing a problem at all. Therefore, when the female partner senses that her male partner is well connected to the therapy process (tasks and goals) and to me as a person—in other words, likes me, trusts me, thinks I'm smart, thinks I'm fair to him and that this will not be a husband-bashing session—the female partner is more likely to engage fully in the therapy herself. And of course, if she feels she and her husband agree on the value of the therapy, she's also able to relax into the process. In other words, it's often the case, as this study suggests, that women are closely examining the degree to which we therapists make a good bond with their husbands: If we don't, the therapy might end, as she will feel less enthusiastic or be tired of trying to convince her husband to stay engaged.

In a later study on the relationship between the therapeutic alliance, couples' level of satisfaction, and progress in therapy (Glebova et al., 2011), several findings emerged that bear on work with last chance couples:

1. As was found by Knobloch-Fedders et al. (2007), this study found that the therapeutic alliance is established in early sessions—really, in the first session—and, once formed, does not shift much over the course of therapy. As the authors note, "Thus, it may be the case that first impressions matter quite a lot in therapy. For clinicians, this means that the first session, and perhaps even the first phone contact with clients, is essential in creating a working relationship with clients" (Glebova et al., 2011, p. 59).

2. Couples who reported higher levels of relationship satisfaction prior to beginning couple therapy also rated the therapeutic alliance higher; those more distressed reported a less positive alliance. As Glebova et al. (2011) write, "If the alliance is a factor in why clients remain in treatment, then it would appear that only

the 'well' remain and those couples who are most dissatisfied with their relationship struggle the most with alliance in therapy and would be less likely to remain in therapy" (p. 60). This suggests that it is most challenging to form a therapeutic alliance with last chance couples, who are at the height of their distress. They are more likely to quit therapy than are less distressed couples, unless the therapist demonstrates early on that it can be useful.

3. The researchers found that men's relationship satisfaction ratings prior to beginning therapy were more positively correlated with the quality of the therapeutic alliance than were women's satisfaction ratings, and that men's ratings of the alliance were better correlated with changes in satisfaction by session 3 for both the male and the female partners. For women, there was a nonsignificant trend of a different sort: When they reported a better alliance in session 2, that was related to less change in satisfaction—probably because their satisfaction levels had reached a ceiling beyond which it could not improve significantly.

Furthermore, discrepancy between partners in relationship satisfaction was related to therapists' ratings of the alliance: The greater the discrepancy, the less the therapist viewed the alliance with the couple as positive. This makes perfect sense: If one partner seems less happy with the relationship and the other is happier with it, they are less likely to agree on goals or on the value of doing the therapeutic activities suggested by the therapist, leaving the therapist in a dilemma as to how to move them forward. How do you get the partner who says "Everything's pretty much fine!" on board to make the changes that the other feels necessary?

Factors That Affect the Formation of a Therapeutic Alliance

What contributes to the formation of a strong therapeutic alliance? And what factors interfere with forming such an alliance? Tambling (2012) reviewed the literature on "expectancy effects"—the beliefs that people hold about upcoming experiences of any sort—and how these expectations may influence the strength of the therapeutic alliance. A large number of studies has demonstrated that when clients in individual therapy have positive expectations and are hopeful about the potential for therapy to help them, these expectations become self-fulfilling prophesies. Potential clients seeking therapy look for information about the expected process of therapy—essentially, the roles and tasks that both therapist and client will engage in, and the quality of the therapeutic interchange in sessions—as well as the likely outcome or goal attainment of the therapy (relief of symptoms, development of greater psychological and interpersonal skills, greater happiness and life satisfaction).

A positive expectancy is closely related to a sense of hope—not only about hoped-for positive outcomes, but about the hoped-for personal and professional qualities of the therapist. In line with the large literature on common factors (Davis et al., 2012; Sprenkle et al., 2009), clients generally hope to find a therapist who will be "warm, empathic, and experienced/expert" (Tambling, 2012, p. 404). Davis et al. (2012) further specify that the therapeutic alliance is positively affected when clients perceive the therapist to offer a coherent, sensible structure to the therapy. Drawing on early work by Jerome Frank (Frank & Frank, 1993), therapists who engage clients in "credible healing rituals" (therapeutic activities explicitly stated to be important to their improvement) have better outcomes.

Davis et al. (2012) remind us that research comparing different models of therapy has not demonstrated significant differences in outcomes between models, even those established as empirically validated. Rather, as noted above, a growing body of research suggests that it is the qualities of the therapist—and the resulting quality of the therapeutic alliance—that are most strongly related to successful therapy. They write:

> The model-driven change paradigm often deemphasizes the therapist's role in change, instead focusing on the treatment dispensed. The common factors approach, on the other hand, emphasizes that treatment models do not exist in therapy outside of the therapist delivering them, and therefore the qualities of the therapist delivering the treatment are more important than the treatment itself. (Davis et al., 2012, p. 37)

This is not to say that what we do in therapy—our specific techniques—is unimportant. As research on therapeutic effectiveness becomes more refined, attention is turning to the effectiveness of specific interventions or processes in particular sessions, rather than pre-/postanalyses of overall therapeutic outcome (Davis et al., 2012):

> Nuanced findings . . . may provide insight into which processes are at work at which stage of therapy with which types of clients and presenting problems. . . . In other words, the model

(or component of the model) would be selected based on the degree to which it facilitated the requisite process, and the requisite process would be determined by client feedback (Halford et al., 2012—this issue), the stage of therapy, unique issues relevant to the couple's presenting problem, and other variables discovered as research progressed. This client-centered approach would still be empirically informed, but much more flexible and adaptive (and therefore presumably effective) than the dominant "hammer/nail" approach in which a client is expected to conform to the efficacious treatment rather than vice versa (Blow et al., 2007). (Davis et al., 2012, p. 38)

This more nuanced perspective on what contributes to therapeutic effectiveness suggests three other therapist factors that may play a central role: ongoing responsiveness to clients' changing levels of investment and confidence in the change process and in the concerns they bring to therapy over time; flexibility and resourcefulness in addressing these changing degrees of investment and needs; and client-perceived credibility—not only of the therapist overall but also of the therapist's approach to the client's particular needs. The perceived overall credibility of the therapist is established mostly by the referral source's enthusiasm for the therapist, whether that referral source is another professional or a former, satisfied client; the therapist's status in the field as demonstrated by publications and presentations; and even the quality of their website.

However, therapists cannot rest on their laurels—they need in each session to prove that they can be useful in meeting the needs of the specific and unique couple who sits before them. Sadly, I've seen a number of couples who had previously sought help with therapists highly esteemed in the field but felt that they received a kind of generic, packaged treatment that wasn't adapted to their particular needs and style as people. Indeed, research suggests that clients' sense of the credibility of the treatment offered significantly affects their engagement and therapeutic outcomes (Constantino et al., 2018; Devilly & Borkovec, 2000). Clients need to see that the therapist really understands what they are struggling with, who they are as people and their particular admixture of challenges and strengths, and that the techniques offered by the therapist make sense given their specific challenges. When therapists demonstrate that they are attentive to clients' concerns and flexibly adapt their approach to meet those concerns as they evolve and are revealed over time, this strengthens the therapeutic alliance (Stiles et al., 1998).

This probably makes great sense to you as a practicing therapist, but unfortunately, it seems that research often lags behind the well-known commonsense facts of what actually goes on in therapy. As all therapists know, the problems that clients present in a first phone call and first session are often just the surface of what is troubling them. The couple who comes in with communication problems turns out to be struggling with a previously undisclosed affair by one partner, or a secret drug addiction finally comes to light. Partners who present as having impasses in providing a unified front to their children, or major differences in how they think about money, or conflicts around who does more or less of the housework and child care, reveal after several sessions that they have little to no sexual intimacy, a problem they were reluctant to discuss initially or that they had not even yet discussed themselves. The therapist must be ready to adapt their way of working to meet these emerging, newly revealed sources of difficulty.

Here's a clinical vignette from work with a last chance couple that demonstrates the importance of these research-supported principles of therapist responsiveness and flexibility, and of the credibility of one's chosen approach. Tanya, an African American woman, and Ramon, a Dominican American man, married 11 years and together for 13, described their presenting problem as long-standing serious communication issues that entailed high conflict followed by long brooding silences that were leading them both to consider divorce. I suggested that I begin working with them to improve their communication and problem-solving skills, and they enthusiastically agreed to this plan (well, she was enthusiastic—Ramon was not so keen to be doing couple therapy at all, and sat with arms folded and an impassive expression on his face during that first session). Training in communication skills led to a rapid decrease in their level of conflict and improvement in their sense of connection, and to Ramon's sense that therapy would provide practical tools that could actually help them— as opposed to, as he said, what he thought therapy would be—"just a lot of 'blah blah blah.'"

However, this improvement led to emergence of an issue that, for a different reason, threatened the trust and stability of the marriage. Tanya revealed, for the first time to me, her extensive and dramatic history of childhood sexual abuse, which had been the hidden issue affecting her comfort during sex with Ramon. Ramon knew about some of her abuse history, but it had been a long time since they'd discussed it, and he had not known the extent of the abuse she had suffered. Tanya's history came to light in a session after she arrived home from work one night and saw Ramon with their two-year-old daughter

Jessica sitting on his lap, a blanket around her, happily watching a kid's TV show. In their bedroom later that evening, Tanya expressed her discomfort with this scene, which led Ramon to become hurt and outraged that she could imagine that he would be sexually abusing their daughter. Tanya reminded him about her history of childhood sexual abuse, but Ramon only became more offended—"How could you possibly think I'm one of 'those guys'?!" He then said if she really thought this, they shouldn't be together. Tanya experienced his anger as a sign that he didn't care about her and that they still had significant communication issues.

I asked Tanya if she would describe what had happened to her. She had been repeatedly abused starting at age eight by her mother's various boyfriends and male babysitters, and as a teen, had a relationship with a somewhat older man whom she initially saw as a kind and protective figure, but who recruited her into exploitative orgies that she felt unable to refuse. Ramon had not heard some of these details and, while sympathetic and upset for her, still did not understand how she could assume that he would do this to their own daughter. He viewed himself as macho but very protective of women, and especially Tanya. She agreed that he had never exploited her trust and was attracted to him because he was a "strong gentleman" and the first protective man she'd ever been with. This softened Ramon's demeanor somewhat, but far from completely.

I responded to this new crisis by explaining the psychological effects of sexual trauma, which I happen to have spent decades working on (Fraenkel, 2019a; Sheinberg & Fraenkel, 2001), especially the way that trauma survivors can be triggered by seeing something that reminds them of their abuse, even if the stimulus is innocuous. The couple agreed to my suggestion that I have an individual session or two with Tanya to witness empathically and explore her trauma history, to work on containing the impact of trauma symptoms when they got triggered, and to explore her dysfunctional relationship with her mother. These sessions greatly helped Tanya come to terms with her history, as she had never sought psychotherapy for these experiences. She also said understanding more about trauma explained her reactions at times when Ramon insisted on having sex: She would freeze and become uncommunicative—something he had noticed but interpreted as her not wanting to have sex with him in general.

Tanya expressed concerns that Ramon's reactivity and macho style made him a wrong choice for her, despite her report that when they first met and fell in love, he was the first man she felt could be safe and protective. I hypothesized that perhaps she had picked him because he was strong and could be forceful at times, but that he also seemed to be a man who would not abuse or mistreat her, or a child they might have in the future. Based on his loving and protective behavior as an involved father, and Tanya's report that Ramon had never done anything abusive or clearly inappropriate with their daughter, I had no concerns that he might be inclined toward abuse.

I explained the premise guiding Bowen family systems therapy—that unlike Freud's notion that we neurotically pick an adult partner with whom we compulsively repeat the same problematic relationships we had with early parent figures, instead we pick someone similar enough to a problematic parent (or other problematic adult figure) but a less extreme version, whom we unconsciously sense may allow us to master and overcome those old conflictual experiences. I noted that if she had wanted to find a less strong-willed, more compliant and passive man to marry, she likely could have done so. She found this hypothesis extremely helpful in reframing why she ended up marrying Ramon instead of other men who showed interest in her and who were less macho (she was a professional singer involved with the downtown arts and music world, and had encountered many such interested men, but had turned them down).

Individual sessions with Ramon centered on further explaining and normalizing Tanya's moments of being triggered, to help him not to take these personally and get angry, but rather to approach these moments as opportunities to help her heal. This work also allowed us to explore his own history of physical and emotional abuse. His father had abused him and his mother, which had shaped his determination to be a protective husband and father. I empathized with him and applauded his relational goals. I also noted that despite his intentions, his tendency to get quite angry and defensive at times with Tanya might be undermining his own desire to show himself to be "a different kind of man" than he had experienced with his father and that Tanya had encountered with other men. I shared (with Tanya's permission) that she was deeply attracted to his protective style and still saw him that way for the most part. Ramon agreed with these points and was reassured to hear what Tanya had said about him.

In the following couple session, they reported on a powerful moment that strengthened their mutual trust and helped Tanya begin to separate from her history of sexual trauma. One night while they were making love, Ramon stopped and said, "Hey, are you okay? You seem distracted. We don't have to do this if you're not comfortable." In the past, when Tanya would seem removed during sex, Ramon would take it personally and get upset. Tanya told him she was okay, just momentarily tired, but was fine to continue making love—in fact, his checking in with her made her even more desirous. There was a palpable sense of relief and warmth between the two as they recounted this moment.

Tanya also apologized for her reaction to seeing Jessica on Ramon's lap and again explained, in line with their work with me on improving their communication, that she had mostly just wanted to share her being triggered—she didn't mean to imply that he was doing anything improper, even though she understood now how he heard it this way. Ramon gently reassured her that he now "got it" and welcomed her to tell him in the future if she felt worried.

This vignette illustrates the importance of being a resourceful therapist who can draw upon a range of theories, research, and therapeutic techniques to address the issues that emerge over time. Chapter 2 describes my comprehensive, multiperspectival approach to couple therapy that allows maximum resourcefulness and flexibility, and that seems most credible to couples as a result. The vignette also demonstrates the need to have a strong relationship with each partner to respond to each partner's needs around a topic that threatened to dissolve their relationship, as well as a strong relationship with their relationship, to help them forge new ways of interacting and understanding one another.

Here's another vignette that demonstrates the delicate dance of affirming each partner's point of view on their problems and then helping them see how each one's changes in attitudes and behavior will promote change in the other. This delicate dance is central to sustaining a couple's sense of the credibility of our approach to working with them. George and Alice were a white Jewish American couple in their mid-60s. Married for over 40 years and with two grown children, they had been deeply unhappy from the very beginning. Although both felt they should have left the relationship earlier, they'd had their first child soon after marriage and felt committed to preserving the family for the sake of the kids. George felt chronically rejected by Alice. He loved to talk and share his feelings, and she was quiet and reserved—in their marriage, although not with friends and at work. Alice was a lawyer in a leadership position in a community advocacy organization, deeply committed to her work, which was at times challenging and required long hours. George was a high school guidance counselor who became a professional life coach and structured his practice to allow for plenty of time with Alice and the kids. He happily did most of the domestic chores, including cooking and cleaning. But he felt lonely and wished for more intimacy with Alice. In a classic instance of the pursuer-distancer pattern, the more he asked for talk time with her, the more she resisted.

When I started seeing Alice and George, they were as polarized as a couple could possibly be. George was verbose and expressive—in fact, he repeated himself over and over—while Alice sat impassively listening to his complaints about her, with an absolutely blank face. For years, George had criticized her devotion to her work, frequently asking her how many sick days and vacation days she had not used (which he wanted her to use for time with him), and complained that she did not put their relationship first. Alice felt affronted by these critiques, leading her to retreat further into her shell.

Simple suggestions about carving out some joint time for connection failed. Exploration of their respective families of origin revealed that George had felt deprived of attention by his parents and had, not surprisingly, picked a partner with whom he would face the same challenge of getting attention in hopes of mastering that childhood experience (rather than being with a woman who seemed equally interested in close connection). As a child and teen, Alice had been discouraged from pursuing her intellectual and social justice passions and career, and part of her intense interest in work was to correct for the disapproval she experienced from her parents. Although George fully supported Alice's work passions and was proud of her dedication and competence, his request that she cut back on the time she spent on work was enough to elicit in Alice the old script of her parents discouraging her career ambitions. The partners found these interpretations interesting, but increased understanding of the roots of their needs did not result in change.

I then further empathized with George's sense of emotional abandonment—which initially triggered a look of resentment toward me from Alice—but then quickly validated Alice's feeling that her devotion to work was being seemingly denigrated by George in his attempt to get more attention from her—which led George to look a bit deflated, as if I had withdrawn my support for his position. I suggested that George had imposed a perspective on priorities that simply did not square with Alice's passion, and that it should be possible for her to be deeply devoted to her work and still make some time for them—but not until George stopped critiquing her.

I proposed a visual metaphor—that they were each on separate islands, and were not likely ever to live completely on the same island, but could meet on a joint island periodically to connect. I asked them to envision what they could do on that island. They decided they would take an exercise class and an online course. But I reiterated to George that unless he ceased critiquing Alice's work life, she was not likely to get on the bridge to their joint island. Somewhat surprisingly, he balked at this and said, "I understand what my 'ask' is—what I need to do—but what is Alice's 'ask'? What is she needing to do?" Alice, who had been more engaged than ever before, immediately retreated to her blank-face posture. I said, "George, I'm not sure what you're confused about here—you need to stop nagging her and critiquing her if she is to come toward you and onto the island!"

I invoked another metaphor—that of planting seeds in a plot of earth. If a gardener continues to check on the seeds multiple times a day and turn the earth while the seeds attempt to gestate, they will not grow. I suggested he needed to engage in this experiment of meeting on the island and seeing what could grow there. Alice looked relieved; George finally seemed to understand. The couple began to meet on their island and slowly developed a sense of connection and pleasure that had been missing for most of their marriage—albeit one that did not fully meet George's desire for intense engagement. However, my hope was that despite not fully meeting his intense attachment and intimacy needs, he would come to be satisfied with a "good enough" connection (to paraphrase Winnicott's 1971 notion of the "good-enough mother"), and thereby overcome his family-of-origin issues.

This vignette demonstrates the reality of working with couples in which both partners are highly sensitive to whether the therapist supports them. Supporting one partner at length without confirming support for the other will quickly lead to disengagement of that partner, and possibly quitting the therapy. The therapist must move deftly back and forth between opposing views, showing appreciation for both, and then side with the relationship, requiring each partner to take steps toward the other. And as in this case, sometimes it is necessary to suggest that one partner start the circular process of change. George felt it a bit unfair that he needed first to stop critiquing Alice in order for her to step forward, but she simply did not feel safe offering herself if it meant risking another attack from him claiming that she wasn't giving enough.

The Special Challenges of Creating a Therapeutic Alliance With Last Chance Couples

The research on the therapeutic alliance suggests that how we, in the very first session, form a working relationship with both partners in a last chance couple—one or both of whom is strongly considering ending the relationship—may determine how engaged they become in the therapy process, or even whether they return for a second session. Last chance couples are the most distressed of any couple that presents for therapy and, by definition, the most ambivalent about pursuing it. Therefore, we must pay special attention to forming a strong therapeutic alliance, one that aligns with each partner on their often quite different assessments of the problems, goals, tasks, and level of satisfaction they feel about the relationship. Especially challenging is to form a relationship with the partner whose goal is to save the relationship, as well as with the other partner, who typically seeks to end the relationship as amicably as possible. Glebova et al. (2011) suggest that when there is a large discrepancy between partners in pretreatment relationship satisfaction, the therapist should pay special attention to this discrepancy, given that these differences in satisfaction level predict the quality of the therapeutic alliance. The authors note, "couples who are highly distressed and conflictual, in essence do not share an alliance that allows for adaptation and change. They may approach the relationship with a therapist with the same level of distrust as they have with each other, thus making establishing a working alliance with these couples more difficult" (Glebova et al., 2011, p. 63).

Attention to these different satisfaction levels between partners, validating and accepting each partner's point of view, and yet finding a way to experiment with possibilities of change is at the heart of work with last chance couples. What is not useful is to try to change the more negative partner's views without providing them with new data that comes through these experiments. Much as I endorse generally the strengths-based foundation of most approaches to family and couple therapy (Walsh, 2012), techniques such as narrative therapy's focus on eliciting the "subordinated story" and "unique outcomes" representing the relationship's positive qualities and stories of earlier, better times, or solution-focused therapy's attempts to unearth "exceptions" to the problem, tend to irritate the partner who has pretty much decided that the relationship is mostly negative (whatever the earlier love story might be) and worth leaving (Fraenkel, 2019b).

The gender differences identified by Knobloch-Fedders et al. (2007) about what aspects of the therapeutic alliance are most related to progress reveal another of the core challenges in working with last chance couples, at least those in which partners are cisgender and heterosexual. If it's the case that a woman's sense of the man's alliance with the therapist is crucial to her engagement in therapy and to progress, and if she needs to sense a strong alliance with her husband about the therapy in order to engage in progress-oriented goals and tasks, what happens when it's the woman who wants to leave the marriage? Although there are no statistics yet on the percentage of last chance couples in which it is the woman or the man who is expressing the desire to end things, my experience of 30 years suggests that it is roughly 50-50—as many women as men raise the specter of divorce. So when it is the female partner who expresses the desire to end the relationship, the role of persuading the other partner to try therapy—usually held by the woman—now falls on the man's shoulders. If they've held the typical socialized gendered pattern in which the woman is relegated to attending to the quality of the relationship and addressing issues ("pursuing") and the man tends to withdraw from her attempts to get him to the table (Christensen & Heavey, 1990; Gottman & Gottman, 2018), last chance couples in which the woman is fed up and ready to leave put the onus on the man to try to convince her to stay and work things out. And it creates special challenges for the therapist—especially a male therapist—to develop a therapeutic alliance that will not be perceived as taking sides with the husband to keep the wife in a marriage she wants to exit.

HOW TO BUILD A GOOD INITIAL THERAPEUTIC ALLIANCE IN THE FIRST SESSION

The process of establishing a strong alliance with last chance couples perfectly illustrates the distinction I discuss in Chapter 2 between what science provides as guides to therapy and what the craft of our field provides (Doherty, 2012). As my review of the literature shows, science indicates the importance of establishing a warm, genuine, empathic, and structuring relationship with each partner, with the relationship as a whole, and fostering an alliance between the partners. But science so far does not provide much guidance on how to do this, especially given the wide variety of couples, issues, motivational levels, and other factors that distinguish one couple from another. It's not enough just to be a nice, kind person who cares about people. That's certainly necessary, but not sufficient in order to engage those qualities across the many challenges last chance couples present therapists to connect well with them.

The steps to form a good initial therapeutic alliance with a last chance couple are as follows:

1. You must validate each partner's desires for the future of the relationship, which may mean both partners' deep ambivalence about

staying together, or one partner's wish to leave and the other partner's wish to stay.

2. You should state that in general, you are inclined to help couples improve the relationship and stay together. Unless you specifically describe your work primarily as divorce counseling (Lebow,
2015)—helping couples separate as amicably as possible with a
subsequent referral to a divorce mediation specialist—you should
note that you generally work to help people stay together when
couples are not in the last chance moment. However, you should
say that you will work with the couple to decide which direction
they want to go. That said, you should invite the couple to tell you
if they perceive you to be inadvertently pressuring them to stay
together. You should note that you will enthusiastically work with
the couple to explore the potential of the relationship to improve,
but initially only to help them empirically evaluate whether they
should stay together or end the relationship. You should request
the couple not to misinterpret your enthusiasm for the change
techniques as pressure for the partners to preserve the marriage.

3. The therapeutic contract—a statement of how you will work
with the couple—must be tentative and developed collaboratively, meaning that each session will end with jointly evaluating
whether it felt useful and whether you addressed the partners'
concerns as much as possible in one session. There should be no
automatic assumption that the couple wants to return for a subsequent session. The couple, especially the ambivalent partner,
should be invited to think after the session about whether they
want to return.

4. You should outline a plan of action in the first session. This plan
should include imparting specific practices or tools to help the
couple experiment with possibilities—to see if improved communication, small steps toward restoring pleasure, apology rituals,
and other practices will lead the couple to reevaluate their relationship's potential. As I discuss further in Chapter 2, it's important to let last chance couples know from the outset that you will
offer them concrete practices to create change, and to reassure
them that you will not engage in a protracted exploration of their
history before offering them strategies for improvement. Even in
the first phone call or online consultation, and then again in the
first session, describe your model as an action/insight approach,
in which you will first suggest research-based techniques for
changing their style of interaction, and then will explore their
respective family- and culture-of-origin experiences and learnings

to help them uncover the sources of their emotional sensitivities or triggers and the beliefs they acquired about relationships that get activated in their current relationship. The initial emphasis is almost always on suggesting new forms of interaction, as couples are impatient to see whether you can help them actually change, not just understand what went wrong and why.

5. You should introduce the notion that the couple can enter a liminal space—a space between staying together and ending the relationship. You should suggest that for a few weeks, discussion about whether to end the relationship be suspended so that the couple can experiment with the relationship's potential. Explain that continuing to raise the strong possibility of dissolving the relationship serves to pull the rug out from under their efforts, making it difficult to assess for themselves whether their efforts to change are leading in a positive direction.

6. However, especially to reassure the ambivalent partner, you should cast these experiments in improvement as *nonbinding*. This means that even if the relationship improves, the ambivalent partner should feel free to reassert their desire to end things. Without this reassurance, the ambivalent partner is not likely to agree on the tasks and goals that constitute two thirds of the therapeutic alliance, for fear that improvement will invalidate their desire to end the relationship.

These steps are critical to forming an emotionally safe, productive, beginning therapeutic alliance with a last chance couple. Notice that I deliberately avoided the adjectives *strong* or *successful* in describing this initial alliance. This is because the only way the alliance will be perceived by the couple partners as strong or successful is through observable evidence over the first few sessions that you understand their experience, that your plan for helping them works, and, most importantly, that you actually did what you said you would do. Remember that one or both partners come to you feeling that promises each made when they first committed themselves to one another—promises of a loving, passionate, cooperative life together—have not been kept. They are now equally suspicious about whether your promises will be kept. There's no way to convince them that you will follow through and execute the approach you outlined until they witness you do it, or that the practices you enthusiastically recommend lead to some improvement, even if the improvement is incomplete. As one man said to his fiancée after a session in which I helped them devise a new balance of time in intimate conversation, time with family, and time engaged in solo activities, "It all seems great in theory—but I can't relax and be confident until I see if it actually works." I supported his reticence, as it provided further energy for the couple to make the change happen. As I often say to couples, "The rubber has to hit the road before you feel confident that these plans will make things better."

THE CRAFT OF CONNECTING: DETAILED TIPS FOR DEVELOPING A THERAPEUTIC BOND

The six steps described above mostly center on two of the three core components of the therapeutic alliance: establishing agreement on goals and agreement on tasks, as well as a framework for pursuing these goals and engaging in these tasks when one or both partners are highly ambivalent about the relationship and about engaging in therapy. But what about the third component of the alliance, the emotional bond or connection between the therapist and the couple? Although many psychotherapy authors, from client-centered therapy creator and early psychotherapy researcher Carl Rogers onward, have emphasized the importance of the common factors of therapist warmth, genuineness, and empathy in establishing the bond aspect of the therapeutic alliance (Davis et al., 2012; Sprenkle et al., 2009), little has been written about specific practices for connecting with clients in general, and couples specifically. In work with last chance couples, it can at times be challenging to sustain a bond that includes genuineness, warmth, and empathy, as it's not uncommon that one or both partners have done things to one another, or to others, that violate a partner's values, or sense of safety and integrity. As Winnicott wrote about individual therapy, the "bad behaviors" of the patient can arouse understandable revulsion and even hatred in the therapist (as discussed in Tuber, 2008). It is critical that the therapist acknowledge and examine whether these feelings of revulsion stem from their own unresolved (in psychoanalytic terms, unanalyzed) psychological issues, or are realistic, objective reactions to the distasteful, hurtful, and even unethical behavior of the patient. Otherwise, the therapist may be unconsciously biased and act out their revulsion against the patient.

One whole category of last chance couples centers on those in which a partner has had an affair (or multiple affairs) and persistently lied about it, has perpetrated violence toward the partner, has engaged in persistent overuse of alcohol or drugs and frightened or angered the partner and children with this addictive behavior, has gambled or in other ways threatened the couple's financial well-being, or engaged in other behaviors that pose a threat to the partner's physical and emotional well-being. These value and safety violations toward the partner may also violate the therapist's personal and professional values. Likewise, high-conflict couples may use language and nonverbal behavior that is offensive to the partner as well as to the therapist, including language that insults the partner (or the therapist directly) in terms of their gender, sexual orientation, gender identity, age, race, ethnicity, level of education or intellectual abilities, religious, political, or social belief system, and other aspects of social location and identity. As two of my earlier vignettes illustrated, one or both couple partners may also directly challenge the therapist's competence or devalue the entire field of psychotherapy.

Here are some practices I've refined over decades to help build the bond, starting in the first session.

1. Admiring and showing interest in couple partners' work and other areas of competence

Unless the couple is in such a state of crisis that they would not feel relaxed enough, the therapist should start the first session by asking each partner what they do during the day. Usually this will mean asking about their work lives and careers. I open this up by saying, "Before we get into the challenges you two are facing right now, I'd like to ask you each about what you do during the day." Ask them what they do, how they got into that type of work (which often involves a brief history of their academic background), and what they like about it (when they like it). When one partner has left work and is a full-time parent, ask about their work and career prior to becoming a parent. (In cisgender heterosexual couples, it is usually women who have stepped partially or fully away from work to raise young children, and asking them only about parenting can implicitly suggest that their work and career are not important.) I also ask each partner, "When you think about yourself as a person—your talents, strengths, sensitivities, capacities—what do you bring of yourself to this work when you feel you're doing it at your best?" Clients like this question, as it suggests the therapist is interested in their strengths, especially given that they come to couple therapy feeling deskilled and incompetent in many ways about the relationship. Oftentimes, these strengths— being a good communicator, forming trusting relationships with clients, being highly organized, creative, solving complex problems, and so on—can be transferred to improving the relationship.

Most importantly, these questions allow the therapist to show genuine interest and excitement about the clients' areas of interest and expertise. The therapist can express respect and even genuine amazement about what the client does in their work life. If the therapist at one time considered the client's career but decided they didn't have the talents for it, telling that story can implicitly communicate the message, "While I may be an expert in relationships and you feel ashamed about not doing so well currently in this domain, you have skills and talents I don't have, that I admire, and that I have wished for." This can have the effect of helping discouraged clients feel a sense of self-esteem in relationship to the therapist. It can also diffuse the potential for a client, especially one who holds a position of power in the workplace, to challenge the therapist or question their competence when doing so comes from the client's difficulty not being in charge and feeling they must submit to the therapist's expertise. The therapist is acknowledging that the client is a "master of the universe" in their work domain, which can reassure an anxious client that they are respected despite having relationship difficulties.

For instance, Tony was a working-class man with an undiagnosed learning disability who barely graduated high school, but he was a gifted boiler mechanic. His wife, Linda, told me in the initial call that he was anxious about starting therapy, because "he's not so good with words." In our first session, I expressed my admiration for his skill set, noting that I get too anxious when something like a boiler is malfunctioning to do anything to repair it, and am not so good sorting out all the issues that might be going on with mechanical devices. Tony smiled, sat up a bit more in his chair, and told a few stories of particularly challenging boilers in large buildings that other mechanics had not been able to repair. It became clear that he was considered a master boiler mechanic, one who often mentored beginning mechanics and was called on to solve particularly tough cases.

Likewise, with a client who was an architect, I noted that as a kid I was deeply interested in architecture and even took some architectural drawing classes, but when I heard that you had to be good at math to be an architect, I dropped it. Subsequently I learned that engineers are the ones that handle the math side and had regrets about not pursing that field. This led the client to laugh and confirm what I'd learned, but she also seemed pleased that I was so admiring of her work. We talked a bit about our favorite architects. She recommended I check out some architects that I'd never heard of, and I sensed that she realized through this discussion that I truly was interested in what she did so well and, more importantly, was open to hearing her point of view, which transferred smoothly into our work together.

Starting sessions with these questions also provides an opportunity for the therapist to observe how one partner responds when the other is talking about their work. Do they smile and even offer a statement of admiration—"She's an amazing lawyer"; "He's a genius mechanic"? Or do they look uninterested, or even express annoyance—"Yeah, he brings his lawyer side home—I often feel I'm on trial," or "Well, if she treated me half as well as she treats her patients, we'd be doing better!" As Gottman (Driver et al., 2012) notes, couples that engage in "positive sentiment override"—expressing positive feelings even during conflict—do better than couples who do the opposite, inserting negative affect and deflating their words into otherwise positive moments. Observing these interactions gives the therapist a beginning hint of whether there exists at least a modicum of mutual admiration and appreciation, another variable from Gottman's research that strongly predicts relationship happiness. Although research has not investigated this, mutual admiration between partners likely strengthens the partner-to-partner aspect of the therapeutic alliance and their motivation to improve the relationship.

2. Dealing with doubts about therapy and challenges to the therapist's expertise

Some clients are highly suspicious of the entire field of psychotherapy. Based on films and other media portrayals, they may view it as endless "talking about my mother" and not leading to actual changes. Emphasizing the focus on learning new tools and skills often assuages these concerns. Other clients may express skepticism about whether therapy can help them, given how long the couple has been struggling, especially if they've had unsuccessful attempts at therapy. Asking them about those therapy experiences and distinguishing what you will do with them from what they experienced previously often reassures them.

When a partner is particularly confrontational about the therapy, folding their arms and saying something like, "I just don't believe in this therapy stuff," as I illustrated in one of the vignettes in the introduction, I often find it disarms them when I express my own doubts. I'll say something like, "Well, of course I believe it does work for many people 'cause I've seen it work, else I would have gone back to drumming in wedding and Bar Mitzvah bands (which I did, for years), but I come to each session with my own skepticism and doubt, which keeps me sharp. And of course, I don't know that what I will offer you will be helpful to you, but I will do my best. And that also depends on what you put into it. Let's see what happens!" This statement combines several elements that assist in establishing a warm, empathic, and genuine bond when working with a challenging client: nondefensiveness, humility about the process and prospects of therapy, validation of their concerns, and a touch of self-effacing humor.

Often these sorts of critical statements by clients are also infused with the issues mentioned earlier in working with a client who is powerful in their work domain—an alpha male or female or master of the universe—and who has difficulty taking direction from others. With one client (described in the introduction)—a multimillionaire whose first words to me were to question the usefulness of therapy (and which he delivered with an air of smug self-assurance)—I said something to this effect, noting that he was used to giving directions, not taking them. By the end of the session in which I had quickly identified the fundamental problem patterns in their relationship and taught him and his wife communication skills, he looked at me appreciatively, and with a slight smile but still an air of superiority, used a complimentary term from the world of finance: "I'm impressed—on the upside," and we laughed.

3. Connecting with partners whose behavior has violated values and safety

As I noted briefly earlier, as therapists, we must be prepared to work with people who have done emotional or physical harm to others and who have violated basic relationship values of honesty, commitment, trust, safety and protection, integrity, kindness, and compassion. We may feel disturbed by their behaviors and, when working with couples, can then be pulled emotionally to side with the offended partner. These situations challenge us to locate the humanity of the offending partner and find ways to empathize with their experiences, even when we disapprove of their behavior. We must do this so that we can sustain a systemic, relational perspective on the couple, wherein we identify the problematic behaviors that the nonoffending partner has engaged in that might have stimulated (but not caused) the offending partner's behavior, or that at least occur alongside these behaviors even if not directly contributing to them.

In this regard, I was fortunate early in my career to be the sole man in a team that developed a family-based approach to incest (Fraenkel, 2019a; Sheinberg & Fraenkel, 2001), as I was asked by my colleagues to work with the male family member who had perpetrated sexual abuse on his female child, stepchild, or sister. I had to find a way to connect with these teens and men, understand the sources of their behavior, and make them feel cared about, despite not only the egregious harm they had caused the abused child, but the emotional harm and relational trauma they caused for other nonoffending family members (mothers/partners, siblings), rupturing the entire family.

This work, and my work with partners who cause harm or violate the safety of the other, led me to develop a few key therapeutic strategies. First, we must remember that this person is a human being who also suffers, and in most cases, their behavior is a problematic attempt to decrease their suffering and get their needs met. We must remember that our role is to be a therapist, not a priest, rabbi, imam, lawyer, judge, or police officer, and that our best hope of helping them change their behavior—for their sake and others—is to identify and empathize with their suffering and to guide them to nonharmful ways of being in relationships.

Second, drawing upon the work of Goldner et al. (1990; Goldner, 1998) and their feminist-systemic-psychodynamic integrative approach to working with interpersonal violence, the therapist must take the position that although the partner's actions may be a response to the other partner's problematic words and behavior, the partner who has engaged in value- or safety-violating behavior is 100% responsible for choosing to behave in this manner rather than in other ways that do not threaten the safety and values of their partner. Effective therapy must adopt a view that some aspects of the couple's difficulties can be understood as circular, back-and-forth patterns in which both partners play a part and must change, and other aspects—the choice to violate values and safety—involve a linear, one-way misuse of power that is not caused by the other partner, and this "power-over" behavior needs to end (Knudson-Martin, 2013; Knudson-Martin & Mahoney, 2009).

As I discuss again in detail in Chapter 6, closely related to this stance is the need to distinguish between finding a psychological explanation for the value/safety-violating behavior versus excusing the behavior. Whether it's acts of physical violence, threats and emotional intimidation, affairs, persistent drug or alcohol overuse, misappropriation of money, or other violations of safety, commitment, and trust, there is always a psychological reason underlying the behavior, and always other ways the partner could choose to respond to their needs and issues. Therapy in part centers on engaging the partner in a frame-by-frame review of times when they chose to act in value- and safety-violating ways, empathizing with their pain and struggles, and locating the moment when they could have chosen another course of action. Examples of better, nonabusive choices include talking to their partner about their unhappiness, loneliness, and desire to have sex or emotional intimacy with someone else; finding ways of self-soothing other than substances; taking a time-out or leaving the home if they feel compelled to act in violent or intimidating ways; learning anger management skills; and engaging in structured communication skills to express their needs in a modulated manner. This therapeutic exploration helps partners eventually take 100% responsibility for their behavior if they haven't already. The alliance-building practices described in the present chapter are at the core of how the therapist establishes a warm, genuine, and empathic relationship with partners who have violated relationship values and safety, enabling them to look nondefensively and honestly at their behavior, apologize, and make a genuine commitment to avoid such behavior in the future.

4. Connecting across therapist–client differences in culture and social locations

The field of couple and family therapy has become increasingly attuned to the impact of racism, ethnicism, classism, sexism, hetero-sexism, and other forms of oppressive beliefs, behaviors, and institutionalized socioeconomic practices and policies that discriminate against and oppress people in various intersectional social locations (Boyd-Franklin, 2003; Falicov, 2017; McDowell et al., 2017; McGoldrick & Hardy, 2019; Pinderhughes, 1989; Walsh, 2012). Along with the need to understand how individual, couple, and family psychological and relational difficulties are related to these forms of oppression (discussed more fully in Chapter 2), therapists need to inquire about people's cultural backgrounds and affiliations, and the beliefs, customs, rituals, and practices that inform their identities, coping skills, and approach to relationships (Falicov, 1998, 2016, 2017; Walsh, 2009).

Couple partners may come from similar backgrounds but often also have social locational differences. For instance, in one couple, both partners were second-generation Indian Americans (born in the United States to parents who immigrated from India), both grew up in the same area of New York, and both were highly educated, but differed in their family of origin's social class—she upper-class, he lower-middle class. This class difference led to differences in their expectations about who should take care of domestic chores: She didn't give them much thought, as her parents had a full-time housekeeper, whereas he was used to doing chores at home, and ended up unhappily shouldering these chores in their relationship. Likewise, partners may differ in how they relate to and position themselves to their shared culture of origin, for instance, an African American couple in which both partners were raised lower-middle class and were involved in the Christian church. But as an adult, one partner left the church and gradually embraced pantheistic and more New Age spiritual beliefs, while the other still felt connected to his Christian religious beliefs. This resulted in a number of conflicts, including around sex: The woman, who had embraced pantheistic beliefs, wanted to experiment with polyamory, while the man felt uncomfortable doing so.

Given the kaleidoscopic mixtures of social locations, cultural backgrounds, and degree of connection people hold to their cultures, it is impossible to achieve so-called cultural competence, a term that implies being adequately familiar with the experiences and meaning systems held by people from various locations and cultures. Rather, the therapist needs to adopt a stance of "cultural sensitivity and curiosity"—asking questions of clients to learn from them about their unique intersectional and culturally informed experiences (Hardy & Bobes, 2016).

Forming the therapeutic alliance always involves connecting to clients who differ from oneself in some or many ways. Therefore, virtually all therapy relationships are cross-cultural or cross-locational in some fashion. Even if one shares many aspects of location and culture with one's clients, there are inevitable differences that often need to be recognized and bridged. For instance, I am a white cisgender heterosexual highly educated upper-middle-class Jewish American (third generation) raised in New York and Boston and originally lower-middle class in early childhood, but I was raised nonreligious although immersed to a great degree in Jewish culture. Working with Orthodox Jewish couples, who also vary as a group in terms of their degree of observance (for instance, Modern Orthodox versus Hasidic), I always have much to learn about their cultural practices and the couple's specific relationship to and interpretation of their culture. Working with Jewish couples who, like me, were raised nonreligious and middle class, I have much to learn about those who now are quite wealthy and inhabit the "1%" in social class, with all its many privileges and some unique problems. Working with a Jewish husband who was a staunch Republican Trump supporter, whereas I am a left-leaning liberal Democrat whose grandparents were socialists, I had to find ways to bridge our differences so that he trusted and felt respected by me. Working with nonreligious upper-middle-class highly educated Jewish couples from the South, or from the Midwest, I've found it important to understand and bridge with their particular cultural niche and styles of interacting, quite different from my Northeastern upbringing (they being more polite and reserved than I'm used to as a New York City and Boston-bred Jew).

Here's some tips about how to build the alliance across these inevitable cultural and locational differences and similarities.

Just Ask

Inquiring about the couple partners' respective social locations and cultures and how these inform their beliefs about relationships is central to forming the alliance, as well as to assessing areas of difference between partners when these exist. Demonstrating genuine curiosity helps couples feel that you see them and are interested in their unique realities. For instance, in working with the African American couple in which one partner had left the church while the other remained faithful to Christ, I asked them how they experienced their issues as an African American couple with different views on religion and sexuality. Just asking this question led the couple to feel more comfortable with me: They said they appreciated that I, as a white therapist, would be curious about their somewhat different forms of African American identity and how it shaped their relationship challenges.

Share One's Enjoyment and Partial Knowledge of the Other's Culture

Just as expressing enthusiasm for and genuine curiosity about couple partners' respective work lives and interests can build a sense of warmth and respect central to the therapeutic bond, sharing one's genuine enjoyment of others' cultures can lead couples to feel respected and appreciated. Obviously (I hope), this needs to be done with a smile and a sense of humor, as a small break from the seriousness of your work with the couple, and not with an awkward "tourist in another country" naivete that goes on and on. For instance, with Indian couples, somewhere in the process of exploring their cultural background, I will often mention, with a kind of humorous tone, that for years I've cooked Indian food and even make my own *rasmalai* from scratch (rasmalai is a classic Indian dessert made with fresh cheese, sugar, rose water, cardamon, and cream, and is quite a time-intensive endeavor). Couples are inevitably impressed and laugh, saying even their mothers don't make rasmalai.

With African American couples, I sometimes will throw into the conversation, at an opportune moment, that I'm a professional jazz and funk drummer, or mention some of my favorite African American musical artists, or even, when talking about sex, adopt a Barry White bass voice and say something about "making love" using his dulcet tones. The experience of a white therapist who knows in some depth and honors their cultural references and even can be cute and silly in expressing his appreciation of their culture, rather than being overly earnest or offensive, can increase a couple's comfort. Of course, this must be done in a way that avoids people feeling that their culture is being mocked. It must be done with the greatest respect. These actions essentially provide a playful, safe way to acknowledge differences, which further opens a back-and-forth about their cultural background and experience. However, if you don't feel comfortable knowing how to achieve this approach of respectful and playful mentioning of your appreciation of another's culture, or if playfulness is not your strong suit, best not to try these moves until you've gotten some supervision on it.

One example of this sort of playfulness about differences, initiated by the couple and that involved me answering questions about my social location, occurred early in my work several years ago with a low-income, highly educated African American couple, James and LaShonda, in which LaShonda's mother, Betty, was highly critical of her parenting of their eight-year-old daughter Dominique, and had even contacted ACS (the Administration for Child Services, the New York State agency that investigates alleged child abuse). When I asked the couple what Betty's allegations included, LaShonda noted that years ago as a toddler, Dominique had pulled a hot cup of tea off the kitchen table and burned herself, but LaShonda had brought Dominique immediately to the emergency room (where, as often happens with African American couples, doctors started an investigation through ACS, which was summarily dismissed). More recently, LaShonda related, Betty had criticized her cooking, declaring vigorously, "Your green beans taste like wax!" This led James to laugh uproariously and comment that this type of critique was typical of his mother-in-law, and he had started audiotaping their calls "so that the next ACS worker who comes to visit us will hear her craziness."

I suggested that perhaps they could invite Betty to a session, and they both expressed doubt that she would come. I offered to invite Betty directly. They then paused and LaShonda, with a half smile, said, "Well, that might work, because you're Jewish—you are Jewish, aren't you?" I smiled and said, "Yes I am. . . . How would that help?" James said, "Well, in her generation, you know, Jewish doctors are seen as wise, smart, caring . . . " I smiled and said, "Oh really?" James teasingly said, "Yeah, not so much in our generation, but in her generation for sure." LaShonda then countered, "But when she sees that you are younger than she is, it might not work—how old are you?" I said, "46," and she said, "Yeah, that might be a problem." We all laughed, and in the end, they decided against inviting Betty to a session. Instead, we talked about how to engage her in a more supportive, less competitive manner with Dominique and their young son, Tommy.

Are these sorts of moves and moments unorthodox by traditional psychotherapeutic standards? You bet! Are they effective? Definitely, and partly because they are unorthodox. Couples come to therapy often with a stereotyped expectation of couple therapy and therapist behavior. In this script, they will describe their problems; the therapist, speaking in a serious, professional, somewhat distant tone, will weigh in on their issues and provide some guidance; and the couple will leave the session with some useful ideas and practices to improve their relationship. All well and good, but frankly, boring and not fully engaging. I believe that the distinction between a good and a great therapeutic experience with couples hinges on the quality of the therapeutic bond, which in turn determines how engaged the couples are in the process. I interpret the research-based dictum to be genuine as not limited to telling clients what we really think about their problems. In fact, I sometimes withhold my concerns about their prospects as a couple, to give them an adequate chance to experiment with possibilities and discover their potential for themselves. But to create an emotional bond with the couple, they need to see us as lively human beings who respond to their unique reality, including their cultural backgrounds, with deep emotional involvement, interest, respect, and, as appropriate, a sense of humor.

Sharing a few areas of personal pleasure about a couple's culture of reference is quite different than oversharing about one's personal life. I believe that therapists must be extremely circumspect about sharing aspects of their own relationships and psychological challenges. I think that it's only appropriate to do so when couples are not comforted in hearing about research findings on common challenges such as the transition to parenthood, balancing work time and couple time, and the need to insert novel leisure experiences when their usual menu is no longer generating a sense of closeness. At these moments, I may share that "I've been there, like most couples," and took action to rectify the problem. Couples are inevitably grateful to hear that their therapist has also struggled with these generic stressors, and that can inspire them to take steps to address these issues. But couples generally do not profit from hearing the details of the therapist's own struggles. Our personal struggles can help us appreciate and understand those faced by the couples we see, but keep them as informational backdrop to your work. Metaphorically, I think of our similar personal challenges and how we overcame them as the strings of a multistringed guitar, allowing their stories and emotions to resonate fully within us. We don't need to show them our guitar.

THE CREATIVE RELATIONAL MOVEMENT APPROACH: A DESCRIPTION OF THE CHANGE PROCESS FOR COUPLES

The field of couple therapy is replete with models that describe techniques for assisting couples to change (Fraenkel, 1997, 2009, 2022; Gurman & Fraenkel, 2002; Gurman et al., 2015). Most of these models include imparting skills or other suggestions about changing interaction patterns that the couple is instructed to enact between sessions—so-called homework or intersession activities. However, any couple therapist will tell you that one of the greatest challenges is getting couples to follow through and do what you are suggesting they try. Couples often come back after a productive session in which you taught them research-based communication and problem-solving skills, or activities designed to enhance their mutual respect, or to increase their sexual pleasure or emotional connection, and report that they "didn't do the homework." They offer a wide range of reasons for not following through: The activities made sense but felt awkward, forced, and not spontaneous. Or the activities almost seemed emotionally irrational, given how negatively they feel about each other. Or they describe how they just don't yet feel motivated enough to treat each other better. They wonder how they can experiment with restarting their pleasurable connection or a more respectful dialogue when they've spent years feeling alienated, angry, lonely, and doubtful that the other has any positive intentions toward them. Or they wanted to try the communication techniques but were too negatively aroused to do so (even though one part of the technique always includes what to do to decrease negative arousal). Or they list any number of circumstances that interfered: a hectic work week, issues with a kid's schooling, an ill older parent who needed tending, and so on. Although all these stressors are real, and the therapist should empathize with them, if the activities were designed to be relatively brief, they don't really constitute valid reasons for not following through.

Much has been written in the couple therapy literature about the need to "shake up the system" and address "resistance" (Anderson

& Stewart, 1983). Whole schools of couple and family therapy were based on the assumption that the "homeostatic mechanisms" (the need to maintain a stable state) in couples are so powerful that the couple needs to be outwitted through paradoxical techniques such as slowing down progress and prescribing the symptom, which were intended to provoke the couple to rebel against the therapist by doing the suggested activity (Haley, 1987; Madanes, 1981; Selvini Palazzoli et al., 1985). In my early training, supervised by an expert in strategic couple therapy, my supervisor actually called in to the therapy room from behind the one-way mirror and suggested that I tell a couple who engaged in repetitive fighting that they should set their alarm clock for 3 a.m. and wake up and fight at that time, because their unconscious minds would be more available and they could then express their deepest concerns. They looked affronted, didn't like this suggestion at all, and it didn't lead to less fighting—just to me needing to repair our now slightly damaged relationship with my charm and humor!

Instead of viewing couples as resistant, I've come to realize that we therapists don't prepare them adequately for what it will feel like to initiate change. We need to provide them a descriptive theory of change that anticipates the sorts of challenges to change that I listed above. This led me to develop the Creative Relational Movement theory of change (Fraenkel, 2019b). Providing this theory to couples explains why we believe it's important for them to enact new ways of being with each other, adjusts their expectations about how trying new things will go, and builds the couple's sense of confidence in us, strengthening rather than damaging the therapeutic alliance.

Let's examine the actionable meaning of the words in this Creative Relational Movement approach to change.

Why Creative?

Creativity is defined as "the ability to transcend traditional ideas, rules, patterns, relationships, or the like, and to create meaningful new ideas, forms, methods, interpretations, etc.; originality, progressiveness, or imagination" (Dictionary.com, n.d.). To *create* is "to make or bring into existence something new" (Merriam-Webster, n.d.a). Distressed couples need to try new ways of being with one another, because either they never developed satisfying patterns, or memories of happier days seem so remote and blurry, shaded by years of dissatisfaction and disappointment. Over time, partners have each accumulated a metaphoric "mental forest of tall dark trees" that block the sun—negative attributions or assumptions that the partner doesn't and can't love them, is trying to control them, and has no respect for them, and negative beliefs about the relationship's potential (Bradbury & Fincham, 1990; Bradbury et al., 2000). Albert Einstein once said that "imagination is more important than knowledge. Knowledge is limited. Imagination encircles the world" (Viereck, 1929, p. 117). Unfortunately, last chance couples are typically so mired in negative views of each other and the relationship—their partial and often distorted "knowledge" about their partner and the accounts of their history together—that they literally cannot imagine a preferred way of being. They can speak in general of wishing for better communication, effective problem solving, satisfying intimacy, and fun. But if asked to do an exercise such as the solution-focused miracle question—"Imagine you go to sleep tonight and in the morning, you wake up, and all the problems you've described have magically disappeared. How would you know? What would be different?"—they find it hard to get beyond these general wishes to envision what better communication and intimacy would look like.

Rather than engaging in an often-futile attempt to help couples identify and revive their strengths when they vehemently declare these don't exist or did so long ago that these feel irrelevant to their present moment, the therapist accepts their narrative of despair and disempowerment and suggests that they need to get creative, to forge a new path toward their hopes. But how can they do so in a dark forest of negative feelings and beliefs?

The phenomenological philosopher Martin Heidegger (1962), whose ideas were a forerunner of existential-humanistic therapies (Schneider & Krug 2017), provides a useful framework for personal change. His philosophy centered on the German concept of *Dasein*, or being-in-the-world. He was concerned with the problem of how people create a meaningful life and expand their lives in novel, preferred directions. He argued that to escape the power of our existing constructions or beliefs about what is possible, we need, metaphorically speaking, to enter *eine Lichtung*, or a clearing—as in a lighted space in a dark forest. The only way to enter such a clearing is to act in novel ways that are not based on our existing beliefs. We can then observe the results of our interactions with the world and revise our sense of who we are and what is possible.

In an early article, the cocreator of narrative therapy, Michael White (1991b), referenced cognitive psychologist Jerome Bruner's (1986) distinction between the "landscape of consciousness" and the "landscape of action," noting that changes in one can lead to changes in the other. However, whereas narrative therapy tends to start the process of change by examining clients' restrictive, "problem-saturated" stories or "totalizing descriptions" about themselves, locates and expands their preferred but "subordinated" stories (memories) of competence and other positive qualities, and then encourages them to take steps in the landscape of action to support those reemerging preferred narratives, I find that the first step with last chance couples must be in the landscape of action, which then begins to build a new, or renewed, positive sense of the couple's identity.

As I noted earlier, the existentialist psychologist Rollo May (1975) emphasized the role of courage in forming and expanding relationships. He also spoke of the need for courage to create something— whether that be in the domains of the arts and literature, science and technology, social policy, or personal life: "A curious paradox characteristic of every kind of courage . . . is the seeming contradiction that *we must be fully committed, but we must also be aware at the same time that we might possibly be wrong*" (p. 20, emphasis in original). He elaborated, stating:

> Commitment is healthiest when it is not *without* doubt, but *in spite of* doubt. To believe fully and at the same moment to have doubts is not at all a contradiction: it presupposes a greater respect for truth, an awareness that truth always goes beyond anything that can be said or done at any given moment. (May, 1975, p. 21, emphasis in original)

Couples will naturally have doubts about whether the suggestions of the therapist will work for them, or whether they will have the emotional resources to enact the suggested activities. Rather than viewing these doubts as resistance, the therapist should validate their doubts and even share their own "wait and see" stance. Even interventions with strong scientific support for their effectiveness and years of success with other couples may not work, at least initially, with the next couple. Taking this stance of "try it and we'll see" with the couple strengthens the therapeutic alliance—we join with them in their doubts and encourage them to experiment nonetheless. The therapist of course will have more confidence about particular interventions than will the couple. Couples need not believe fully or be fully committed in order to try a suggested activity. It is the therapist's role in the alliance to hold more of the enthusiasm for an activity initially, based on previous success with it and, if available, research showing its effectiveness. Trying the techniques first during sessions allows the therapist to coach the couple to learn and eventually master them, but the therapist should also note, "Let's try it this week, see how it goes, and we'll tweak it as necessary. And if it really doesn't do the job, we'll try something else!" Couples are greatly reassured when the therapist echoes their doubts and still suggests they try, often paired with pointing out that their usual way of interacting clearly has not worked. Some alternative must be created.

Why Relational Movement?

I believe that, despite its usefulness and empirical support, the theory of behaviorism has an aesthetic problem. My experience as a psychology professor and therapist has revealed that many people have negative associations to the term *behavior*. As a graduate student in a psychodynamically oriented clinical psychology program in the 1980s, I heard several professors cast aspersions on behavior therapy. Terms like "surfacy" (as opposed to deep), thin (as opposed to rich and nuanced), simplistic (as opposed to complex), open to symptom substitution (as opposed to creating structural personality change), and the like indoctrinated me into a view that psychoanalysis was the superior approach. Behavioral terms such as reinforcement, punishment, shaping, negative practice, black box, and extinction are not exactly warm and fuzzy (Newman et al., 2003). Just compare these to the language of psychoanalysis: dreams, free association, interpretation, subjectivity, and the unconscious, as well as the famous photos of Sigmund Freud's consulting office, with a couch covered in rich tapestries and cultural artifacts cluttering his desk—in contrast to psychology textbooks' usual photos of behavioral experiments with rats and dogs in cages receiving shocks, or scenes from backward mental hospitals where tokens were given to people with chronic mental illnesses so that they could get cigarettes in exchange for compliant behavior.

Similarly, humanistic therapies use language more appealing than behavioral terms: self-actualization, growth, human potential, and unconditional positive regard. In my classes, I start the section on behavioral and cognitive–behavioral therapy with a questionnaire that asks students to rate on a scale of 1 (cold) to 5 (warm) (a scale based on early cognitive research on the "semantic differential," the dimensions on which we organize meaning and experience; Osgood et al., 1957) terms from psychoanalysis and behavior therapy, and psychoanalytic terms are invariably rated much warmer. I then propose that behavior theory and therapy has an aesthetic problem—the terms are unappealing and do not reflect how deeply humane and effective behavioral approaches are. When they hear the term *behavior*, students—and also clients—often have an immediate association to times when a parent or teacher admonished them about their misbehavior.

The terms we use as therapists have the capacity to engage and excite our clients or to turn them off. Therefore, although I base much of my approach to working with couples on research and interventions from cognitive–behavioral theory and therapies, I substitute the term *relational movement,* or at least *interaction,* for *behavior* when talking with couples. The term *movement* connotes dance, walking and running, and change. New relational movements mean activities in which the couple moves together in more positive ways, enacting a novel dance of connection. Emotionally focused therapy (EFT) pioneer Susan Johnson (2019), an accomplished tango dancer, often refers to the "tango" of couples' emotional attunement and interactions, as well as the tango of couple therapy.

The Importance of Nonverbal Meaning

Along with this focus on relational movement, I emphasize to couples that movement, and motion, are meaningful—even without the addition of words. Much of the research of Gottman and others has documented the negative emotional effects of nonverbal behaviors such as grimaces, eye rolls, gaze aversion, shoulder shrugs, and voice tone (Driver et al., 2012). Over the past few decades, the field of couple and family therapy has moved toward a greater focus on listening to clients' words—their narratives and constructions—and away from the field's initial focus on observing interaction. The implicit premise is that only words convey meaning—a notion in philosophy known as the Whorfian hypothesis, or sometimes the Sapir-Whorf hypothesis, after the anthropologist-linguists Edward Sapir and Benjamin Lee Whorf, who popularized the theory. It holds that our understanding of the world and ourselves in it is fully determined and mediated by the language we use (Koerner, 1992).

However, along with being rejected by later linguists such as Noam Chomsky (and even earlier thinkers, such as Plato and Kant), this theory ignores the enormous literature on the meaningfulness of nonverbal behavior, not only in humans but in other animal species, as well as the power of the nonlinguistic arts—music, dance, powerful wordless moments in theater, and the visual arts—to convey meaning. People convey meaning through voice tone, pitch, volume, tempo, and rhythm, hand gestures, and facial expressions, as well as whole body movements, not only through narratives and other verbal expressions. It is critical for couple therapists both to listen to partners' words and to notice these nonverbal means of interaction, to comment upon problematic aspects of nonverbal relational movement, and to create interventions that help couples reshape their nonverbal expressions. A strong therapeutic alliance is necessary to share these observations with couples, as people are sometimes a bit self-conscious when their facial expressions and style of speaking are pointed out. But ultimately, couples appreciate this feedback, because it shows that the therapist is attentive to the details of how they interact, and changing these aspects of interaction can greatly improve their relationship in a manner more powerful than the words they speak.

For example, Josh was president of a growing tech startup company and a former high school debating champion. He tended to speak loudly and quickly and in a gravelly monotone. His wife, Rachel, was a writer and was also extremely verbal. However, Josh's verbal outpourings often silenced Rachel, although often not intentionally. He would then become surprised and frustrated when she withdrew with an expression of resignation on her face. When I pointed out the impact of his style of speech, Rachel expressed gratitude to me with tears in her eyes, and said, "It's true, Josh. I feel firehosed by your words." Josh reminded us of his background as a debater, and I noted, "Well, that style was highly successful in the debate forum, but it is not working here, because you two need to stop debating and instead start listening to each other and finding consensus. The goal is not to win an argument."

Slightly embarrassed but appreciative that I pointed this out, Josh noted that this style was so well practiced that he didn't even notice when he used it. He believed his style garnered praise from his staff but, on closer review, acknowledged that he'd often received feedback that they weren't always able to remember what he said, and then couldn't follow through with his requests without reminders. As with my work with people prone to anger (see the vignette of Bahir and Sarah, in Chapter 4), I said that I was sure this style of talking worked well in certain contexts, but clearly was not working with his wife.

He agreed to a few sessions where I used a metronome to demonstrate the typical speed of his prosody, and then set the metronome to a slower speed and had him practice speaking at this slower pace. I also referenced great orators such as President Obama (whom both partners greatly admired—Josh had met him once), who not only spoke more slowly than Josh but also used a wider range of voice tones (high and low pitches, louder and softer volume) and pregnant pauses to allow listeners to absorb his words. Drawing on my background in music, I also connected with Josh's enjoyment of jazz to help him hear an analogue to his speech style and an alternative style. I played two examples of jazz trumpeters—Dizzy Gillespie, known for his rapid-fire solos (the musical version of Josh's verbal firehosing), and Miles Davis, known for his more relaxed and spacious sound. I shared two quotes commonly attributed to Miles (the exact source is hard to find! It's part of the jazz community's oral history/lore), who was famous for his use of silence: "In music, silence is more important than sound," and "Music is the framework around the silence."

Josh was intrigued and asked me to recommend some Miles Davis recordings to serve as a musical model for how he needed to revise his speech patterns. I recommended the classic album *Kind of Blue*, which is often held up as the premier example of Davis's sound and silence approach (and happens to be the best-selling jazz album of all time). Josh's speech style changed, and his and Rachel's relationship greatly improved.

In my earlier-described work with George and Alice, a turning point occurred when, after a few sessions to gain their trust and to help George speak less from resentment and more from his vulnerable feelings, I pointed out that Alice remained absolutely stone-faced and expressionless even when George finally expressed in a heartfelt, nonblaming way his desperate sense of loneliness. The words were slightly different from before, but most different was his tone. I said, "Alice, George is finally dropping his whiny barbs at you and just speaking from his heart about his loneliness, yet your face suggests that you are entirely unmoved."

Alice initially felt criticized by me and almost left the session. I responded that I could understand that she felt criticized, and apologized for that effect, but that my intent was just to point out her part of their extreme pursuer-distancer pattern. Her impassive facial expression was part of what drove George to provoke her into speaking through what she called his "passive-aggressive behavior." She calmed down, and then said in a tone of desperation mixed with frustration, "It's just been years of hearing his complaints that I'm not doing enough, not connected enough, that I work too much and am depriving him. I'm so sick of it!" Looking now at George, I said, "Can you understand what Alice is feeling? You want her to come forward to you, but she's terrified that if she does but not enough to satisfy you, you will resume the barbs to provoke her to connect, which will only make her withdraw again." George looked initially upset by this comment on his interactional style, then thoughtful, and finally concurred. I suggested that it would take some time with him avoiding his whiny resentful tone for Alice to trust that he would not critique her. Alice looked grateful for my comments. This work on the non-verbal exchanges between them set the stage for the intervention describe above, meeting on an island where they could finally enjoy one another.

In yet another couple, Samantha was a Jamaican American woman and Phil a white American man. Both were highly accomplished business consultants and argued incessantly about every aspect of their lives together. Much of their relationship centered on their unpleasant nonverbal dance. However, to her credit, in one session after many months of therapy pointing out these interactions and teaching them communication skills (which they rarely used), Samantha led off in a positive tone, listing her hopes for the summer (of 2022, as the pandemic had started to diminish). The couple had been staying in Florida, initially to get away from New York City when the pandemic first hit. Now they were planning to move back to New York in the fall, where they needed to find a new apartment close to their children's new school, and before that, she hoped to take the family (her two young daughters and a son) to see her estranged father for the first time, go to Disneyworld, then travel up to Phil's parents' home in New England for a month so that the kids could spend time with those grandparents and Phil could see his parents. To my surprise, she also said that she hoped they would book a hotel in a week to celebrate their anniversary.

Phil listened silently, eyes fixed on the floor, with a dour facial expression. I asked him to comment on Samantha's ideas. He put his head in his hands, and in a voice tone that combined bitterness, disdain, and anxiety, took down each one of her ideas, with the central theme being that it would all cost too much, that he was at the breaking point with work, that he was considering taking a job at another company whose conservative politics he abhorred but where his salary would be higher so he could accommodate Samantha's expensive plans and higher spending habits. As he spoke on and on—albeit apologizing for going on and on—Samantha's face gradually fell, and then she softly said, "Can I take a break? I need to get some air," and left for five minutes.

Having worked with Phil individually on changing his facial expression and voice tone, with little lasting impact, I quietly said, "Well, this approach to expressing your concerns clearly isn't working, as we've known for some time. Your negative voice tone, your head in your hands, staring at the floor . . . right?" Phil nodded glumly in agreement. Drawing in an admittedly provocative way on his long-standing passion for protecting the civil rights of African Americans (after college, he had taught elementary school in the Deep South), I said, "I'm not saying you're Derek Chauvin here [the white policeman who killed Black man George Floyd by pushing his knee into Floyd's neck for nine minutes in May 2020, leading Floyd to say repeatedly, "I can't breathe!," which sparked protests about racism around the country], but your way of talking sucks the air out of the room, and Samantha can't breathe." My comment hit hard, as I intended it to. "Phil, as we've discussed for months, this does not work. There are other ways you can express your concerns, mostly by you and Samantha just looking at her desired plans and the money that's available." Samantha came back, and Phil finally looked at her, apologized, and they decided to construct an accounting of their available funds and then decide which trips they could and could not take.

In these three examples, it was essential first to establish a strong, trusting working alliance so that I could take the risk of pointing out couples' problematic nonverbal behavior. Pointing out behavior sometimes makes partners uncomfortable and can result in a rupture or breach between the therapist and clients, so the therapist must quickly do a bit of alliance damage control, apologizing for the unpleasant part of the impact of their comments, clarifying their positive intentions, and exploring the vulnerable feelings of each partner that drive their problematic vocal or gestural style. Sometimes it is useful before making such a comment to apologize in advance and anticipate that a partner will feel affronted by one's comments.

In yet another example, in working with the couple whose case is described in detail in my article "Love in Action" (Fraenkel, 2019b) on last chance couple therapy (and appears again in Chapter 7), Michael was a successful lawyer and was overusing alcohol, often spending a week in bed with hidden bottles of vodka, which his wife, Ana, the head of a hospital nursing department, would inevitably find. Their young children frequently asked Ana why "daddy was sick." Ana felt desperate and ultimately angry about Michael's drinking, which he either denied or minimized. The couple had been referred by Michael's addictions psychiatrist, who was also prescribing him an antidepressant and Klonopin for anxiety, a benzodiazepine that often interacts powerfully with alcohol. Michael attributed his drinking to feeling unloved and unappreciated for all his hard work—not only by Ana but by his boss and colleagues. He pointed to Ana's anxious style of talking about his drinking and her lack of warmth. He also complained bitterly that she did not allow him to interact much with the children or participate in their care. Ana haltingly tried to tell him that she was frightened by his alcohol use and was trying to minimize

the kids' exposure to him when he was drunk. When he acknowledged his drinking, Michael nevertheless said that it didn't show and
that, because it was vodka, the kids couldn't smell it on his breath (a
common but unfounded reason that many alcoholics move from other
forms of alcohol to vodka).

There were many important interventions I did with this couple, but
one was gently and apologetically to confront Michael about his nonverbal behavior. "Michael, I know that this might make you angry, and I
apologize for that, but I don't think you fully hear yourself and how bitter your tone is when you speak to Ana. I hear that you feel unloved and
unappreciated by her, but the way you're delivering the message—with
so much bitter anger and no eye contact—puts her on guard and makes
her feel anxious and defensive. The words alone are hard enough for
her to hear, but the harsh music of your voice makes them that much
harder to take in. I wonder if you could tell her how you feel, but in
a different tone." As predicted, Michael initially sulked after I said this
but sat quietly for a few minutes. He then looked directly at Ana, with
an open facial expression, and said in a sad and almost apologetic tone,
"Ana, I feel so unloved and unappreciated by you. I know the drinking
is pissing you off and scaring you, but I do it because I just can't stand
my life sometimes. I need a break, and it's the only way I can get out
of my head for a while." Still tentatively and on guard, Ana nevertheless responded with a bit more warmth than I'd seen previously, saying,
"Michael, I know you're under stress and depressed, and I do appreciate all your hard work. But I'm scared to death about your drinking
and that we won't make it through this. And it hurts me when you
blame me for all your stress and for your drinking. I'm trying my best
to hold things together." Michael looked pensive, paused, and then said,
"You're right. I really have to stop, and it's not your fault that I drink.
But I have to get some sign from you that you still love me." Ana teared
up and said, "I do still love you—that's why I haven't just left."

This was an important turning point in their relationship, and in
our work together. Once again, I had banked on the strong alliance
I'd made with both partners in the initial few weeks, including their
sense of the credibility of what I had been offering them—an action-
focused approach that helped them change how they interacted,
including a focus on the nonverbal aspects. Anticipating a possible
rupture with Michael when I confronted him not only on what he said
but how he said it, apologizing for the likely impact on him and being
ready to repair the breach if necessary, helped him to feel a sustained
connection to me, and to understand my willingness to take a risk in
confronting him.

One last and somewhat outrageous vignette about the importance of establishing a strong alliance to allow the therapist to point out problematic behavior. Saul was a 62-year-old highly successful, wealthy, and aggressive businessman born and raised in, as he described it, a "tough Jewish family in Brooklyn." He was married to Ginnie, a soft-spoken woman in her late 40s from Tennessee. They had a son and a daughter, 14 and 16 years old. In one session, Saul got angry at Ginnie and called her a "fucking c*nt." She was appalled, as was I. I said firmly, "Saul, we don't talk like that in here, sorry." He grumbled and did not really apologize, but stopped using that sort of language.

I had met the son and daughter in a previous session—they were good-looking and fashionably dressed, adorable but with an air of privilege and entitlement, clearly disconnected emotionally from their father and aligned with their mother. They reported how their father would often insult their mother, and that Mom rarely voiced a retort, which they found irritating.

In an individual session with Saul after the one where he used foul language toward Ginnie, he complained loudly and bitterly about how his kids didn't show him love, respect, and appreciation. In a distinctly old-style "tough" Brooklyn Jewish accent (which is, by the way, quite similar to an Italian Brooklyn accent—you've heard it if you've ever watched movies like *Goodfellas* or *Moonstruck*), Saul said, "I don't get it, Doc! I take these kids to Paris for a weekend of shopping and concerts, and they show me no love!" I paused, looked at him steadily, and asked, "Really, Saul? You don't get it?" He replied, "No, I have no clue!" I said, with a faint, knowing smile, "Well, maybe it's because you call their mother a fucking c*nt and other insults at home. What do you think?" He paused for two seconds, looked at me with irritation, and said, "Fuck you, Doc!" I replied, "Fuck me?? Fuck you, Saul!" He burst into laughter, and said, "You know, Doc, this is why I like you and trust you. No one else talks to me straight like you do!" I laughed as well. Saul never insulted Ginnie again, and he apologized to his kids for his past behavior.

The Five Premises of the Creative Relational Movement Approach

To sum up the Creative Relational Movement approach in a manner that is brief and reassuring to couples as they embark on the process of change, there are five premises to share. It is often useful to share these premises along with the first set of suggested new activities, in the first session.

1. Insight does not automatically lead to new action

Psychodynamic and humanistic psychotherapies (and intergenerational approaches to couple therapy) presume that people first must achieve insight into the roots of their problem patterns in order to initiate new action. These roots may be difficult experiences growing up in their respective families, or in previous relationships, or intrapsychic conflicts that result in anxiety. In therapy with individuals, understanding these sources of problems typically takes several sessions (often over a period of months) of in-depth exploration. When working with two people, the time needed doubles. Furthermore, it has long been assumed that once clients achieve insight, they will automatically know what they need to do to engender new experiences.

As a therapist with years of enthusiastic training and experience in psychodynamic therapy, I must confess that I've rarely seen change occur automatically once people achieve insight. In addition, the destructive interactions in which couples repeatedly engage—despite insight gained from their individual psychotherapies and against their better instincts—over time develop an automaticity or functional autonomy. Our emerging understanding of the role of the limbic system, particularly the amygdala, in detecting or anticipating possible danger and readying us for fight or flight suggests that the insight gained through higher cortical brain functions and the rational judgments issuing from the prefrontal cortex become overwhelmed by the fundamental need to protect ourselves (Fishbane, 2013), despite our best intentions.

Therefore, the Creative Relational Movement approach holds that insight is not necessary and not even usually effective enough to automatically result in interactional change. Rather, couples need to engage in new action that makes sense and see what transpires. Interestingly, once the couple establishes new, nonconflictual, and more enjoyable relational movements, they are better able to gain insight into what drove their problematic patterns. New patterns provide a kind of safe platform above the mess of their past styles of relating, from which they can look down and examine those patterns and their sources in experiences and beliefs from their families of origin, cultural backgrounds, previous relationships, and internal, intrapsychic conflicts. Moreover, when therapists explore each partner's family and culture of origin before establishing new patterns of interaction and increased empathy, partners may even weaponize what each other discloses about their painful early histories. ("You see? It's your messed-up relationship with your mother/father that's causing all our problems.") For many couples who've been in previous, failed therapies that focused more on achieving insight, hearing this premise is greatly reassuring and distinguishes how you will work with them from what they experienced before. It is an important step toward building a sense of therapeutic credibility.

2. Change often feels awkward, artificial, and even irrational at first

High-conflict couples who are taught the Speaker-Listener Technique—in which one partner speaks for 10–15 seconds using "I" statements, and the other partner repeats back what they heard—inevitably see that this technique is preferable to their destructive ways of communicating about problems. However, they usually note that the technique feels artificial and awkward. Likewise, when partners try making one statement of appreciation or admiration to each other each day (an activity supported by Gottman's research), they see its value and often note that they've longed for such comments for years, but given how angry and disaffected they've felt, it seems almost irrational and certainly not spontaneous. Couples often feel similarly about my 60-second pleasure point activity—doing six 1-minute-or-less fun, pleasurable, or even sensual activities across the day. That these suggestions come from the therapist only adds to the feeling that they are prescribed rather than coming from the partners' own spontaneous initiative.

The therapist should normalize these feelings by saying that any new behavior—whether a new way to swing a tennis club or baseball bat, a new approach to playing a musical instrument, or getting familiar with a new computer keyboard or software program—will feel artificial and awkward at first, but with practice becomes natural and effortless. Ask the couple to reflect on times when they had to learn some new behavior and how it felt. This will bring home the point in an embodied fashion.

As to the activity not feeling spontaneous—especially one designed to elicit warm feelings—again suggest that there's no way to restart positive, affectionate interactions spontaneously when they've been alienated for so long. They must start somewhere, albeit feeling a bit forced, and over time these activities will emerge more spontaneously. In addition, you can suggest that the basic suggested *form* of the activity—making a statement of appreciation, doing one-minute pleasurable activities—may not feel spontaneous or improvisational, but that the *content* of what they insert into the form can be completely spontaneous. As a jazz musician since age 14, I have the benefit of drawing on my years of playing music where the chord changes and basic rhythm of a tune are essentially the same night after night, but what soloists do with those chord changes and rhythmic base can vary enormously. (You're welcome to borrow from my musical expertise or, better yet, draw upon your own metaphors from activities outside of psychotherapy that make the point—sports, arts, and so on.)

As to the activity feeling irrational, the therapist should say, "Of course it does! You've been living in such pain with each other for so long, and have held such negative views of each other for so long, that trying to treat each other more respectfully and lovingly will of course not make sense in terms of your *emotional* logic, even if you see that these activities make sense and you believe the research supporting them." Remind them that if they did only what makes sense in terms of how negatively they feel, they would just continue treating each other badly. You can add, "So this is a moment where you need to step away from the tall forest of your negative feelings, and step into a clearing where the light can shine on new possibilities, by acting exactly the opposite of what your negative feelings and predictions tell you to do."

3. Motivation is not necessary for change

When partners state that they don't feel highly motivated to try new things, empathize with this feeling, but remind them that the only way they can really assess the potential of the relationship is through the emotional results of observable action. They need to ignore their low motivation and follow the words of the popular Nike commercials that suggest people take action. Have them reflect on whether their motivation for everyday activities—going to work, exercising, doing the housework, taking care of the kids—is always high. They will quickly concur that their motivation for these activities fluctuates wildly, but for the most part, they still show up. Ask if they've noticed whether motivation usually increases once they engage in the activity. Almost always, they will answer "yes." I sometimes share my experience of practicing the basic patterns of drumming—called rudiments—for over 50 years. Exciting? Not really. Boring? Kinda. Do my hands feel better once I start? Always. This is a moment in which the therapist can usefully share something not so personal from their life to help couples feel that they are not alone. You can also note that, somewhat surprisingly, there is little research showing that motivation levels are well correlated with therapeutic outcomes.

4. The importance of nonbinding creative experiments with possibility

As I've described above, change occurs primarily through experiments in possibility. Emphasize that the activities you are suggesting should be viewed as an exploration of how it feels to be different with one another, but that improvement does not necessarily mean that one or the other partner will still want to stay in the relationship. This is a critical frame to establish, to make it emotionally safe for ambivalent partners to try new things, so that they do not feel they will be trapped in the relationship by progress.

5. Change efforts need to be linked to time

The couple needs to create "rhythms of relationship," regular times of the day and week when they engage in change practices. Once again, the language we select to convey ideas is important. Avoid the term *scheduling*, because that term conjures up the multitude of work and other obligations that need to be put on the calendar. Instead, *rhythms* connotes music, the beating of the heart, the rotation of the planets, the seasons. Couples are much more likely to sign on to creating rhythms of intimacy than to schedule sex, a date night, or statements of appreciation and admiration.

In sum, creative relational action or movement must occur that partners can observe. Only such novel action can generate new feelings and thoughts about the relationship and its possibly more propitious future. In the words of Alcoholics Anonymous, "It is easier to act yourself into a new way of thinking (and I would add, feeling) than to think yourself into a new way of acting" (Alcoholics Anonymous, 2001, p. 366), sometimes phrased, "You can't think your way into better living, but you can live your way into better thinking" (Tolin, 2006, p. iv). And just as the AA program advocates a step-by-step, one day at a time approach to maintaining sobriety—a process that initially feels extremely awkward, artificial, and even irrational given how much the person in recovery wants to drink, and for which the recovering person experiences wildly fluctuating degrees of motivation—therapists with last chance couples must behave like a steady, supportive sponsor, encouraging couples to stick with new practices long enough for them to feel more natural and automatic. I often tell couples that "successful marriage is largely a motor skill"—a set of relational habits that partners engage in automatically, with minimal thought and effort. But to create new habits of relating takes practice, just as it takes practice to meditate, learn an instrument, swing a golf club or tennis racket, establish a healthier diet or exercise regimen, or any other activity.

Fishbane (2013) summarizes the evidence that our brains have the capacity for neuroplasticity—as our social interactions change, we can lay down new connections and pathways in the brain, and these pathways are central to the development of new, automatic habits. But these new pathways only develop through practice. Just understanding the value and the research behind the interventions we suggest isn't sufficient: Such understanding is a prefrontal cortex function, whereas new, automatic interactional patterns require changing the limbic system, the hypothalamus (memory center), and the motor cortex—all lower brain functions that drive most of our daily behavior. Malcolm Gladwell (2008) famously reported that "phenoms" (outstanding achievers) in any skilled activity require 10,000 hours of practice. Couples don't need to aspire to having a phenomenal relationship—"pretty good" is often good enough! But even "pretty good" requires lots of practice.

THE THERAPIST AS A COLLABORATIVE EXPERT

There has been much disagreement in the field between those who advocate that therapists should take a more directive approach—teaching research-based skills, sharing observations of couple interaction patterns and making strong suggestions about how to transform those patterns, eliciting strong emotions, and the like—and those who advocate a less hierarchical, more collaborative, clients-as-the-experts approach that limits therapist activities to asking questions meant to elicit insight or preferred narratives. In fact, both approaches are needed, but at different moments in the course of therapy. Greater directiveness is usually required early on when the last chance couple feels most hopeless, is engaged in destructive conflict, and is in crisis, with a shift to less directiveness as the couple's crisis decreases and the therapist's focus is to launch them into independence from therapy.

Although this initial directiveness is necessary for therapy with most couples regardless of their level of distress, it is absolutely essential with last chance couples, because they demand evidence that things might change. Such change simply does not emerge through insight and certainly not through repeated bitter, mutually blaming recitation of painful stories of dysfunction and disappointment.

As I noted earlier, the venerable Vietnamese monk Thich Nhat Hanh has said, "The best way to take care of the future is to do our best to take care of the present moment" (2006, p. 233). His form of engaged Buddhism provides a useful philosophical perspective that integrates well into couple therapy. The approach to therapy described in the Creative Relational Movement approach and this book more generally is all about taking care of the present moment, toward creating a better future.

In short, this book advocates a flexible integrative stance—that of a collaborative expert. The vignettes shared above, and those in the remainder of the book, illustrate the nuances of this stance through clinical vignettes.

Leaders in the field of couple therapy and research such as the late Al Gurman (2011) have long suggested that researchers need to consult more with therapists in developing their research protocols so that their findings can actually inform clinical practice. Instead, researchers often bemoan the challenges of getting clinicians to sign on to their empirically supported approaches (Chambless & Ollendick, 2001). A whole body of research efforts is dedicated to what is known as translational research, or research on how to most effectively disseminate empirically supported treatments. But the more recent developments in research described above that focus on understanding the centrality of the therapist's attentiveness to couples' shifting needs over time, and flexibility and responsiveness in meeting those needs with an approach different from the one used initially, highlights the importance of the common factors in therapy and of tending to the therapeutic alliance. As I have argued (Fraenkel, 2019b) and describe in the next chapter, these findings also support adopting an integrative approach to couple therapy that can draw upon multiple theories or perspectives on the source of couple's challenges, and a wide variety of techniques or therapeutic practices to address those challenges.

CHAPTER 2

THE THERAPEUTIC PALETTE INTEGRATIVE APPROACH TO ASSESSMENT AND INTERVENTION

IN THIS CHAPTER, I DESCRIBE an integrative approach to couple therapy refined over 30 years. There are four major reasons for working integratively: (1) The complexity and wide variety of issues that couples bring to therapy; (2) the lack of empirical evidence that any one approach is superior to another and the finding that many couples who receive empirically validated treatments, which are typically single-theory approaches, do not sufficiently improve or sustain improvement; (3) the need to respond to couples' ideas about what they believe will be most helpful to them, and their reticence to engage in certain approaches, sometimes due to previous negative experiences in couple therapy; and (4) most importantly, the need to be flexible, responsive, and creative in our work, to be ready for anything a couple brings to us for assistance.

In addition to describing how to integrate the variety of theories and techniques/practices in the cornucopia of perspectives available in the couple therapy field, I describe how to integrate ideas and materials from outside of psychotherapy and psychology more generally. There is a strong case for occasionally utilizing the perspectives of the arts and humanities, which form a complementary stream of observations about the human condition (Fraenkel, 2020; Wilson, 1998).

Before diving in to examine the factors that lead to distress and dissolution of relationships and how to work with couples, it is important to articulate what it means to be in a healthy, happy romantic intimate relationship.

THE GOAL: ROMANTIC LOVE IN THE HEALTHY AND HAPPY COUPLE[1]

At the broadest level, healthy couples engage in kindness, compassion, collaboration, effective communication and problem solving, pleasurable activities, and mutual responsiveness. Given the broad cultural differences in beliefs about intimate bonds, it may be presumptuous to advance a unified, prescriptive description of the nature of romantic love. Nevertheless, based on extensive research and clinical theory about what distinguishes happy from unhappy couples, and what predicts stability or relationship dissolution over time, a view of healthy couplehood and romantic love is herein proposed. I acknowledge that this research and theorizing has mostly been conducted based on couples in North America, South America, and Europe, and may therefore be culturally biased. However, it has also been influenced by my work with couples living in the United States whose countries and cultures of origin include South Asia, East Asia, Africa, and the Middle East. I also acknowledge certain ethical biases—namely, that partners should be able to have equal voice (ability to express their perspectives, needs, and feelings) and equal power (Knudson-Martin, 2015), including the ability to decide together who has more power or "say" around particular issues (for instance, when it is mutually agreed that one partner will take the lead on organizing finances or on establishing routines for a baby). I recognize that my approach to working with couples would not be well suited for people who adhere strongly to patriarchal perspectives and are not willing to explore the limits of these perspectives.

Love is borne from initial attraction in some admixture of physical attraction and shared intellectual and aesthetic interests and curiosity about the world; shared social, spiritual, religious, or ethical values; and curiosity, excitement, and enjoyment about differences between the self and the other, as well as caring about the well-being of one another. As the relationship progresses, movement from a *Me and*

---

1   This section appears in different form in Fraenkel, P. (2022). The therapeutic palette integrative approach to couple therapy. In J. L. Lebow & D. K. Snyder (Eds.). *Clinical handbook of couple therapy* (6th ed., pp. 339–361). New York: Guilford Press. It is printed here with permission from Guilford Press.

You relationship to one of *We* becomes important—a sense of shared identity that does not subsume the individual identities of each partner but adds another conjoint layer to the couple. This We identity plays a role in a wide range of decisions and necessary compromises by each partner, such as how to spend time, the nature of leisure activities, how to parent, choices about shared purchases, and many others. The degree to which partners experience a sense of We-ness is significantly correlated with relationship satisfaction and stability (Buehlman et al., 1992).

Attaining a sense of We-ness requires each partner to get to know the other's mind—a process termed "mentalization" (Asen & Fonagy, 2012, 2021; Jurist, 2018). Knowing one another's minds—including how the partner views oneself—provides the space to find areas of commonality that become central to the We identity, along with acceptance of differences, which can also be part of the broader sense of We (as in, "we are similar in these ways, we are different in these other ways, and we accept those differences"). A related process is attaining a degree of intersubjectivity (Benjamin, 2017), wherein shared understandings and feelings form the basis of the relationship, which then recursively reshape each individual's intrapsychic life, such that each partner's individual identity is reconstructed to include being part of a We. Similarly, Solomon (2017) suggests the importance of developing "relational self-awareness"—people getting to know themselves and how they are in relationships, which is an ongoing process based on experiences in intimate relationships that can reshape the overall nature of the We. From an existential psychology perspective, love and intimacy require "social courage . . . the courage to relate to other human beings, the capacity to risk one's self in the hope of achieving meaningful intimacy" (May, 1975, p. 17). Partners need to continue to attend to the quality of the relationship and put energy into it. May (1975) writes, "It is the courage to invest one's self over a period of time in a relationship that will demand an increasing openness" (p. 17).

Romantic love also requires behaviors that build and maintain trust (Gottman, 2011)—which, depending on the needs of each partner, can include ending friendships with ex-lovers or at least bringing those partners into the joint friendship circle, restrictions on time spent alone with people who might stimulate romantic or sexual desires and opportunities, and openness about one's whereabouts when apart and one's times for arriving home. Trust is sustained through acts that encourage emotional attunement and safety, such as listening empathically and compassionately to each other's upset about issues other than the relationship (and of course, about one's upsetting behavior in the relationship) and avoidance of aggression, intimidation, or other forms of undue, undesired forcefulness, including in sex. Over time, a deep, reliable friendship becomes a central part of an intimate couple-hood (Gottman, 2011).

Flexibility in each partner's expectations about the course and content of a life together is also important, as partners go through inevitable disappointments and changes in work and other endeavors that may have financial or geographic repercussions for the couple, as well as illnesses and disabilities. Periodic refreshing of the couple's menu of leisure activities is necessary, as research suggests that couples who have a balance of regular activities that bring pleasure and occasionally introduce novel joint pursuits sustain more pleasure and satisfaction over time (Aron et al., 2000).

ADDRESSING THE WIDE RANGE OF COUPLE CHALLENGES[2]

Like all couples, last chance couples typically present with a wide range of challenges. As Snyder and Mitchell (2008) noted, "couple therapists confront a tremendous diversity of presenting issues, marital and family structures, individual dynamics and psychopathology, and psychosocial stressors that characterize couples in distress" (p. 354). Among other difficulties, last chance couples often engage in problematic patterns of communication and show an inability to solve problems effectively, patterns that often started early in the relationship (Driver et al., 2012; Fraenkel & Markman, 2002; Markman, Rhoades, et al., 2010). They engage in high levels of negative expressed emotion and lower levels of positive emotion (Gottman & Gottman, 2018; Markman, Rhoades, et al., 2010)—or sometimes, conversely, present in an emotionally disengaged, withdrawn style. Whether high conflict or low connection, last chance couples display a lack of emotional attunement and trust (Gottman, 2011). Partners often have developed "negative attributions" or beliefs about the motivations underlying each other's behavior (Bradbury & Fincham, 1990; Bradbury et al., 2000). These negative attributions usually infuse struggles around power, closeness and care, respect and recognition, a sense of personal safety

---

2 This section appears in different form in Fraenkel, P. (2022). The therapeutic palette integrative approach to couple therapy. In J. L. Lebow & D. K. Snyder (Eds.). *Clinical handbook of couple therapy* (6th ed., pp. 339–361). New York: Guilford Press. It is printed here with permission from Guilford Press.

and integrity, trust, commitment, and acceptance (so-called hidden issues, which are often not so hidden; Markman, Stanley, et al., 2010). There is usually a lack of affection, kindness, compassion, mutual responsiveness, attention, and care, as well as problems with sexual intimacy and other forms of intimacy.

Couples often have different ideas about the balance of work and relationship time, or different levels of job-imposed pressures, and different preferences regarding how to allocate nonwork time between time alone with the partner versus with children versus with friends or extended family versus alone (Fraenkel, 2011; Fraenkel & Capstick, 2012). They may differ greatly in how they approach money, parenting, domestic chores, religion and spirituality, cultural differences (even when they essentially share the same cultural background), and other aspects of a life together. They may face any number of stressors for which they have inadequate joint coping skills (Bodenmann & Randall, 2020)—financial difficulties (across the socioeconomic spectrum), job loss, and legal issues, including those related to immigration and naturalization, problems with their living situation or home, health problems or disabilities of their own or experienced by their children or aging parents, their children's behavioral and academic issues, difficulties launching young adult children into independent living, adjustment to immigration and the new country (including language skills), and many other challenges. They usually report an absence of regular pleasurable leisure activities and sources of shared enjoyment, and often report different preferences for how they want to spend leisure time (Fraenkel, 2011).

Along with these problems in the present, partners usually come to their relationship with memories of negative, even traumatic, experiences from their respective pasts. Many of these experiences occurred in their families of origin, where they also witnessed problematic models of intimate relationships between parents, grandparents, and other family members, which they either then repeat in the current relationship or try to avoid (Fishbane, 2019; Gratwick Baker, 2015; Papp & Imber-Black, 1996; Scheinkman & Fishbane, 2004). Other painful experiences from the past may include problems in school and learning; with peers, including bullying, and attacks or rejection based on race, ethnicity, social class, appearance, stature and body type, disabilities, sexual orientation and gender identity, and more; the challenges of coming out to family and peers about gender identity and sexual orientation; and failed prior intimate relationships, to name a few. These negative experiences and learnings from the past may influence how they respond to one another when something the partner says or does (or doesn't say or do when a certain response is desired and expected) triggers a painful memory. What they saw and experienced in their families growing up and childhood more generally may establish problematic maps, scripts, and expectations about how to negotiate conflict, a lack of capacity for self-soothing, and little sense of how to soothe and take care of their partner, what they desire in terms of expressed affection, their attitudes, desires, and level of comfort with sex, and other aspects of what is preferable and possible (and not possible) in an intimate relationship.

Many couples also bring differences between partners based on cultural backgrounds and the intersecting social locations of gender, gender identity, sexual orientation, race, ethnicity, social class and education, age, immigration history and citizenship status, primary language, ability or disability, religion, spirituality, and ethics, and other aspects of identity. As noted in Chapter 1, even couples who share a social location or cultural background may differ on how they relate to those locations and cultures. For instance, one Bengali American couple had quite different upbringings—she was extremely close to her family and valued long visits with them during which they chatted about their lives and feelings, whereas he was raised in a more (as he called it) British Bengali family, where there was no discussion of feelings, and conversations were limited to the father asking him about his schoolwork and thoughts about intellectual topics. He found time with her family barely tolerable, as he felt uncomfortable engaging in "small talk." As a result, she and her family felt he looked down on them.

In an Italian American couple, both raised in the same Italian neighborhood in Brooklyn, he sought to distance himself from that culture, which he associated with the Mafia-related activities of some of his family, whereas she wished to spend every weekend with her close extended family. A successful physician, he also wished to separate himself from his working-class culture, whereas she was comfortable in that world. This difference was unresolvable, and they divorced. In yet another example described earlier—an African American couple in which both partners were raised in similar religious, socially and sexually conservative lower-middle-class households—she had become interested in Eastern religions and spirituality and wished to experiment with polyamory, whereas he was intent on remaining close to his roots and focused on demonstrating that he could be a responsible, hardworking Black man, different from his father, who had become an alcoholic and was not responsible to his family.

When partners come from different cultural backgrounds and are of different social locations, they often have experienced different levels of oppression or privilege in the broader society, which may infiltrate the relationship and contribute to power struggles between partners (Knudson-Martin & Huenergardt, 2010; McDowell et al., 2017). For instance, in one couple in which the wife was a liberal white woman from an upper-class family, raised in the South, and the husband was a mixed-race Latino African American who grew up poor in New York City but became a successful criminal lawyer, disputes about how to handle their nine-year-old daughter's misbehavior at school (he spoke firmly to her about changing her behavior, whereas she was more gentle and wanted to reinforce the daughter's positive behavior) led the wife to threaten to call the police if he spoke "harshly" (as she saw it) to the daughter again. The husband was outraged that his wife would consider putting him, a Black man, at risk of a police intervention and potentially jeopardize his law career, that she was so insensitive to his own upbringing, in which he was beaten for misbehavior (something he never did with the daughter), and that she seemed not to realize how their mixed-race daughter put herself at risk of being labeled as a problem at school. Her level of automatic unexamined white privilege, including her assumption that she knew best how to parent, was quite striking and was addressed in the therapy.

Partners also often have different ideas about their future goals. If not yet married, they may differ on whether to become more formally committed to a life together. They may differ on whether or when to have children, their financial goals, whether or when to move from an apartment to a separate home, and whether or when to retire. Chapter 8 addresses these sorts of couples that diverge in their "projected life chronologies" (Fraenkel, 2011).

RATIONALE FOR AN INTEGRATIVE APPROACH TO COUPLE THERAPY

Each of these difficulties and more represent potential targets for intervention. The wide range of difficulties couples bring strongly argues for an integrative approach to couple therapy—one that addresses present issues in how partners think, feel, and interact, that addresses the influence of the past on the present, and that recognizes how divergently partners may construct their preferred future. Whereas other approaches to couple therapy tend to focus either mostly on present-oriented patterns, or on revealing the link between past experiences and the present, or on the future, the Therapeutic Palette (TP) integrative approach is designed to help therapists flexibly traverse these different time frames. Likewise, whereas other approaches tend to focus mostly on cognitions (beliefs and narratives), emotions, or behavior, the TP systematically addresses all aspects of partners' psychological functioning and ways of responding in the relationship, including neuropsychological contributions to their reactivity (Fishbane, 2013), addressing their arousal states, emotions, beliefs, narratives, and interactional behavior in a fluid, combinatory manner.

The TP is one of several integrative approaches to couple therapy. Since the mid-1990s, the field of couple therapy has moved steadily in the direction of integration, combining theories and associated practices that provide couples practical tools for changing interaction patterns (for instance, cognitive–behavioral couple therapy, CBCT), those that provide insight and mutual understanding (intergenerational and psychodynamic therapies), and those that elicit powerful, healing emotional experiences (emotionally focused and experiential therapies) (Fraenkel, 2017; Gurman, 2015; Kelly et al., 2019; Lebow, 2014; Nielsen, 2016b; Pinsof, 1995; Pinsof et al., 2018; Scheinkman, 2008; Snyder & Mitchell, 2008; E. Wachtel, 2019). From an integrative perspective, no one approach suffices: Couples need action-, emotional/experiential-, and insight-oriented interventions, and therapists must be familiar with the essential theoretical bases of these interventions to conduct a thorough multidimensional assessment and create an integrative treatment plan. As Gurman (2015) notes, "The major virtue of integrative approaches is an enhanced understanding of human behavior and thus enhancement of treatment flexibility" (p. 193). An integrative therapist can shift from one approach to another when the initial approach fails to produce sufficient change (Pinsof, 1995; Pinsof et al., 2018).

Limitations of Single-Theory Empirically Validated Approaches

Research on empirically supported or "validated" single-theory approaches such as CBCT and emotionally focused couple therapy (EFCT) has found that although a significant number of couples improve in highly controlled, randomized studies (Baucom et al., 2015), many do not move from the distressed to the nondistressed/happy range of relationship satisfaction (Bradbury & Bodenmann, 2020). Long-term follow-up studies show that couples who receive these treatments often do not sustain their gains (Bradbury & Bodenmann, 2020). Moreover, the highly controlled conditions (usually an academic setting) necessary for randomized clinical trials have been criticized for not being "ecologically valid" or generalizable to treatment conducted in normal, community/agency or private practice settings (Bradbury & Bodenmann, 2020; Wright et al., 2006). Participants in such trials are typically screened carefully, and those who present with serious psychopathology (including drug or alcohol use disorders), who are strongly considering divorce, or where couples have engaged in interpersonal violence (among other common issues) are not accepted into the treatment protocol, unless these conditions are a focus of the treatment. Yet as couple therapists, we see couples with all these excluded issues.

Moreover, there is a selection bias in that couples are told at least the general nature of the approach to treatment they will receive, are therefore positively predisposed to this approach, but also have the option to decline participation. In contrast, therapists in regular practice settings need to find a way to accommodate to the couple's desires for a particular approach and aversion to other approaches lest they lose clients. To be bluntly realistic about it, therapists working in agencies or private practice need to secure clients to make a living and must therefore find a way to engage a wide range of couples, whereas the work of therapists who see couples in academically based treatment studies is either funded by a grant or is part of their graduate training; they can afford to turn away couples who do not fit the inclusion criteria of a treatment study or who do not wish to engage in the particular form of treatment offered.

Importantly, in order to conduct an empirically validated approach successfully, therapists must receive extensive training in the approach. In carefully controlled studies, researchers do periodic adherence checks on whether the therapists are following the manual. Therapists working in nonacademic settings may not be able to avail themselves of this training in an empirically validated treatment due to cost, time, or availability, and are not likely to have an independent auditor of their work's adherence to the manual.

Additionally, although these approaches have amassed a fair amount of empirical support, studies have not been conducted that demonstrate one approach to be superior to another. Some couple therapy approaches—for instance, psychodynamic, intergenerational, solution-focused, and narrative—have not been subjected to much empirical study, yet they have gained decades of anecdotal/clinical support. Davis et al. (2012) note that "although reliable differences in treatment models may be discovered, we believe it is unlikely that one model will be shown to be universally more effective than others" (p. 37). This point suggests that although there are excellent, research-supported approaches that help many couples, the field still needs innovative approaches that provide the most comprehensive treatment for the wide range of couples and challenges they present. Furthermore, no treatment outcome research has focused specifically on which approach is most useful in working with last chance couples, including mixed-agenda couples (Doherty et al., 2015).

The Research Basis of the Therapeutic Palette: Evidence Informed Versus Empirically Validated

Wachtel (2010) has noted that therapies can be "based on evidence" and founded on "respect for evidence" (p. 215) without meeting the more rigorous gold standard needed to establish an approach as empirically validated. Sexton et al. (2011) describe several levels of evidence-based practice, with Level One ("evidence informed") being therapies supported by research that demonstrates the effectiveness of component interventions, and that target aspects of couple or family functioning identified through research as areas of risk, without the full therapy approach having been subjected to empirical testing through open or randomized clinical trials.

The TP is one such evidence-informed approach. Although its effectiveness has not been evaluated through empirical studies, the TP approach is based as much as possible on research about the variables that distinguish happy from unhappy couples, and that predict from happy newlyweds which couples will sustain satisfaction and stability over time and which will end up dissatisfied and often divorced (Bradbury et al., 2000; Buelman et al., 1992; Driver et al., 2012; Gottman & Gottman, 2018; Markman, Rhoades, et al., 2010). And despite the critical review presented above about single-theory empirically validated approaches, the TP draws upon techniques that have been demonstrated in those approaches and others to be effective such as communication skills and problem-solving training (Baucom et al., 2015) and which form the basis for approaches that foster dyadic coping (Leuchtmann et al., 2018), as well as similar research from relationship education programs designed for nondistressed couples (Halford, 2011) such as the Prevention and Relationship Enhancement Program (Fraenkel & Markman, 2002; Markman & Rhoades, 2012; Markman, Stanley, et al., 2010). It also draws upon techniques developed from basic research on happy versus unhappy couples but not yet tested in randomized clinical trials, such as Gottman's (Gottman & Gottman, 2018) techniques of encouraging partners to respond to each other's "bids for attention," make regular statements of appreciation and admiration, provide mutual soothing, and being open to each other's attempts to influence them.

Research on the need for novel leisure activities in sustaining couple connection and pleasure over time forms an empirical basis for various TP pleasure-building interventions (Aron et al., 2000; Coulter & Malouff, 2013; Strong & Aron, 2006). Findings on the neurophysiological correlates of conflict (Fishbane, 2013; Levenson & Gottman, 1985) and the demonstrated effects of mindfulness practices on reducing anxiety and depressive symptoms and increasing open awareness, attention, and emotion regulation (see reviews by Atkinson, 2013; Baer, 2003; Jahnke et al., 2010) as well as emerging findings on the impact of mindfulness on intimate relationships (Adair et al., 2018; Atkinson, 2013) form the empirical basis for introducing mindfulness and other self- and other-soothing techniques. As is discussed in detail in Chapter 1, research on the importance of establishing the therapeutic alliance in a first session and the challenges in doing so informs the TP's high focus on creating a trusting, confident working relationship with couple partners (Knobloch-Fedders et al., 2007; Pinsof et al., 2018).

In line with Gurman's (2015) functional analytic integrative approach, "any variable that can be shown to influence treatment outcome is considered to be both scientifically and clinically important" (p. 193). At the same time, the TP approach incorporates theory and techniques that have demonstrated effectiveness in particular cases but have not been tested empirically. As Dan Siegel (2015) writes in his foreword to a book by Julie and John Gottman, "In IPNB (interpersonal neurobiology), we say that our approach to mental health needs to be consistent with science but not constrained by it. What this means is that we draw on science as a starting place, but acknowledge that as specialists of the mind, and the mind being the source of subjective experience, we can never fully measure this core mental feature" (pp. xi–xii). Similarly, the TP approach is informed but not constrained by science. It is based as much as possible on scientific findings about variables related to couple health and happiness as well as couple intervention science, and also utilizes techniques that have garnered a substantial history of usefulness or have strong theoretical support but have not been tested empirically.

Responding to Couples' Ideas and Preferences for Therapy Approach

Another important reason for adopting an integrative approach is that couples often come with their own preferences and theories about

what they need. Some couples want to focus on changing their problematic interactions and have little patience for exploration of family-of-origin experiences. Others may believe that such exploration of
their respective childhood experiences is essential to resolving their
present conflicts. With many clients, it often seems that their preferences for a particular approach to therapy aligns with broader beliefs
about how change occurs and problems are managed—for instance,
being more action oriented and wanting quick results versus believing change occurs first through patient, slow, careful examination of
thoughts and feelings leading to insight.

Cultural and social-locational aspects of the couple may also influence a couple's request for a particular approach and avoidance of
another. For instance, Boyd-Franklin (2003) and Falicov (1998) have
noted that African American and Latinx couples (respectively) are
often concerned about sharing aspects of family history that might be
judged negatively by the therapist and contribute to the stigmatization
of people in those communities, and so prefer a more action-based,
here-and-now problem-solving approach. They may also feel a great
deal of urgency to restore a positive relationship and avoid divorce,
lest they be judged negatively by family and community, or may want
effective parenting strategies with a teen who through misbehavior at
school or in the streets is at risk for the sorts of racial and ethnic pro-
filing many Black, Indigenous and other persons of color experience.
In contrast, mostly white, intellectual or artistic urban upper-class
couples (a cultural group in itself) may believe that psychoanalytic
theory and exploration of deep issues is the way to approach their
presenting problems. Additionally, couples who had an unsuccessful
experience in couple or individual therapy may declare that they want
a different approach from the one the prior therapist(s) took.

From the perspective of the TP, it is important to understand and
honor the couple's preferences for a particular style of therapy. This
is crucial for establishing a strong, respectful, collaborative therapeutic alliance. However, if warranted, the therapist should suggest that
other approaches might be useful at some point.

CORE PRINCIPLES OF THE THERAPEUTIC PALETTE
INTEGRATIVE APPROACH

The TP approach is designed to equip therapists to work with any couple irrespective of their presenting problems and level of distress, their
cultures and social locations, and is maximally flexible and responsive

to the moment-to-moment needs and opportunities for intervention they spontaneously present. Most other integrative approaches stipulate applying a set, logical sequence of theoretical perspectives and their techniques—for instance, always starting by addressing problematic forms of interaction, then moving to intergenerational sources of reactivity, individual psychodynamic conflicts, and so forth (Nielsen, 2016b; Pinsof et al., 2018; Scheinkman, 2008). In contrast, the TP approach involves keeping several theories and their associated practices in mind simultaneously and shifting or circulating from one to another, even during one session (Fraenkel, 2009, in press). Metaphorically, each theory provides a different lens or vantage point on the couple, and the more lenses available simultaneously, the more the therapist can notice the range of factors affecting the couple at the same time.

The shifts among different perspectives and techniques are based in part on the openings or "affordances" couples present. The notion of affordances comes from perceptual psychology (Gibson, 1979) and social psychology (Good, 2007), and refers to how people (and other living beings) notice opportunities for adaptive action in their environment Therapy can be construed as a sort of social environment or relational ecology, and the TP suggests that therapists be highly attentive to the affordances provided by couples through the language they use to describe their moment-to-moment experience of the therapeutic process. This sensitivity to the openings couples present enhances the couple's sense of the therapist's responsiveness and attunement, which as I noted in Chapter 1 is found to be a significant factor in the therapeutic alliance (Kramer & Stiles, 2015; Stiles et al., 1998).

For instance, when teaching couples CBCT-based communication and problem-solving skills, it is common for one or the other partner to reflect on how different these ways of talking about issues are from what they witnessed in their families growing up, or from their cultural traditions. This opening provides an opportunity at least briefly to explore each partner's family- and culture-of-origin experiences. If it seems important to return to working on honing communication skills, the therapist can note that they can return to these important family and cultural themes in a subsequent session, or, if the couple seems to have developed at least preliminarily the new skills, it might make sense to transition in that moment to a more extensive exploration of those family and cultural experiences. In contrast, a couple that wished initially to review various traumatic experiences in their long marriage and who reported that they generally did not have problems communicating might end up engaging in high-conflict interchanges about their differing accounts of the past, and this can be a moment for the therapist to suggest that some work on communication skills might be useful. The therapist states the idea of shifting from one approach to another explicitly, rather than simply launching into the new approach, and the decision to shift is made collaboratively with the couple.

For instance, with a couple in which one or both partners spontaneously reflect on how different the communication skills being taught are from what they saw their parents do, or who reflect on how different these ways of talking are from their culture(s) of origin, the therapist can say first, "Tell me more about that," and after the partner speaks a bit about what they witnessed and learned in the past, can say, "I'm wondering if we should pause on the communication skills for a bit and talk about what each of you saw your parents do during conflict—what do you think?" Or with the couple that explicitly says they do not think they need to learn some structured communication skills—that they generally communicate without conflict—and yet are demonstrating a conflictual style as they talk about their troubled past, the therapist might say, "I know you said that you communicate fairly well, but I'm noticing that you've gotten into some heated disputes about what happened a few years ago—would you be open now to learning some less harsh ways of discussing your different memories of those events that allow you to hear each other's different points of view?" Likewise, with a couple in which one partner says that the communication skills being taught are not enough to assist them and spontaneously talks about how "demons appear" when the partners are apart that get them thinking negatively about one another, the therapist might see an affordance in that language (the partner's anthropomorphizing a tendency to think negatively) for introducing the narrative therapy practice of externalizing (see Fraenkel, 2009, for a case vignette in which this was successful, described briefly in Chapter 7).

Engaging the couple to sign on to the shift in methods strengthens the sense of collaboration between the therapist and couple partners, and models for the couple attentiveness to their own process, as well as resourcefulness in utilizing a variety of psycho-relational tools to address their issues in the future, both between sessions and long after therapy has ended. In the spirit of relationship education (Halford, 2011; Leuchtmann et al., 2018; Markman & Rhoades, 2012), one major goal of couple therapy is to equip the couple with a new set of tools. However, from an integrative perspective, the toolkit should go beyond the usual CBCT-based set of relationship skills and include practices (including ways of thinking about and concep-tualizing issues, not only action-oriented tools) from a wider variety of models, including family of origin, psychodynamic, attachment based, reflective functioning, narrative, and experiential, among oth-ers. To paraphrase a metaphor often used to describe the limitations of single-theory approaches to therapy, not all challenges in a couple's life can be fixed with a hammer: They need a range of tools to work on the multiple levels of their difficulties.

THE THREE PRIMARY COLORS IN THE TP APPROACH

Metaphorically speaking, the therapist draws upon three primary colors in constructing a fluidly integrative approach to therapy: time frame focus, level of directiveness, and change entry point. Each of these primary colors or orientations to couple therapy, and how to use them flexibly, are described below.

Time Frame Focus

Single-theory approaches—or as Pinsof et al. (2018) call them, "mono-chromatic theoretical models" (p. 33)—tend to focus on one time frame in couples' lives. Some focus assessment and intervention pri-marily on the present patterns of interaction (structural and strategic couple therapy, CBCT, integrative behavioral couple therapy, EFCT, acceptance and commitment therapy). Some focus primarily on each partner's experiences as children and teens in their respective fami-lies and cultures of origin and the impact of these experiences on the current relationship (intergenerational couple therapy, object relations couple therapy, mentalization-based couple therapy), looking for his-torical sources of current sensitivities, vulnerabilities (Scheinkman & Fishbane, 2004), or what partners often refer to as triggers or but-tons that get pushed. These approaches focus largely on identifying the (variously termed) internalized maps, beliefs or themes (Papp & Imber-Black, 1996), working models, schemas, scripts, or object rela-tions (Siegel, 2015b) that live on in conscious and unconscious beliefs about how relationships should or should not go, and accompany-ing emotional sensitivities. As noted earlier, in some instances, the partners wish to repeat what they experienced and saw modeled, or repair and reverse what they experienced (Gerson et al., 1993). Other approaches focus on each partner's constructions and preferences about the future (solution-focused couple therapy; Hoyt, 2015). Of all the single-theory approaches, narrative therapy takes an approach that spans all three time frames, guiding couples to describe their constraining current story of problems and deficits, examining the historical roots of this story, and supporting them as they construct a future preferred story that builds upon the past positive, subordinated story of their relationship.

In the TP approach, it is recognized that all three of these time frames need therapeutic attention. The chronological flow of time itself is viewed as a construction (Fraenkel, 2011), with only the present moment actually available for change efforts. The past no longer actually exists but is powerfully represented in present-day beliefs, memories, learned behaviors, neuronal pathways, and readiness for particular sorts of emotional reactions. The future likewise is represented by beliefs, fears, or hopes about what the next day (or week, month, or year) will bring. Changes in the present bifurcate the present from the painful past and change the relationship of the present to the imagined future, as long-standing patterns stretching back in time can only truly be constructed as the *past* when they are substituted with new patterns of thinking, feeling, and interacting. New images of the possible future only become possible with changes in the present that distinguish the present from the past.

Over time and repetition, these new, healthier and preferred patterns become the couple's new past and narrative, and as they plan to enact these new patterns in the present moment they are creating a new, preferred future, which when enacted in the present quickly add to their new past. In some sense, although they can recount endless negative experiences and locate them in a date and time, couples caught in destructive patterns have no past—only a long present that stretches back over days, months, and years. Thus, in practical terms, the only time frame in which new action, feeling, and emotion occurs is the immediate moment, but these changes must address partners' memories and embodied, repetitive ways of interacting, as well as their hopes for the future. Put more simply, how couples think, feel, and interact in the present moment both creates their new histories and also determines how they create their near futures.

The choice about which time frame to focus on in the therapy encounter initially is determined by two main factors: the couple's level of distress, and their beliefs about what would be most helpful. With most last chance couples, in which at least one partner is no longer firmly committed to being in the relationship in the long-term future and is fed up with the patterns that have traveled across time from the past to the present, the therapist must introduce experiments in possibility that, if successful, start to loosen the couple's sense of hopelessness about the future and their preoccupation with dissatisfaction about the past. Moreover, the variety of crises that often finally propel last chance couples to seek therapy—the revealing of an affair, an incident of violence, yet another drunken binge by one partner, or, simply, the often hard-wrought statement by one partner that they've finally "had enough"—means that the therapist must help the couple negotiate this crisis and help them take some form of action that will provide the ambivalent partner(s) a beginning sense of hope that things could change.

However, as noted above, some last chance couples come to therapy believing that the road to improvement must involve detailed discussion of their history and coming to terms with their painful past—which, if they have never done this successfully, in a sense is also a new form of present-moment interaction. Other couples may want to focus primarily on discussing in detail their degree of alignment in their future goals. The therapist should work with whichever time frame the couple seems most open to initially, mindful that all therapeutic work occurs in the present moment and can transform the couple's relationship with their history and their possible future. Over time, all three time frames are addressed in a comprehensive couple therapy.

Degree of Directiveness

Single-theory approaches tend to use a particular level of directiveness, from low to high (Fraenkel, 2009). Techniques that represent low levels of directiveness include questions that elicit feelings and thoughts, search for and mobilize existing strengths or "subordinated positive narratives," and that explore family- and culture-of-origin history. Techniques representing higher levels of directiveness include psychoeducation about relationship risk factors; teaching research-based relationship skills such as structured, nonconflictual communication; problem solving; making positive, affirming, appreciative statements toward one another; teaching couples apology rituals; advising them on how to balance better work time and relationship time, providing a convincing rationale for one partner to take on more of the domestic and childcare responsibilities; advising the couple on strategies for coping with health, financial, child-rearing, and other challenges; and suggesting various pleasure- and intimacy-building activities. With high-conflict last chance couples (Type 1 scenario), or those in which one partner's values and/or safety have been violated by the behavior of the other partner (Type 2), a higher degree of directiveness is called for initially and always welcomed by couples. Those whose major issue is their discrepancies around goals for the future (Type 3) and those who present as extremely disconnected and want to make sense of a painful or disappointing past that has led to a loss of passionate intimacy (Type 4) may be served better initially by a less directive, more insight-oriented approach, although the "last chance" crisis often leads the couple to request concrete, action-oriented suggestions.

However, over the course of therapy, couples who need more directive input initially to move beyond a crisis state will benefit from less directive, more exploratory methods to understand the preexisting, historically and culturally based beliefs and emotional sensitivities that contributed to disharmony and ruptures. Likewise, those who prefer to start with less directive methods typically find that they need more direction from the therapist to move beyond mutual understanding and toward actual change in their relational patterns. In other words, however the therapy begins, eventually all couples need both action- and insight-based techniques and interventions that range from high to low directiveness to reach the best therapeutic outcomes.

Change Entry Point

The change entry points are interactional behavior, cognitions (depending on the model, terms include beliefs, attributions, schemas, scripts, narratives, theories of mind), emotions (including expressed emotions and attachment styles), and physiological arousal/interpersonal neurobiology. Single-theory approaches tend to focus on one or two entry points, privileging these in formulating the salient challenges couples face but neglecting or at least de-emphasizing other important aspects of partners' engagement in difficulties. For instance, although contemporary CBCT and integrative behavioral couple therapy have evolved to incorporate more attention to emotion, the theories that guide evaluation and intervention are historically drawn mostly from the study of behavior and cognition (see Baucom et al., 2015). Likewise, EFCT strongly emphasizes attachment and emotional expression; and intergenerational and narrative approaches tend to emphasize memory and constructions. No approach centers solely on physiological arousal and interpersonal neurobiology, and only recently has this focus been integrated into other theories, especially CBCT, but often as a second thought rather than as a major focus of assessment and intervention (Fishbane, 2013). Fishbane (2019) has more recently described an innovative integration of intergenerational theory and neurobiology.

Of course, all these aspects of functioning co-occur simultaneously and mutually influence one another in a circular manner. Human beings interact, think, feel, and are physiologically aroused in particular ways, all at the same time, and in a dynamic, evolving fashion. The words and nonverbal communications of one partner set off thoughts, feelings, and physiological responses in the other, which then influence how the other partner responds interactionally. Feelings and arousal prompt thoughts that prompt interactional behavior, which then results in feelings, arousal, confirmation of negative attributions, and a behavioral response from the other partner, and the cycle results in escalating conflict or withdrawal.

Therefore, a comprehensive couple therapy must address all aspects of human functioning, and it is propitious to do so in all or most interventions. Quite simply, when partners describe an instance of problematic interaction, the therapist can ask each partner how they felt during it, including their level and quality (positive versus negative) of general physiological arousal; what they were thinking about the other and the relationship before, during, and after it; and the history and source of those interactions, thoughts, and feelings. Or when partners lead off in a session by expressing negative thoughts about each other, the therapist can ask, "And how do you feel and what do you do when you're thinking about [them] that way?" Or when they express a negative emotion or state of arousal, the therapist should explore the associated thoughts and behaviors and how these aspects of experience and being in the moment reinforce each other, both within each partner and between them. Likewise, in observing couples, the therapist must attend to the couple's style of interaction, their stated or apparent (but unstated) beliefs, and their likely feelings and arousal states based on nonverbal expressions and signs (facial expressions, voice tone, rate of breathing, flushed faces, agitated movements, and the like). In sum, a thorough assessment of the matrix of variables that lock partners into difficult behavior and stances toward one another must incorporate a focus on interaction, cognition, emotion, and arousal.

On the other hand, couples present with different affordances regarding which change entry point they prefer to focus on and are most ready to address. A highly intellectualized couple or partner that has difficulty experiencing emotion might need to be engaged first on their thoughts and beliefs, then gently encouraged to locate the emotions and physiological arousal accompanying their beliefs, and then helped to see how these beliefs and emotions influence and are influenced by the nature of their interactional styles.

In contrast, a highly emotional couple might need the therapist, in the style of Murray Bowen, to say, "Tell me what you're thinking, not what [or along with] what you're feeling." Bowen, one of the founders of the intergenerational approach to couple therapy, believed that distressed, reactive couples need to cultivate two related forms of what he called "differentiation"—intrapsychic (the ability to separate thoughts from emotions, and to privilege thoughts over emotional reactions) and interpersonal (the ability to respond calmly and thoughtfully to a perceived provocation by the partner rather than automatically and impulsively) (Gratwick Baker, 2015). In that spirit, the couple that goes into battle mode in session and exchanges mutual barbs will need to be interrupted lest the session feel unsafe and like nothing more than doing what they do at home, but at a financial cost paid to the therapist. Each partner needs to be asked, "Okay, let's slow down for a minute—tell each other how you're feeling and what you're thinking that's fueling this exchange." I often tell couples that they need to "say" or speak their feelings rather than "doing" or demonstrating their feelings in action.

When teaching couples new patterns of interaction, the therapist should check in with each partner to find out whether these new ways of relating resulted in a change in how they think and feel about each other, as well as in their levels of physiological arousal. The therapist can then help couples gain greater awareness of the ways in which interaction styles, emotions, physiological arousal, and beliefs mutually reinforce one another and, in moments of distress, ricochet as if each element sends a pinball to the other within and between them. Vicious cycles among these elements of experience can be avoided and transformed into virtuous spirals by a positive change in any one element.

ASSESSMENT: CORE CONCEPTS FROM SPECIFIC APPROACHES TO COUPLE THERAPY

My experience teaching family and couple therapy has been that after exposure to the third major approach, students become anxious about how they can possibly master all of these models and become resourceful integrative therapists (Fraenkel & Pinsof, 2001). Although it is advisable for students to become familiar with the details of each approach's history of development, specific theoretical concepts, and range of techniques, in actual practice, it is not necessary to keep all these details in mind. Nor is it necessary to undergo extensive training in each model to avail oneself of the most important foci provided by each approach. The following list of core concepts drawn from each single-theory approach, written as a series of assessment or hypothesis questions for the therapist to attend to, is designed to guide the TP integrative therapist in assessment and in deciding on the focus of interventions without a sense of overwhelm.

Following each list of core concepts are lists of interventions special to those single-theory approaches. The details of how to implement these interventions are described in later chapters, especially Chapters 4 and 5 on high-conflict last chance couples.

Please note that in many cases, the specific language used to describe these assessment foci and interventions is not drawn exactly from previously published work by the respective creators of the various theories. Instead, they are my own formulations, based on my distillations of the theories and techniques as I use them in therapy and teach them.

Note that there is overlap among many of the theories regarding the foci of assessment and intervention. For instance, most theories include concepts having to do with the degree of experienced and preferred closeness, the degree of closeness and involvement partners have with people outside the relationship (extended family members, friends, and others), the degree of experienced and preferred balance of power, and so on. The original schools of family therapy were developed largely without knowledge of each other—or at least, without much interest in each other (for instance, structural family therapy or SFT, Bowen's intergenerational family systems theory, experiential therapy, the Mental Research Institute, CBCT). Once the creators of these approaches learned of or had to confront each other's work at conferences and through reading each other's publications, there was intense competition for students in training programs—the so-called guru phase of the field (Fraenkel, 2005), which Imber-Black (2011, p. 270) called "the model wars." This period of competition for allegiance of students and professionals deterred a process of collaboratively coming together to formulate a consensual systemic theory of couple therapy (Fraenkel, 2005; Gurman & Fraenkel, 2002; Imber-Black, 2011). A good example is the obvious dimension of closeness/connection: Minuchin's (1974) SFT described this as a dimension with "enmeshment" on the high end and "disengagement" on the other, whereas Bowen's intergenerational family systems theory (Kerr & Bowen, 1988) termed these two poles "fusion" and "cutoff." This overlap in concepts and targets for intervention is yet another argument for an integrative approach, so that the field can work from fewer, consensually accepted concepts, and attain the pragmatic/scientific (and aesthetic) goal of parsimony—the smallest number of concepts that explain the largest number of events (Kuhn, 1986). In the lists of core concepts and assessment foci for each theory presented below, I have generally eliminated redundancy across the theories.

Assessment Is Ongoing and Intertwined with Intervention

Whereas some approaches to couple therapy conduct a thorough assessment prior to beginning the treatment phase (Baucom et al., 2015; Gottman & Gottman, 2015a, 2015b), in the TP approach, assessment and intervention occur in an intertwined fashion. Certainly, the therapist must get a sense of initial targets for intervention before leaping into the couple's lives with suggestions. But especially with last chance couples, in which one or both partners declare that they have only committed to one session and want to see if the therapist can offer something useful (and that their partner will respond) before returning for a second session, intervention needs to start in that first session based on the information gathered so far. This occurs especially with couples who have had disappointing couple therapy before, usually with the therapist spending too much time getting into their problematic history without offering techniques and other ideas for change.

Other prominent couple therapists agree with this approach to ongoing intervention as opposed to a full assessment up front: Pinsof et al. (2018) note that they adopt an approach of "partial and progressive knowing" and that "assessment (what we call 'hypothesizing') and intervention are two co-occurring processes that span the course of therapy. In IST (Integrative Systemic Therapy), there is no assessment or intervention phase. Both are ongoing from the first phone call to the last goodbye" (p. 43). Likewise, Doherty (1995) writes, "In the complex mosaic of explanations for human problems, there are plenty of issues therapists can choose to emphasize at different points in therapy" (p. 86).

This approach of "partial and progressive knowing" makes sense in terms of the TP's notion of affordances or openings presented by the couple to explore and work on particular issues. At the onset of therapy, last chance couples are in a crisis around whether to remain together or not. As I've noted repeatedly, for most last chance couples, action-oriented, here-and-now issues must be addressed before they are able and willing to explore their respective family-of-origin influences and other aspects of their histories. Once the couple is less reactive and agrees to slow the pace toward the decision to separate, they become more open to this sort of historical, insight-oriented exploration.

In addition, how couples respond to the therapist's suggestions and interventions reveals issues that could not readily be assessed without trying new ways of interacting or otherwise relating to one another. For instance, although at the outset a couple might indicate that they feel quite disconnected from each other and lacking in any pleasure, the extent of their alienation gets revealed when they feel they cannot engage in even minimal positive activities suggested by the therapist, such as doing six 60-second pleasure point moments with one another across the day—hugging, holding hands, giving each other a brief neck massage, or even nonphysical activities such as telling something funny from the day, looking out the window together, sharing a piece of pie, and so on (Fraenkel, 1998b). Exploring their reluctance to engage in such minimal activities provides the therapist a better sense of just how afraid and hopeless the partners feel about having any sort of positive connection.

Likewise, the degree of negativity experienced by the couple is revealed when they engage successfully in an intervention—for instance, they practice the communication skills taught them, and yet report that they made no progress. The therapist can note just how powerful their negative view of their relationship is that they devalue legitimate progress, and explore what keeps them from seeing and feeling that they took some objectively positive steps. In addition, sometimes incidents that the couple reports from the prior week as a sign of things worsening—for instance, a fight they had about how generous to be with their liquor with friends when they entertain—can be recast as a sign of progress from the period when they were so on edge with each other that they could not have such an open and normal disagreement.

An Integrative View on Core Activities of Couple Therapy

Before launching into the specific points for assessment and specific techniques from each model of couple therapy, let's consider some of the core activities of couple therapy shared by most models. As I described in Chapter 1, the common factors approach to integration has focused largely on qualities of the therapist and therapist–client relationship that are important and a key to positive outcomes across all models of therapy (Sprenkle et al., 2009). From the TP perspective, there are also commonalities across most models in what therapists do in terms of therapeutic activities on a session-to-session basis (Fraenkel, 2022). These include:

1. Questions and comments (in some models, based on observations in session, in some, based only on the couple's narratives of their lives outside the session) about sequences of behavior, thought, and emotion (including physiological states).
2. Witnessing and empathizing with each partner about their suffering in the relationship and unhappy emotions due to other issues (work, health, finances, etc.).
3. Questions and comments about the couple's existing resources that may be underutilized and positive aspects of their previous attempts to solve problems.
4. Drawing out and understanding the historical and cultural sources of unexpressed beliefs, perceptions, feelings, and arousal states.
5. Suggesting new, preferred ways to interact and new ways they could see and feel about each other based on changes in behavior. In some models (CBCT, EFCT) these suggestions are based on research on effective interventions; in some they are based on accumulated clinical wisdom about what has helped other couples.

A Note on General Principles of Clinical Assessment Interviewing

Note that assessment/hypothesis questions are not usually the questions to be asked directly to the couple. Rather, the therapist asks the following sorts of simple questions to elicit each partner's perceptions and narrative examples that illustrate those perceptions.

First, "I'd like each of you to tell me what challenges or difficulties you're experiencing in the relationship and that you want my help with." Then get examples by asking, "Tell me about a time when that happened." Ask for "video descriptions"—meaning a detailed account of a time or times when the problem occurred (two examples are good to start to get a sense of the patterns across time, place/setting, and topic)—how the incident started, what happened next, and next, and next, and how it ended, and how they were feeling and what they were thinking as the incident transpired.

This is in contrast to asking directly the hypothesis/assessment question in a yes/no format: for instance, "Do you fight often?" "Do you have problems with intimacy?" "Do you agree on most issues?" "Do you both contribute to household and childcare?" Avoid these sorts of questions, as they do not provide much information. If you want to get a sense of how couples function around these sorts of common themes, ask instead, "How do you two typically handle differences around various issues?" or "Tell me about how intimacy goes in your relationship," and then ask for examples. As my wise professor Irving Alexander at Duke often intoned in our assessment class, "Go to memory." Yes/no questions elicit general opinions; as a therapist, you want to hear detailed descriptions of what happens between the partners and how they think and feel as they interact: These accounts, which often differ between partners, provide the data upon which successful, targeted interventions work to create change.

When partners describe wildly divergent accounts of incidents in their lives—for instance, one describes critical and contemptuous communication while the other thinks they communicate pretty well, or when one describes feeling insulted by the other during a party with friends and the other believes they treated the partner just fine, this discrepancy points to the need for consensual, coordinated action, so that they emerge from future experiences with the same memory of how it went. Partners often want the therapist to judge who was right and who was wrong in these sorts of differently remembered incidents. Unless one partner is reporting egregiously problematic behavior that threatens the safety of the other, such as violence or excessive drinking, and where it is important to at least tentatively validate the concerns of the partner reporting these behaviors, I will usually note that we are dealing with the "wish there was a headcam" problem—they report quite different accounts of an event, I wasn't there and there's no video, and therefore I cannot ascertain objectively what transpired. Rather, what's necessary is to avoid these sorts of interactions going forward and to have partners use these moments to commit to preventing them. In other words, these moments in which one partner felt hurt or offended by the other and the other doesn't recognize or acknowledge their own behavior provide a compass for traversing the territory ahead, where they will aspire to avoid such hurts and insults and use effective communication skills to address them in the moment.

Second, ask about any elements of experience (thoughts, emotions, arousal states, perceptions) that the partner has left out of the description. Most of the time, partners will begin by describing a distressing interaction—either a type of interaction that's happened repeatedly (e.g., "When I'm upset about something, he never wants to talk" or

"When I approach her for sex, she always rejects me") or a specific interaction that happened on a particular day and time ("The other night I saw him texting and asked him who he was texting, and he finally admitted that he's having an affair" or "She yelled at me the other night for not loading the dishwasher the way she likes it"). Ask about the accompanying thoughts, feelings, and arousal levels. Sometimes, partners will lead off with their general thoughts or feelings ("I just feel so angry at him all the time" or "I just don't think I love her anymore" or "We seem to have such different goals for our lives, we've grown apart"), and then the therapist should ask for descriptions of the interactions that have contributed to the development of those feelings and thoughts over time.

Structural Family Therapy and Basic Family Systems Theory

Although there are a few theories of couple therapy that are based on fundamental ideas from systems theory (Fraenkel, 1997), SFT (Colapinto, 1991; Minuchin, 1974; Simon, 2015) is widely considered the clearest, most comprehensive application of systems theory to couple (and family) therapy. Structural family therapy is also the systems approach that has accumulated the greatest amount of research support, although usually as a function of these concepts being assimilated into other approaches where there was more empirical study of couple processes and therapy outcome (like CBCT and EFCT), and also in approaches designed for family therapy rather than couple therapy (for instance, multidimensional family therapy; Liddle, 2014; brief strategic family therapy; Santisteban et al., 2006). Therefore, where there is redundancy across systems-based theories, I've generally listed systemic concepts in this section on SFT. I've also included in this section the important lens of gender (Goldner, 1985; Hare-Mustin, 1978; Knudson-Martin, 2015) and gender identity in this section, especially regarding the distribution of power between partners, and have considered a multicultural lens on such issues as distribution of power in different domains, desired degree of connection with extended family, and other issues that may vary across cultures.

1. Preferred Degree of Closeness/Connection

   a. To what extent are partners satisfied with the degree of closeness, intimacy, affection, involvement, and connection between them?

   b. To what extent do partners agree on the balance between sep-
       arate activities/autonomy for each partner versus joint activity/
       togetherness?
   c. How do partners respond to each other's requests for affection
       and other forms of intimacy?
   d. How do partners make those requests—with or without threat,
       with or without emotional strategies (for example, if the partner
       doesn't provide requested affection, does the partner request-
       ing unfulfilled intimacy sulk and withdraw as a punishment,
       or berate the partner for being cold, unloving, or emotionally
       underdeveloped)?

2. Preferred Degree of Power Sharing and Methods of Asserting
    Power

   a. To what extent do partners share power and influence?
   b. How satisfied are partners with this balance of power?
   c. When partners hold different degrees of responsibility and
       influence over decisions in particular domains (finance, child-
       care, scheduling social events), is this differential power arrived
       at consensually or established by fiat, with one partner assert-
       ing greater power without agreement by the other partner?
   d. To what extent is degree of power in cisgender heterosexual
       couples influenced by partners' gender beliefs?
   e. In Queer couples, are differences in power related to whether
       one or the other partner is out (for instance, in a gay male cou-
       ple where one partner is not out and the other is, and the latter
       threatens to out the other to family and colleagues as a means
       to hold greater influence), or to the particular gender identity
       of each partner (for example, does a bisexual cisgender male
       have more power than his nonbinary trans partner who was
       assigned female at birth)?
   f. To what extent do partners resort to intimidation, aggression,
       or violence to assert dominance?

3. Boundaries

   a. To what extent do partners agree on the acceptability of close
       relationships with people outside the couple (extended family,
       friends, past lovers/partners, work associates, neighbors)?
   b. To what extent do partners agree on how much time to spend with
       people outside the couple relationship (friends, extended family)?

c. To what extent do partners agree on how much information to share about the relationship with these people, and on how much influence others outside the relationship should have on decisions and activities of the couple (for instance, how much do they agree on taking advice or direction on parenting from their own parents, who are now the grandparents, or on financial decisions)?

d. Does there appear to be a coalition between one partner and someone outside the relationship against the other partner (for instance, a husband in coalition with his mother against the wife; a wife in coalition with her sister against the husband), or inside the immediate family (for instance, between a father/husband and son against a mother/wife?) How does that coalition affect the degree of closeness and balance of power between the partners?

e. Are other people regularly playing a role in stabilizing or destabilizing the couple's level of closeness? Does a partner who is not getting enough connection or affection from the other seek it from someone else, thereby temporarily relieving the relationship from conflict but often also resulting in conflict about the partner's relationship with someone else (at the extreme end, another romantic involvement/affair?) This pattern was called a triangle in Bowen's intergenerational family systems theory, but because it is not really about family-of-origin historical influences on the current relationship and is more about current patterns, I believe it fits more coherently into the SFT notion of boundaries, coalitions, and perceived boundary violations.

f. To what extent do partners struggle around one or the other partner's degree of involvement in extrarelational activities and endeavors: work, exercise/sports, community groups, hobbies, or even therapy or 12-Step communities?

4. Circular Conflict Patterns. One of the major theoretical innovations from systems theory was the notion of circular patterns in couple and parent–child interaction. This was in contrast to the prior linear conception of one partner affecting the other, or a parent affecting a child, in a one-way causal direction. The notion of circularity in human interaction recognizes that in most cases, when there are problems in relationships, all participants play a role in sustaining those problems, and all share equal responsibility for changing, even if one person's behavior starts the sequence. The major exception to this formulation in couples is when one partner initiates violence or intimidation against the other. The partner who exercises this high degree of force is often empowered to do

so by larger societal beliefs about gender and power, with more power afforded cisgender heterosexual men than women (Goldner et al., 1990; Knudson-Martin, 2015; Knudson-Martin & Huenergardt, 2010), or gender identity and power discrepancies within the Queer community (for instance, as noted earlier, an out gay man may wield greater power than a closeted gay man by threatening to out him; or a Queer cisgender heterosexual female partner who wields greater power toward her trans woman partner who was assigned male but has transitioned to female; Fraenkel et al., 2022). Holding to a circular conception of intimidating or violent relationships disregards these larger narratives about gender or gender identity and power and treats the perpetrator and victim as equally responsible for the abuse, which unwittingly reinforces the perpetrating partner's view that it was the other partner who elicited and caused him/her/them to behave in an aggressive fashion. Three major circular patterns occur often in couples, which are revealed in the couple's narrative about their problematic interactions:

a.   Pursuer-distancer (also called the demand-withdraw pattern): One partner attempts to engage the other in conversation or nonverbal interaction (e.g., affection), the other pulls away (giving verbal or nonverbal signs that they do not want to engage), leading the first partner to increase the intensity of the attempts to engage the other, leading to further withdrawal by the second partner, and on and on, resulting in conflict. Research has demonstrated that in cisgender heterosexual couples, women usually are in the role of pursuer and men in the role of distancer (Christensen & Heavey, 1990). However, from a feminist perspective, I suggest that the pattern be reconceived and relabeled the distancer-pursuer pattern, because in my experience, the first attempt toward engagement by the so-called pursuer is often quite appropriate, and the behavior escalates only because the distancer withdraws from this reasonable request for engagement, thereby initiating the problem pattern. Conceptualizing the pattern this way avoids the implicit and sometimes explicit description of the pattern as that of a "nagging wife" and a beleaguered husband. In addition, feminist couple therapists have repeatedly pointed out the larger societal beliefs that women are responsible for attending to the quality of a relationship, and are thrust into the unwelcome role of having to always be the one to identify problems and raise issues, leaving the man the freedom either to engage or not engage.

b. Blamer-placater: One partner blames the other for problems, and the other takes full responsibility for the issues, even when this is not accurate, rather than taking responsibility only for their part and asking the other partner to do the same.

c. Overfunctioning-underfunctioning: Due to lack of skills in a certain domain (for instance, housework, managing finances), depression, incapacitation due to drug or alcohol overuse, legitimate physical disability or health issues, or simply due to obstinate failure to assume equal responsibility (once again, often informed by gendered beliefs, with men refusing to do their part and expecting women to handle childcare and household responsibilities), one partner does not contribute to daily and weekly tasks, and the other has to take up the slack, albeit grudgingly. The more one takes over, the less the other does, which often exacerbates the psychopathology or other individual factors that led the underfunctioning partner not to contribute equally.

5. The Couple's Relationship With Larger Systems

a. To what extent is the couple involved with larger systems such as medical, legal, employment, and educational institutions?

b. To what degree does the couple struggle with challenges and pressures coming from these involvements?

c. To what extent does the couple work as a team to address these issues? Or is there resentment on the part of one partner for the other's issues with larger systems?

d. The Couple in the Larger Society. To what extent are couple partners and the couple as a unit affected by the impact of racism, ethnicism, immigration and citizenship status, classism, and other forms of oppression based on partners' social locations and cultures?

Figure 2.1 depicts the core concepts of closeness and power/hierarchy in systemic/SFT theory. The two core relational dimensions of power (symmetrical/equal to asymmetrical/unequal) and closeness/connectedness (high to low) are orthogonal, meaning that they are in principle independent of one another (Wood, 1985). A couple can have high closeness and symmetrical power sharing, high closeness and asymmetry between partners in power, low closeness and symmetrical power, and low closeness and asymmetrical power between partners. However, in reality, the placement of the relationship on these two dimensions and how they operate in couples are often related and affect one another. For instance, when one partner dominates the other, this often results in decrease of closeness and connection; conversely, when partners drift apart, one partner may attempt to assert power over the other in order to get emotional/relational needs met.

Note that I avoided the original SFT conceptualization of closeness as varying from enmeshed (extremely and problematically high) to disengaged (extremely and problematically low). Years of research using a questionnaire called the FACES III that was designed based on SFT and the circumplex model (Olson, 1986) did not reveal the theo-

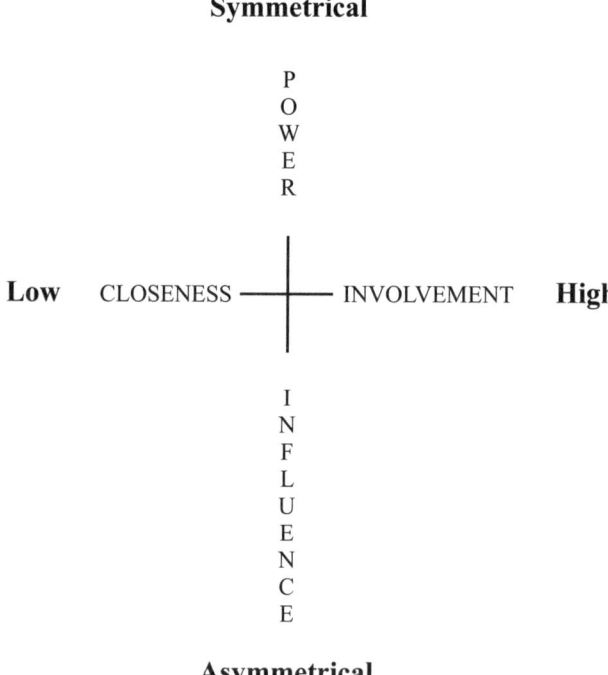

Figure 2.1   Map for Assessing Power and Closeness in Couple Relationships
Source: Reprinted by permission from Springer Nature: Clinical Social Work Journal, (Fraenkel, P. [2009]. The therapeutic palette: A guide to choice points in integrative couple therapy. *Clinical Social Work Journal*, 37, 234–247.) Copyright 2009.

retically predicted curvilinear, or inverted U curve, linking the highest level of closeness (in the circumplex model, closeness/connection is termed *cohesion*) to relationship difficulties (Cluff et al., 1994). In the circumplex model's conceptualization, healthier relationships have a level of closeness/cohesion that is high but not too high: As cohesion reaches higher levels, it was predicted that it would be associated with a decrease in relationship satisfaction (and thus, a curvilinear function). But overall, research has shown that the higher the degree of closeness, the more satisfied partners are in the relationship—rather than extremely high closeness being associated with problems related to enmeshment (Cluff et al., 1994).

In addition, there is a wide variety across cultures in what level of closeness is preferred between partners, with many cultures endorsing extremely high levels of closeness, but some endorsing lower levels. Therefore, what is important in assessment is to understand each partner's preferences for level of closeness, and the family-of-origin and culture-of-origin sources of their desired level. Although one or both partners may indeed feel the relationship is overly close—with partners overly involved in each other's emotions, minds, and behavioral choices (enmeshment), or overly distant and disengaged, my reconceptualization of the closeness dimension as simply varying from high to low leaves open a wider range of possibilities for what high or low closeness signifies in terms of a couple's sense of satisfaction and relational health. The same considerations apply to the couple's relationships to extended family, friends, and others—one partner may desire extreme closeness with her family of origin and see this as culturally normal, whereas the other partner may find this level of closeness with extended family excessive, even when partners share a similar cultural background. The two couples mentioned earlier—one in which both partners had roots in traditionally close Italian American family culture but had different desires as adults for degree of involvement with extended family, and the other, an Indian American couple in which the wife desired a high degree of closeness with her family, which the husband found suffocating—illustrates how important it is not to assume pathology at either end of a relational continuum, but rather to explore each partner's preferences.

Core Techniques of Structural Family Therapy

1. Enactments of problem patterns and especially, of more adaptive, preferred patterns: SFT focuses on creating meaningful changes in the therapy hour through having couples try new ways of relating. In last

chance couples, it is usually not necessary to ask them to demonstrate through an enactment the problem pattern—couples generally do so spontaneously!

2. Building intensity: Minuchin emphasized the need to craft an interventionist statement to couples in a manner that will be memorable, and around which the couple will be more likely to reorganize their interactions outside the session (Minuchin et al., 2014). He frequently used metaphor, dramatic therapist voice tone and pace (usually, quiet and slow), and other methods to emphasize the importance of his message. In a later section of this chapter, I discuss how to utilize products of the arts and humanities to achieve memorability of therapeutic communications such that they go beyond plain "psycho-prose" (Fraenkel, 2020). Appropriate humor can also be used to make a therapeutic message more palatable and memorable.

3. Discussions about concrete steps to reset patterns of closeness, power, and boundaries, including addressing coalitions between one partner and someone outside the relationship: Explore these themes and suggest changes and compromises.

4. Unbalancing: At times it is necessary to side more with one partner temporarily in order to support their voice. With last chance couples, in which partners carefully monitor whether the therapist supports their respective positions, this poses some risks to rupturing the alliance with the partner whose perspective is not equally validated. The therapist needs to establish a strong alliance with both partners before engaging in unbalancing, and even with a strong alliance, must be ready to revalidate the other partner's view and experience of the relationship issues after unbalancing. This is a delicate dance, well illustrated by the vignette of George and Alice.

Unbalancing is especially important when one partner is afraid of the other (for instance, when one partner has engaged in intimidation or violence) or has felt in other ways that their values or safety have been violated, as when one partner has engaged in an affair, or is engaged in overuse of alcohol or drugs. For instance, with Michael, who was abusing alcohol, and Ana, who was trying to keep the kids, extended family members, and Michael's work colleagues from knowing about Michael's drinking, I acknowledged her anxieties and resentment about Michael's persistent, disabling drinking. When he objected by saying that his drinking was due in large part to feeling unloved and unsupported by her, I noted that although they each undoubtedly contributed to their conflicts, "the problem with alcohol is that, like all liquids, it spreads quickly," and that his drinking was affecting everyone in the family. I noted that in order for me to be able to see and work with each of their contributions to their problems, he first needed to make a commitment to controlling his drinking. I also noted that whatever Ana was doing to make him feel unloved and unappreciated, it likely was at least amplified by his drinking, noting metaphorically that "alcohol is flammable." This intervention settled him down and was part of convincing him to enter an outpatient treatment program, which he later came to value.

Cognitive–Behavioral Couple Therapy and Integrative Behavioral Couple Therapy

The assessment foci listed below are drawn from a wide range of studies on the patterns of interaction that distinguish happy from unhappy couples, and that predict better or worse relational outcomes over time from groups of happy newlyweds (see the basic research, especially the concise summary of research from Gottman and associates in Driver et al., 2012; also Bradbury et al., 2000; Markman, Rhoades, et al., 2010; and see the summary of theory and research that forms the basis of CBCT in Baucom et al., 2015).

1. What is the overall balance of positive to negative interactions and thoughts/feelings? Put another way, "partners' subjective satisfaction with their relationship is a function of the ratio of rewards derived to costs incurred by being in the relationship" (Baucom et al., 2015, p. 24). To expand on this general issue, assess:

    a. Positive versus negative statements in communication and problem solving (see below for specific forms of negative affects and statements).
    b. The degree to which partners offer positive statements (compliments, respectful recognition of achievements, warm affection) versus negative statements (distancing, disrespecting, disaffirming, critical and contemptuous comments) to one another about each other's personality, appearance, behavior, beliefs, ideas, and preferences, work or other accomplishments, and contributions to their shared life.
    c. Positive reciprocity: When one partner does something nice for the other, or says something nice to the other, does the other

reciprocate with positive gestures and statements? Or is one partner more of the giver and the other the taker?

d. How regularly do the partners engage in enjoyable leisure activities in which they can share a positive experience and talk about it with pleasure?

2. Do the partners positively reinforce each other for the behaviors they want to see the other do more of, or do they criticize each other for the behavior not being frequent or extensive enough, or done not quite right?

3. How does the couple typically talk about problems? Do they engage in the following well-researched problem patterns (Markman, Rhoades, et al., 2010; Markman, Stanley, et al., 2010):

a. Escalation (repeated exchange of negative affect, especially criticism, contempt, and defensiveness—three of Gottman's "Four Horsemen of the Apocalypse," found to be strong predictors of distress and divorce [Gottman & Gottman, 2018; Driver et al., 2012]).

b. Withdrawal (including stonewalling, the fourth of Gottman's Four Horsemen: freezing the musculature of the face and flattening voice tone).

c. Invalidation (putting down the partner's point of view, feelings, or behavior, or an underresponse to a partner's upset).

d. Negative interpretations (attributing negative motivation or intent underlying the partner's behavior—usually around themes of being unloving and uncaring, attempting to control or hold power over the partner, disrespecting the partner, violating the partner's integrity in terms of personal ethics, comfort, or safety, being untrustworthy, showing a lack of commitment, and lack of acceptance—so-called hidden issues or larger relational themes; Markman, Stanley, et al., 2010).

e. Does the couple engage in the classic withdrawer-pursuer pattern (as described above, one partner bringing up an issue either gently or roughly, followed by the other partner's withdrawal, followed by intensified pursuit, followed by more withdrawal)?

4. Do they engage in any of what I call the subflavors of escalation—specific patterns that characterize this form of conflict (Gottman et al., 1979)? Namely:

a. Summarizing self syndrome (each partner repeatedly stating their point of view).
b. Yes-but (a variation of summarizing self, starting with the phrase, "Yeah, but . . . ").
c. Cross-complaining (one partner bringing up an issue in a particular domain such as housework, affection, finances, or child-rearing, and the other bringing up a complaint in another domain rather than addressing the issue the first partner raised—as in, "Well maybe I do THAT but you do THIS! So we're even!").
d. Kitchen-sinking—what I call the "deli salad bar" approach, in which the partner lodges multiple complaints in different domains, all at once, like piling on one's plate in the deli salad bar with all sorts of different foods.
e. Three versions of what I call globalizing from specific complaints to general statements about:

    i. The partner's personality (name calling, or character assassination, as in "You're a slob, idiot, cold fish" rather than, respectively, "It irritates me when you leave your dirty underwear and socks all over the bedroom," "It's upsetting when you say inappropriate, rude things to my mother even though you say you want a better relationship with her," "It hurts my feelings when you don't greet me when you come home").
    ii. Always-never statements, or catastrophic interpretations, such as, "You never pick up after yourself," "You're always rude to my mom," "You never greet me nicely."
    iii. Blame: "It's all your fault that we're having these problems."

The following issues have been identified in Gottman's (Driver et al., 2012; Gottman & Gottman, 2018) research as strong predictors of relationship outcomes:

5. Mutual soothing: Does the couple engage in mutual soothing—when a partner is upset about something outside the relationship (work, extended family, health issues), does the other partner use caring, empathic words, touch to calm or reassure each other, or other forms of soothing?
6. Meta-emotions and communication about emotion:

a. What are partners' attitudes/beliefs/feelings about expressing emotions, both so-called negative emotions (the vulnerable emotions of hurt, fear, anxiety, sadness, loneliness, upset, or disappointment, as well as more assertive/aggressive emotions of anger and frustration) as well as positive emotions (excitement, joy, pride, happiness, pleasure)?

b. What do partners do when they feel one or more of these emotions?

c. What do partners do when their partners feel/express one or more of these emotions?

d. How do they respond if the partner wants to talk about their feelings?

7. Responding to bids for attention: How do partners respond to one another's bids for attention—their attempts to engage each other in dialogue? Do partners turn toward (metaphorically, with their attention, and literally, shifting posture toward the other and making eye contact) when one partner seeks connection and focus, or do partners fail to shift toward each other or even ignore the other and turn away (in their attention and, sometimes, physically) in response to a bid?

8. Sharing power/taking influence: To what extent do partners take influence from one another—as shown by considering the other's desires, points of view on a problem, or requests to do something important for the asking partner without argument or protest?

9. Friendship: Some of these issues are not solely identified by CBCT, but because "enhanced CBCT" (Baucom et al., 2015) examines these as part of assessing the wide range of attitudes and beliefs, Gottman's research also focuses on the friendship aspect of intimate relationships, and Markman, Stanley, et al. (2010) also focus on fostering friendship in the Prevention and Relationship Enhancement Program, they are listed here:

a. Do the partners demonstrate the interest, respect, and care afforded a close friend?

b. To what extent do the partners have shared passions and interests that can provide activities and stimuli for leisure time and topics of conversation (intellectual interests, preferences in books and other reading materials, music and other arts, films and TV watching, sports and exercise, dancing, yoga, hobbies, the state of the environment and planet, politics and other issues about the world, etc.)?

10. Shared values: Again, these areas of focus do not fit neatly in one or another theoretical orientation, but I've put them here because

of CBCT's broad focus on partners' cognitions, especially beliefs. The issue of degree of shared values is of course also central to working with partners from different cultural backgrounds and social locations:

a. Moral, religious, and spiritual: To what extent do the partners share similar values—in terms of politics, religion, spirituality, personal ethics—and how do these values inform how partners treat each other and others (including strangers, such as people who provide services to the couple—nannies, waiters, doormen, taxi drivers, and so on)?

b. Does the couple have shared aesthetic tastes, preferences and values? Especially in terms of architecture and style of home to live in (house, apartment), décor, preferences for having stuff (memorabilia, souvenirs from trips, clothes) or simplicity? Do they share similar sensibilities in terms of clothing, dress, and other aspects of personal appearance? This theme of aesthetics is one that has garnered little attention in the research literature but is extremely important and often a source of intense disagreement between partners.

11. Expectations and standards for relationship/acceptance of differences: Some of these points overlap with previously discussed themes. Do the partners have realistic, reasonable beliefs and expectations about the characteristics of intimate relationships, or are some of their expectations and standards extreme and unreasonable? Do they understand that couple partners typically have a mix of shared beliefs and differences, or do they expect each other to be mirrors of themselves and aligned in all desires and points of view (about child-rearing, financial issues, standards of tidiness and home upkeep, frequency of sex and what is pleasurable or not in sex, and all other aspects of living a life together)? How do they handle differences around these issues, as well as personality differences—in temperament, volubility of speech, degree to which the partner expresses feelings, degree to which each partner wants and needs expressions of affection, degree to which each partner is comfortable feeling and expressing anger? Do they share sensibilities about the amount of appropriate ambition in their respective work lives and careers? Are there certain differences that they've learned to accept and accommodate to? Or do they try to coerce one another to adopt their perspective through conflict, especially criticism and contempt? For instance, in one well-to-do white cou-

ple, Tim was an investment banker early in his career, making about $300,000 a year. His wife, Angela, bitterly and contemptuously criticized his income, noting that some of his colleagues made well over a million dollars a year. When he pointed out that he came from a wealthy family in which his brothers didn't even work and his father had never worked and supported the family on trust fund money (the father's father had made the family fortune), and that at least he was trying to "make something of [himself]," Angela responded dismissively, in a voice dripping with disgust, "You're not a man. . . . You're a boy!" Integrative behavioral couple therapy, created by Jacobson and Christensen (1998) and refined by Christensen and colleagues (2015) focuses on assessing the degree of agreement and disagreement on these sorts of issues, and added to traditional behavioral couple therapy the important issue of helping partners find a balance between requesting change from one another versus accepting differences.

Core Techniques of CBCT and Integrative Behavioral Couple Therapy

1. Communication and problem-solving skills (described in detail in Chapter 4)
2. Skills to identify larger themes ("hidden issues"; Markman, Stanley, et al., 2010) of power, closeness, respect, integrity, trust, commitment, and acceptance (also described in Chapter 4)
3. Suggesting activities that increase positive exchanges and decrease negative exchanges
4. Shaping: teaching partners how to positively reinforce one another for beginning changes each makes that the other desires, rather than holding out on praise and continuing to criticize the partner for less-than-perfect approximations of the desired behavior
5. Statements of appreciation and admiration
6. Responding regularly to each other's bids for attention
7. Engaging in compassionate mutual soothing
8. Talking more about feelings (but not constantly or at inopportune times!)
9. Emotion regulation and modulation practices (decreasing negative arousal through mindful breathing or other practices like Qigong, a movement meditation similar to Tai Chi)
10. Taking more influence from one another, without protestations, and examining partners' expectations and desires for their lives

together—when these expectations differ, they are often the source of refusal to take influence, although such refusal may also be due to gender-based or culturally based beliefs (and other sources of beliefs) about power and who is entitled to influence whom

11. Empathic rather than critical discussions of differences between partners and striving to accept those that are difficult to resolve

Experiential Theories

The major contribution of experiential approaches, including the original work of Virginia Satir (1983), Carl Whitaker (Bumburry & Whitaker, 1988; Keith, 2015), the later, empirically supported approaches of Greenberg's EFT (2011), and Johnson's (2015, 2019, 2020) EFCT, has been to highlight the importance of directly eliciting couple partners' emotions in therapy, and a range of effective techniques for helping them express these emotions in a manner that brings them closer through empathy, rather than setting them against one another. Other approaches such as CBCT and SFT tended to treat change in emotion as a result of change in behavior and thinking; in contrast, experiential and emotionally focused therapies view emotion as the primary change entry point that then leads to changes in thinking and behavior. It is noteworthy that so-called enhanced CBCT (Baucom et al., 2015) now incorporates emotion as a core focus of assessment and intervention, and, as noted above, Gottman's (Gottman & Gottman, 2015a, 2015b, 2018) research and therapeutic methods, which began as more focused on behavior, also strongly incorporate the role of experienced and expressed emotion, as well as meta-emotion (partners' beliefs and attitudes about emotion), likely in part due to the influence of EFCT.

In addition, Johnson's (2019) pioneering integration of attachment theory, which was originally created in psychodynamically oriented developmental theory and research, has been one of the most significant developments in the field of couple therapy. Johnson also incorporates the related theory and research on emotion regulation (Gross, 2015) or, as Jurist (2018) has reconceptualized the concept, "emotion modulation," to connote less controlling or reducing emotion than an internal process more akin to changing the volume and pitch in music. The capacity to regulate or modulate emotion develops in part in the early childhood attachment relationship with a parent, although it can also be affected by biologically based temperament (Kagan, 2010)—with some people being more prone to stronger experiences of affect than others—as well as by adverse life experiences such as trauma, which may result in greater reactivity as well as numbing (van der Kolk, 2014).

Partners also vary in their ability to read and name their own emotions—on a neuropsychological level, to sense the interoceptive cues of emotion—which is a precondition for being able to respond empathically to their partner's emotions (Fishbane, 2015). Partners who were securely attached in childhood and adulthood prior to their current problematic relationship can also develop insecure attachment due to a partner's repeated rejection of their attempts to be close. Solomon and Tatkin (2011) also focus greatly on working with emotion, especially the coregulation of emotion in couples.

Johnson's approach is integrative, drawing as it does on cognitive–behavioral theory, research, and practice, as well as systemic theory and intergenerational theory, and of course psychodynamic theory, especially with the focus on attachment. However, viewed from the broader perspective of the TP, EFCT is treated here as a single-theory approach, because it has been presented (and branded) as a unified approach rather than one that draws from multiple perspectives. Areas for assessment include:

1. Feelings About the Relationship and the Self

   What are partners feeling about the relationship and themselves as part of it? And what do they feel about specific incidents and during particular interactions?

2. Experiencing Emotion

   How does each partner handle their own emotions—allow them or dismiss them (similar questions to those listed above based on Gottman's theory of meta-emotion)?

3. Emotion Regulation/Modulation

   Related to Number 2, how well do partners regulate or modulate strong negative emotions, especially anger? Although the focus of EFCT and other approaches that discuss emotion regulation is largely on what emotion regulation theorists term "downregulating" (calming and soothing upset and anger), it is also important to assess the degree to which partners are able to "upregulate" emotionally— to become aroused and activated. As is discussed in Chapter 3, one of the ways in which partners are frequently polarized is around one partner being more excitable and arousable and the other more calm and seemingly imperturbable—differences that are often an initial source of attraction but can become the source of frustration between partners. Sometimes these differences are related to attachment style (see below), but may also be due to biological temperament, beliefs about the appropriateness of expressing certain types of emotions and arousal levels, and other factors.

4. Emotion Communication

    How well do partners communicate about their emotions? When frustrated or angry, are partners able to access and express the initial, more vulnerable feelings of hurt, fear, disappointment, and sadness that usually underlie anger?

5. What seems to be each partner's attachment style?

    Attachment style influences the degree to which partners can comfortably negotiate the balance between autonomy/individuality and connection/reliance on the partner. There are four major attachment styles:

    a. Secure: The partner is connected to the other partner, comfortable managing their upset emotions on their own to a degree, and can express needs for reassurance and dependency when feeling shaky about the connection, but does so in a nonattacking or nondesperate manner.
    b. Insecure/Ambivalent: Demonstrated by a mix of anger and tearful neediness when the person feels the connection to the partner is threatened or unstable. These people tend to be overly focused on receiving affirmation and reassurance of the partner's love, care, loyalty, and commitment, and issues of trust are often a major theme.
    c. Insecure/Avoidant: Demonstrated by a tendency to dismiss connection needs, and to engage in an exaggerated display of hyperindependence and need for autonomy and separateness.
    d. Disorganized: Demonstrated by a mix of insecure styles (anxious ambivalent at times, avoidant at other times). Often associated with a history of trauma.

Distressed couples often present with one partner being insecure/ambivalent and the other insecure/avoidant. This pairing often seems related to how partners recruit one another to modulate their emotions (discussed in Chapter 3), with the more emotionally volatile insecure/ambivalent partner drawn to the seeming calmness and independence of the insecure/avoidant partner, and the insecure/avoidant partner drawn to the volatile partner because of the latter's capacity for emotion, which the avoidant partner finds enlivening.

Core Techniques of Emotionally Focused Couple Therapy

EFCT utilizes many of the basic techniques of SFT and CBCT. Additional innovative techniques are:

1. Softening: Asking couples to express the vulnerable feelings of hurt, fear, disappointment, loneliness, and attachment-based anxiety underlying anger.
2. Evocative Responding: Moving beyond the particular content of the problems partners are discussing and drawing out emotions, sometimes with "evocative imagery" (Johnson, 2020, p. 87) and with attention to the nonverbal aspects of emotion expression.
3. Heightening: Intensifying partners' experience of their emotions through the therapist's repetition of something a partner said, using voice tone (for instance, a softer, lower tone to intensify a partner's expression of vulnerable feelings, and a louder, higher-pitched voice tone to underline a partner's assertive statements).
4. Empathic Conjecture/Interpretation: The therapist attends to partners' nonverbal and interactional behavior and offers a thought about what they might be feeling.

Many of these techniques (especially 1–3) are similar to SFT's practices of enactments and building intensity, described earlier.

Another experiential technique pioneered by Satir and developed by Peggy Papp is "sculpting"—having each partner arrange themselves and their partner in a "tableau" that nonverbally, visually, and kinesthetically demonstrates how they see the problems, and then changing it to demonstrate what they wish the relationship to be like (Papp et al., 2013).

Family-of-Origin or Intergenerational Theories

The core goal in assessing each partner's family-of-origin experiences is to understand the source of beliefs, expectations, maps, schemas, memories, and emotional sensitivities that partners bring to the current relationship and that shape their preferences for degree of closeness/distance and distribution of power, and their areas of emotional reactivity to the partner's behavior.

1. Observed Quality of Relationships Between Adults

   a. Growing up, what did each partner observe about adult intimate relationships in terms of the two dimensions of closeness/connection/intimacy and power sharing?
   b. What did each partner observe about the process of managing differences and conflict between adult partners: in parents', grandparents', aunts and uncles', and older siblings' intimate relationships?

2. Quality of Relationships With Parents and Other Adult Figures

   What was the quality of each partner's relationships with parents or other people in parenting roles (grandparents, aunts and uncles, informal parents like close neighbors) on the dimensions of closeness/connectedness and power? (Degree of secure attachment developed in childhood is a central focus of intergenerational assessment, but is listed under assessment themes central to experiential and EFCT.)

3. Quality of Relationships With Siblings

   What was the emotional quality and power relationships of each partner with their siblings (if there were siblings) during childhood?

4. Family Attitudes and Practices Around Emotion

   a. Growing up, what were the explicit and implicit messages partners received about experiencing and expressing emotions? For instance, were they encouraged to express a wide range of emotions—both positive, such as excitement, joy, pride, happiness, and pleasure, and negative (or my preferred term, *unpleasant*, as the term *negative* suggests that these emotions should be avoided and have no usefulness), such as the vulnerable feelings of hurt, anxiety, fear, upset, sadness, loneliness, boredom, disappointment, and the more assertive/aggressive feelings, such as frustration and anger? Or did they learn that one or more of these categories or specific emotions was not acceptable or allowed (and why)? This focus overlaps with Gottman's emphasis on exploring partners' meta-emotions—their beliefs about experiencing and expressing affect—and brings a useful historical/exploratory perspective to their current beliefs.

b. If discouraged from expressing vulnerable or assertive/aggressive emotions while growing up, what did they do to handle those feelings?

c. What experiences, if any, did the partners have around being soothed when upset?

This focus (a–c) overlaps with EFT and attachment theory, and emotion regulation theory.

d. To what extent did each partner receive messages in their family that made them feel good about themselves, that bolstered self-esteem, or that negatively affected their sense of self-worth?

e. This often includes how parenting figures commented on children's bodies and emerging sexuality.

5. Family Roles

What roles did each partner play in their families growing up? Soother and confidant for an upset parent, mediator when parents argued, clown to distract the parents and family as a whole from conflict, angry confronter when parents or others did not address issues, rebel, problem child, star, and so on? Satir (1983) also focused on these sorts of family roles and how they get transferred (or avoided) in adult intimate relationships.

6. Abuse/Trauma/Neglect

Did partners experience abuse, neglect, or other forms of trauma in their families of origin or childhood more generally? How was this handled?

7. Family Secrets

Are there family secrets that have led to anxiety about particular issues in the current relationship (for instance, a parent's secret mental illness and hospitalization, accidental death of an infant, a secret second marriage of the father, or children of the father or mother by previous unmarried relationships (Imber-Black, 1999)?

8. Family Culture and Social Locational Experiences of Oppression or Privilege

Although these issues were not discussed in Bowen's intergenerational approach (or any other of the original intergenerational approaches), they fit well within an intergenerational perspective.

a. What was/is each partner's family's cultural background?

b. To what extent was there agreement among family members about following cultural practices, and to what degree did the partners ascribe to or reject their cultural background as a child and teen (and now, as an adult)?

c. To what extent did the family's or family members' racial, ethnic, class, geographic location (urban, suburban, rural, location in the country), citizenship/immigration status, and other aspects of social location afford the family privilege or result in micro and macro experiences of oppression and marginalization? How were these experiences discussed and handled, if at all?

9. Impact of Family-of-Origin Experiences on Beliefs/Expectations/ Preferences for the Current Relationship

How have these experiences (as assessed in Questions 1–4 and 8) influenced each partner's beliefs about what is possible or not possible, desirable and not desirable in an adult relationship?

a. Are they seeking to repeat or avoid what they saw and experienced in their families?

b. How do those family-of-origin experiences affect each partner's degree of reactivity to the other's beliefs and preferences about relationships, and to their expressed emotions and behavior?

c. How similar or different were the partners' family-of-origin experiences?

d. How understanding, compassionate, and empathic are the partners about each other's difficult experiences in their families of origin?

e. Does hearing about each other's experiences in their families growing up lead the partners to have a less or more judgmental attitude toward the other's reactions and desires for the relationship?

f. Does hearing about each other's experiences lead to greater or lesser willingness to adapt to the other's needs and desires?

g. Does exploring their own family-of-origin experiences lead to less reactivity toward the other partner and less insistence on shaping the current relationship based on unresolved family-of-origin experiences?

h. To what extent does it seem that each partner picked the other, usually unconsciously, to master conflicts and themes experienced in their respective families of origin? For instance, if a partner had a highly intrusive (or conversely, emotionally distant) mother or father, and now complains that their partner sometimes behaves in an emotionally intrusive (or distant) fashion, might this be an opportunity to master the original family-of-origin experience?

Core Techniques of Intergenerational Couple Therapy

1. Constructing a problem-focused genogram for each partner: Pick one of the major issues facing the couple and trace its source across generations using a genogram (for details on how to construct a genogram, see McGoldrick et al., 2008). The value of doing the genogram in front of the other partner is that the listening partner develops a more compassionate view of the behavior, beliefs, needs, and sources of emotional reactivity of the other partner.

2. Exploring effects of family-of-origin experiences on present thoughts, feelings, and behavior: Discuss how experiences in and learnings from each partner's families of origin are affecting how they behave and react in their couple relationship, help partners differentiate what they experienced in the past from what occurs in the present, and devise interactions that help partners leave the past experiences behind.

3. Differentiating from family of origin: Coaching each partner to discuss old issues with parents, siblings, or other family-of-origin members, toward the goal of "differentiating" (becoming less absorbed by) from those old experiences, which reduces the likelihood of the partner transferring those conflicts into the current relationship and into their relationship with their own children.

Psychodynamic, Object Relations, and Mentalization-Based Couple Therapies

There is much conceptual overlap (although the concepts are captured in different language) between intergenerational and psychodynamic approaches to couple therapy. For instance, object relations theory essentially examines the impact of internalized images and messages from parents, just as intergenerational theory does. For an excellent integration of psychodynamic, systemic, and behavioral theories and practices, see Nielsen (2016b), as well as Pinsof et al. (2018). The key additional contributions from psychodynamic theory for the purposes of assessment and treatment planning are listed below.

1. Projective Identification

    To what extent do partners seem to engage in projective identification? Projective identification involves a partner repressing and denying (unconsciously) certain affects (for instance, anger, anxiety, and other forms of vulnerability), projecting them onto the other partner, such that over time, this elicits those affects in the partner even when the partner does not independently experience them (Nielsen, 2016a). Often, this occurs when a partner describes an upsetting situation in their life outside the relationship—for instance, with family of origin, or at work—but in an emotionally flat manner, and the other partner gets inducted into expressing the missing feeling, often in an attempt to be empathic ("How can you let your parents treat you this way!" "Why aren't you more angry at your boss?"). The partner who described the situation then criticizes the other partner for overreacting, which then leads to a fight. The psychodynamic premise is that the partner who described the situation without appropriate affect has difficulty feeling that affect, engages the psychodynamic defense of repression, and relies on the other partner to express it for them, but then gets threatened hearing the affect expressed, and so tries to shut it down in the other partner. The defense of displacement also often plays a part in this process—the partner who has difficulty feeling angry at her parents or boss but is comfortable being angry with her partner now can express her anger toward the partner about her anger toward a parent or boss that the partner is expressing on her behalf.

2. Intrapsychic Conflicts

    To what extent do partners seem to be in intrapsychic conflict around sexual or aggressive needs and drives? How do those intrapsychic conflicts shape perception of self and other, and shape reactivity and other interactions between partners?

3. Guilt and Shame

    How do the affects of guilt and shame affect each partner, and how do those affects interfere with optimal couple functioning? Guilt centers on feelings of remorse about one's behavior toward another, whereas shame centers on feeling bad about what that behavior says about oneself and one's self-concept.

4. Mentalization, Reflective Functioning, and Intersubjectivity

An important psychodynamic perspective built on attachment theory and emotion regulation is that of mentalization, and its related notion of reflective functioning (Asen & Fonagy, 2012, 2021; Fonagy et al., 2002; Jurist, 2018). Mentalization and reflective functioning are the ability to know one's partner's mind, their areas of emotional sensitivity, and their usual motivations for actions. I think of it as "empathy plus"—not only being able to empathize with one's partner's feelings in the moment, but getting to know them well enough to understand how they view the world and the relationship, their typical ways of construing upsetting situations, what they need and desire in the relationship (including what they need to be secure and soothed), and generally, what their intentions are in various interpersonal moments.

A related and slightly earlier important psychodynamic theory is "intersubjectivity" (Benjamin, 1995, 2017), in which partners come to form a joint consciousness, which is central to formation of a sense of We-ness or shared identity. Couples in conflict either have never developed much of a sense of their partner as an independent mind with their own feelings, histories, and reactions, or the ability to imagine the other's mind is impeded because of ruptures in the sense of secure attachment between partners (Goldner, 2014). They have either never developed or have lost a sense of We-ness and how their own consciousness is shaped by being part of the relationship—often holding or reverting to a You-against-Me stance (a sense of separate, non-interrelated being) versus a sense of jointness.

Assessment questions around the themes of mentalization, reflective functioning, and intersubjectivity to consider are:

a. To what extent do partners seem to know generally how each other feels, how they view the world and events that transpire between them and around them, and what they need in the relationship to feel secure, safe, calm, and content?

b. Does the couple narrate the story of their lives as one of shared joys and struggles, and use the pronoun We in telling these accounts, or do they view themselves as separate, autonomous beings and consciousnesses without much overlap or mutual understanding? In another interesting convergence between a more cognitive–behavioral-based line of research and psychodynamic theory, the earlier-described research by Buehlman and colleagues (1992), on how couples' oral histories predict better or worse outcomes depending on the degree to which partners narrate their lives using the pronoun We, supports the premises of intersubjectivity theory.

5. Transference and Countertransference

Transference involves a client responding to the therapist in a manner similar to how they responded to parents or other important adult or sibling figures with whom they had conflicts. With two partners experiencing transference to the therapist, there is a lot to examine that can be useful in understanding partners' respective family-of-origin/object relations. However, from a systemic perspective, the most important transferences are those between the partners. Countertransference refers to therapists having responses to clients that are due more to therapists' own unexamined issues from their families of origin, and it is important for therapists to be aware of how they may be imposing their own unresolved issues onto the relationship with clients. Countertransference is distinguished from natural responses that just about any therapist might have with a particular client—for instance, most therapists might get a bit irritated with a partner who constantly criticizes their attempts to be helpful, or feel overwhelmed and anxious with a partner who is always in serious crisis, irrespective of the therapist's own family-of-origin experiences.

Core Techniques of Psychodynamic Approaches

Psychodynamic therapies focus largely on creating insight into the unconscious sources of problematic beliefs, emotions, and behaviors. Therefore, the generic, common techniques listed earlier (questions, comments, observations, with a focus on linking past experiences to present reactions) are the key techniques in these approaches.

Narrative Therapy

The TP is unique among integrative approaches in that it draws upon not only traditional, systemic, so-called modernist approaches, but also postmodern and post-structuralist approaches, especially narrative therapy. It's not surprising that other integrative approaches have not engaged postmodern or post-structuralist approaches, as the latter approaches reject many of the premises and practices of traditional approaches, including behavior theory and even systems theory (White, 1995). At least in their original iteration, postmodern approaches (narrative, social constructionist, constructivist) distinguished themselves from prior approaches by aspiring to be nondirective or nonhierarchical with clients, whereas aside from psychodynamic or object relations couple therapy, other models generally suggest that the therapist needs to take charge and structure the treatment, at least in initial sessions. A corollary of this nonhierarchical stance was rejecting any form of expert, or "nomothetic" knowledge (Fraenkel, 1995)—theory and quantitative research used as a guide to assess or diagnose and guide treatment interventions. Postmodern therapies are viewed as collaborative "conversations" (Goolishian & Anderson, 1992) and focus largely on how partners view their relationship, their accounts (narratives) about how problems developed and are sustained, and seek to bring forth the couples' own ideas about solutions.

Postmodern therapists eschew making observations about the couples' problematic patterns enacted in the consulting office, because those observations are viewed as imposing the therapist's theories, or expert knowledge (White, 1991b). Language is privileged to the exclusion of attending to nonverbal aspects of communication. Each couple is viewed as unique, and so application of the therapist's experience with other couples or research-based knowledge about patterns that characterize distressed versus healthy relationships are not engaged (see Fraenkel, 1995, 2019b, 2020 for a further critical discussion of the postmodern versus modernist stances toward research-based knowledge and therapy). The therapist's expertise is said to be limited to asking questions, although in actuality, introducing clients to such practices as deconstructing problems and externalizing are interventions that clients do not introduce themselves.

Despite the breach between modernist and postmodern approaches, the TP values the important contributions of the postmodern approach, especially those from narrative therapy. In the TP, a distinction is made between things that actually happen in couples' lives—interaction patterns, expressions of emotion or thoughts, family-of-origin experiences, experiences of oppression and other stressors—and partners' subjective perceptions and narrative accounts of those experiences. Much as narrative therapists might reject any link between their approach and that of CBCT, narratives are essentially the same as cognitive therapy's concepts of beliefs, attitudes, perceptions, and schemas. Narrative therapy's emphasis on how couple partners came to view the relationship and their identity as problematic, and the impact of broader cultural/societal and professional mental health practitioners' diagnostic terms (or in "postmodernese," "discourses") is a useful area to explore. The notion that the "problem story" comes to "saturate" or "totalize" the couple's identity and sense of possibility is quite similar to the well-established cognitive psychology concept of confirmation bias—that one's beliefs tend to focus one's attention on collecting data that supports one's beliefs, leading people to ignore data that contravenes those assumptions. As I often note to couples, when it comes to our relationships, we act more like lawyers than scientists—scientists design experiments with methods to collect data that might disconfirm our hypotheses, and only if those data do not surpass the data collected that confirms a hypothesis do we venture that our hypothesis may be true, whereas lawyers tend mostly to attend to data that supports their positions.

In addition, narrative therapy and other postmodern approaches served as an important corrective to the excesses of the stance of therapist as expert diagnostician and interventionist (illustrated most starkly in various paradoxical techniques in which partners were prescribed to do more of the problem pattern that they sought help to change but nevertheless engaged in repeatedly, so as to disrupt the couple's homeostatic processes). This corrective heralded a more respectful approach to clients' own ideas about their problems and preferred solutions. Narrative therapy also offers a powerful, creative technique, that of externalizing—although postmodernists reject the language of "technique," feeling that it connotes an overly instrumental approach, and prefer instead the concept of "practices."

Assessment questions derived from narrative therapy include:

1. How does the couple describe themselves and their problems? Pay special attention to the language used and ask about how they came to use those terms—what are the sources of those terms, and how did they come to describe themselves in those particular ways? White (1992) describes this approach to understanding the history of the naming of the problem (and how various experts and larger social narratives contribute to the naming process) as "deconstructing the problem."

2. To what extent is this problem description crowding out other more positive ways to view themselves? When asked about this more positive, subordinated narrative, how does the couple respond—are they able to describe it, unable to access it, or state

that given the intensity and longevity of the current problems, the positive narrative is irrelevant?
3. Who and what have influenced the maintenance of this problem story and the subjugation of the positive story?
4. How does the problem story affect each partner's individual identity, and vice versa?

Core Techniques (Practices) of Narrative Therapy

1. Deconstructing the problem story: As noted above, questions that focus on how the couple came to view themselves in problematic ways, and the various larger narratives—from family, the media, popular psychology and the culture at large, previous contact with mental health professionals who provide diagnoses or other problem-centered descriptions and labels, and other sources that contribute to this "problem-saturated story" of their relationship that has submerged the more positive story.
2. Externalizing the problem: Giving a creative name to the relationship problem story or aspects of their joint identity that constrain them, and taking action to put the problem story in its place and recover and build upon existing strengths. Often, it's useful to have each partner also give a name to problematic aspects of their respective identities and behavior that come together to create and sustain relationship problems. Giving problems a name— sometimes a bit humorous, like a creature or being from outer space—seems to work by separating the problem from the person who has it, freeing partners' identities as individuals and as a couple from the problem description, providing a space to take action to diminish the problem.

In one couple, a 52-year-old man who had experienced highly demeaning treatment by his mother, especially around a teenaged sexual encounter with another boy, had years of individual therapy to loosen the grip of this traumatic upbringing, with little success. In moments when he felt criticized by his 51-year-old wife, or by his children, he was prone to explosive outbursts quite different from his usual mild-mannered character. These outbursts led his children and wife to feel anxious around him, never knowing when he might explode. The therapist noted that it seemed the vestiges of the trauma at times "flooded" him and led him to act in frightening ways. Encouraged to give the problem a name, he called it "Marcusi," and was guided to catch the moment when Marcusi began to appear and engage in some self-soothing breathing exercises. This practice was highly successful, restored in his kids and wife trust that he could be emotionally steady and predictable, and allowed him to express discomfort with perceived critiques rather than act out his discomfort in the previous unpredictable ways.

Solution-Focused Approaches

Solution-focused theorists consider their approach to be postmodern, because they focus on people's social constructions of their problems and desired solutions (Hoyt, 2015). As noted earlier about postmodern therapies, it could be argued that solution-focused approaches are no more than a linguistic twist on CBCT, with "constructions" being another term for beliefs and schemas. From the integrative perspective of the TP, the main contribution of solution-focused therapy is its strong focus on working with couples to identify their preferred relationship and helping them move quickly toward that desired future. Little time is spent on detailing the problem pattern or its history, and there is little exploration of each partner's problematic past. Instead, the couple is asked to describe their preferred future in as much detail as other approaches encourage couples to describe their problematic present and past.

Although this focus on the future and solutions is a useful contribution and encourages therapists not to dwell on endless recitation of the problematic history, in its extreme version, solution-focused approaches do not create space for the couple to share their painful feelings and have that pain be witnessed by the therapist. Moving too quickly to solutions can lead a last chance couple to feel that the therapist can't handle hearing their history of suffering, and can result in the couple feeling that the therapist doesn't appreciate their degree of unhappiness, which has played a central role in their sense of futility in trying to imagine a more positive relationship and strive for improvement.

Key assessment questions from a solution-focused approach include:

1. How do you see the relationship now?
2. What would you prefer specifically to have happen in your relationship?

Core Techniques of Solution-Focused Approaches

The miracle question: "Imagine that tonight you go to sleep, and while you're asleep, all the problems you've mentioned magically disappear. You wake up and the problems are gone. How would you know? What would be different?" Ask the couple to describe this imagined problem-free relationship in great detail. Then work with them to design initial steps toward that preferred relationship.

Scaling questions: Ask the partners in an initial session to rate their satisfaction with the relationship, or their sense of how negative or positive it is, on a scale from 0 (as bad as they can imagine) to 10 (as positive as they can imagine). When they return each week, and have taken steps toward the preferred vision of the relationship, ask them to rate how they view the relationship now, in light of these changes. Make a big deal about even a one-point shift in the more positive direction. Ask how they made the change happen ("How did you do that?").

A Visual Summary of Multitheoretical Areas for Couple Assessment and Intervention

At this point, you may feel a bit overwhelmed with the range of theoretical vantage points and themes to assess in getting to know the challenges and strengths of a couple. Figure 2.2 summarizes in one diagram the most salient areas for assessment.

INTEGRATING MUSIC, OTHER ARTS, AND THE HUMANITIES INTO COUPLE THERAPY: THE ARTISTIC CRAFT OF INTERVENTION

In addition to integrating concepts and techniques or practices from the wide range of existing couple therapies, it is useful to draw occasionally upon products of the arts and humanities in designing memorable interventions (Fraenkel, 2020). This fits with the therapeutic craft principle described earlier, Minuchin's practice of "building intensity" (Minuchin et al., 2014)—creating interventions that are salient, that travel out of the consulting room and stay with the couple long after the session ends. Johnson's (2020) EFT also makes use of metaphor and imagery to heighten attention to certain feelings and moments, and as was noted earlier, she describes therapy as a "tango." Although as much as possible, couple therapy should be based on the science of couple functioning, and on interventions shown to have empirical support for their effectiveness, there are many micro-moments in

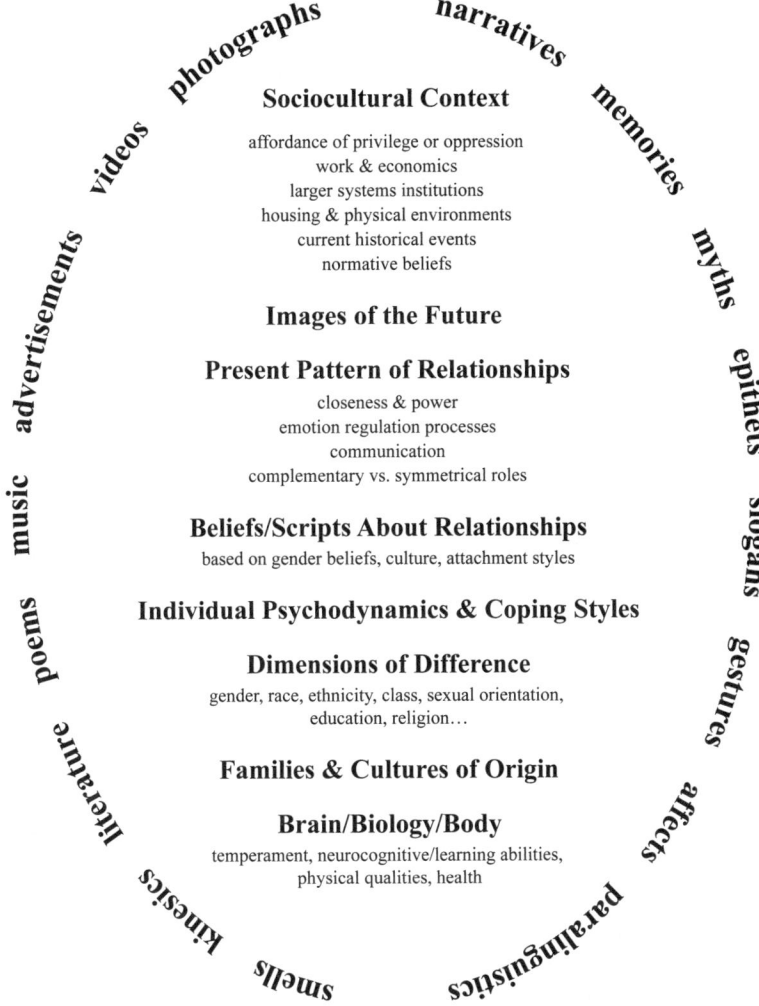

Figure 2.2:   Context and Representations of Selves in Relationships

Source: Reprinted by permission from Springer Nature: Clinical Social Work Journal, (Fraenkel, P. [2009]. The therapeutic palette: A guide to choice points in integrative couple therapy. *Clinical Social Work Journal*, 37, 234–247.) Copyright 2009.

the therapeutic encounter for which there is no empirical support. As Doherty (2012) notes, it is the accumulated craft of couple therapy, more than science alone, that assists therapists to decide choice points of "what words at what time and with what tone and body language" (p. 24). Along with the use of voice tone and phrasing to heighten salience, judicious, strategic use of products of the arts and humanities can provide metaphors and analogies that capture clients' imagination.

The use of the arts and humanities as resources to complement science to understand and intervene in couples' challenges is supported by biologist E. O. Wilson's (1998) consilience theory. Wilson was a distinguished scientist but also appreciated the unique perspectives that the arts and humanities bring to grasping the nuances of the human condition. He argued that the perspectives of the arts and humanities provided creative new ideas that could then be subjected to scientific research. He wrote, "Neither science nor the arts can be complete without combining their separate strengths. Science needs the intuition and metaphorical power of the arts, and the arts need the fresh blood of science" (Wilson, 1998, p. 230). Although my focus here is on what the arts and humanities can bring to the science of couple intervention, indeed, with the growth of digital art, science and technology have begun to have a strong impact on the arts, and the arts have long depicted scenes from great moments in science, and have served as a creative commentary on the process and products of science.

Taking music as an example, the therapist can use music and a musical sensibility in several ways:

1. Playing a song that the therapist feels captures something with which the couple is struggling.
2. Asking the partners to bring in music that captures something of how they are feeling.
3. Attending to the musical aspects of couple interaction: partners' tempo of speaking, volume (in terms of both loudness and amount of speech), timbre (for example, high-pitched and grating versus lower-pitched and soothing), and their paralinguistic (nonverbal) rhythms of interaction (for example, a long pause between one partner's speech and the other's response, which can signal disinterest or disapproval/disgust to the partner who just expressed their feelings; or much cross-talk, in which one partner interrupts and speaks over the other to silence them and take charge of the conversation).

As an example of the first strategy, I have often found that couples who were on the brink of relationship dissolution and now, after several weeks of therapy, have decided to stay together reflect that, even though they are relating better than ever before, they are having a hard time reconciling their improved state with their painful history and feel it almost irrational to go forward together. I ask permission to play a song by jazz-pop singer Michael Franks called "Living on the Inside," a lovely song about a cozy day of intimacy. However, in the second verse, he sings about how the couple used to be preoccupied with their painful past, yet now those memories have receded and become blurry and not important. I play the song and then ask the couple to reflect on how it made them feel. Often, partners are tearful and they get the point—that as they move on together in this better state, they will likely put the troubled past in its place.

Another example: I worked with a couple in which the woman had an affair with someone whom she supervised at work. She went as far as to invite him up to the apartment while the husband was away (and the kids were in another room with the nanny), and had sex with the man in the couple's bed. Needless to say, when the husband discovered this, he was severely traumatized. I describe this case in detail in Chapter 6. But briefly, after months of working with the couple, in which she came to understand how she could have engaged in this affair, apologized repeatedly, and took steps to prevent another such encounter with that man or other men, and after much work with the husband to decrease his trauma symptoms, there were occasions when he would ambush the wife with a nasty comment about her behavior. Straightforward encouragement to him to stop doing so did not change his behavior. In an individual session with the wife, she sadly spoke of being "burned out" by the husband's behavior and how she felt he would never let her forget the affair and allow them move on. In a subsequent session, I finally decided to play an R&B song for his benefit about a man who keeps hurting his partner to the point at which she is completely alienated and done with him. When the song ended, he was wide-eyed and said, "Okay, I get it now," and never taunted her again about the affair.

As an example of the second way of using music, in a case mentioned earlier, Ana, the Dominican American woman married to Michael, the Irish American man who was resistant to acknowledging his alcoholism and getting treatment (and blamed her for his drinking), texted me the titles of two songs that captured how she was feeling: "Vivir Mi Vida" (Let Me Live My Life") by Marc Anthony, which expressed how trapped she felt in the marriage, and a song by Kesha, entitled "Praying," in which the singer says goodbye to her abusive partner and bitterly wishes him well. I encouraged her to play these songs in our next session, which she did. For the first time, Michael understood at a deeper emotional level just how miserable she felt with him. The next day he enrolled in an outpatient treatment program, stopped drinking, and stopped blaming her for his depression and alcohol overuse.

As an example of the third way to use a musical sensibility—attending to the musical aspects of communication—I worked with a couple in which, when angry, the wife spoke loudly, quickly, and in a high-pitched tone toward her husband, who tended to speak in low tones, slowly, and with little expressed emotion. The flatter his speech, the more intense she became. I had taught them communication skills (which they rarely used) and pointed out the pursuer-distancer pattern that repeatedly occurred, to no effect. Luckily, the wife had studied a stringed instrument at a professional level, and I spoke to her as one musician to another, saying that when angry, she spoke at triple forte (very loud), 200 beats per minute (very fast), and in a high-pitched tone, and that this style of expressing herself seemed to have the opposite effect of what she intended: Rather than getting her point across to her husband, he responded almost as if he was turning down the speakers so that he could barely hear her abrasive tone and agitated tempo. She finally understood, and tried making her point slowly, more quietly, and at a lower pitch. He responded positively and, for the first time, acknowledged his responsibility for a situation that upset her.

Other products of the arts—drawings, paintings, sculpture, dance, film—as well as products of disciplines within the humanities, such as poetry, literature, and philosophy, can be integrated in a similar fashion to supplement straightforward prose drawn from psychology and psychotherapy. For instance, with couples who attempt to solve problems too quickly and without adequate discussion, after teaching them communication skills that they do not regularly utilize (usually because these techniques feel too artificial and too slow), I have sometimes asked if I could share a short passage from *The Way of Life* (Bynner, 1944), the classic sixth-century B.C. text of Taoism, attributed to the sage Lao Tzu. The passage speaks to the need to slow down:

> Gravity is the root of grace,
> The mainstay of all speed . . .
> What lord of countless chariots would ride them in vain,
> Would make himself fool of the realm,

With pace beyond rein,
Speed beyond helm?

I amplify the message by first having the partners take turns holding a small but extremely heavy copper ball. They are always surprised by its weight. I reflect on the two meanings of the word *gravity*—both as the force that binds us to the earth and as a way to describe serious situations (as "grave" or "weighty"). The combination of messages brings home the point that for them to address their issues successfully, they need to slow down. Couples are more likely after this artistic intervention to utilize the Speaker-Listener Technique, which slows down problem discussions, in spite of its initial awkwardness.

TP PRINCIPLES FOR SELECTING INTERVENTIONS FROM SINGLE-THEORY APPROACHES

The central approach to intervention in the TP is to encourage last chance couples to engage in nonbinding experiments in possibility. These are activities designed to improve the relationship by providing observable data that may transform partners' attitudes about the potential of the relationship to meet their needs. As noted in earlier chapters, these experiments must be cast as nonbinding in the sense that even if they lead to improvement, one or both partners might still decide to end the relationship. This frame of improvement being nonbinding is critical for engaging the ambivalent partner, who might otherwise be reluctant to try an experiment because improvement would make it harder for them to sustain the argument that supports leaving. For instance, couples might start to enjoy each other more, communicate and solve problems more effectively, and yet one or both partners might feel that they just no longer love the other enough to stay in the relationship. Of all the qualities of relationship, there really are no interventions that can directly change level of love or passion. Reviving love and passion generally come from increasing emotional safety through decreasing conflict, and experiments in mutual pleasure (see especially Chapter 9 for techniques to restart passion and pleasure).

In line with integrative individual therapists Stricker and Trierweiler (1995), and systemic therapists Pinsof et al. (2018), the TP therapist takes the stance of being a local clinical scientist, drawing upon the wide variety of empirically supported concepts about couple health and distress, and, where available, empirically supported interventions, to fashion a treatment that fits the particular set of issues presented by the couple.

Whereas the TP therapist keeps all the major contributing theories in mind as they listen to and observe the couple in order to develop a multitheoretical formulation of their challenges, when it comes to intervention, the therapist must select one intervention at a time. Five principles guide which intervention to select at any one moment. These principles are somewhat overlapping.

1. Degree of conflict
2. The couple's stated preferences for how to work with them
3. Affordances or openings presented by the couple
4. The need to introduce novelty into the couple's sense of what they need
5. The plateauing of a particular technique's usefulness

These are discussed in turn.

Degree of Overt Conflict

By definition, all last chance couples are in conflict about the future of their relationship. However, some present with higher degrees of dysregulated conflict behavior and emotion than others. High-conflict couples require immediate intervention in the first session to decrease their negative expressed affect and to slow down the pace and change the quality of communication, so that both partners feel emotionally safe. Their hopelessness about the relationship is usually largely due to the intensity of their fighting. If possible timewise, in the very first session the therapist should teach them the problem patterns research has uncovered and the CBCT-based skills that research has found effective in eliminating these problem patterns. If not possible, have each partner speak to you in turn while the other listens, and politely but firmly ask that the listening partner please not interrupt or make negative facial expressions if this happens. Couples who present more calmly can be worked with in a more exploratory, insight-oriented manner.

The Couple's Stated Preferences for How to Work With Them

As noted earlier, one of the advantages of being an integrative therapist who can draw upon action-oriented, emotion-oriented, and insight-oriented approaches is that the therapist can match the approach taken to the initial preferences of the couple. For instance, a couple in which each partner has found psychodynamic, insight-oriented individual therapies useful, and who hold a view about change that understanding must precede new action, may request that the therapist work with them in this manner. In contrast, with couples who are not keen to explore their respective families of origin, who may have had a less-than-optimal experience with this approach, and who believe that change occurs through new action, offering them an action-oriented approach is best. As the therapy moves along, the couple may become open to the therapist suggesting a different approach that embodies a different theory of change.

Affordances or Opportunities Presented by the Couple

A switch to a different approach happens most organically when the couple leads the way with the ideas and language they use in a particular moment. For instance, as was noted earlier, a couple that requested an action-oriented approach and is taught the Speaker-Listener Technique may spontaneously reflect on how different this way of talking about problems is from what they saw in their families growing up. The therapist can then ask each partner about what they saw and experienced in their families of origin. Conversely, a highly intellectual couple who preferred the therapist initially to work with them to review their long history of negative experiences and come to consensus about what caused them may see themselves get into problematic styles of communication during the session, which provides an affordance to suggest that the therapist teach them some communication skills.

The Need to Introduce Novelty Into the Couple's Sense of What They Need

Closely related to the previous principle, just as single-theory approaches to therapy are limited in their appraisal of couples' problems and the techniques available to help them, couples' theories about change and their beliefs about what useful therapy looks like may limit their ability to see other factors that contribute to their difficulties and may forgo therapeutic strategies that do not fit their theories. It is the therapist's responsibility to describe how an approach that the couple may not initially find aesthetically or practically appealing could be useful.

For instance, one highly intellectual, artistically oriented couple—one could actually call them rather effete and snobbish—believed that psychoanalysis was the only viable approach to change and openly stated, with a demeaning sniff, that the cognitive–behavioral approaches that I suggested would provide an important set of techniques to avoid their classic high levels of escalation were "surfacy" and "too simplistic" and implied that these techniques were quite beneath their refined psychological capacities. Weeks of psychodynamically oriented treatment did not change their problematic patterns, and I once again suggested teaching them some communication skills. To appeal to their artsy conceptions of themselves, I noted that these techniques were essentially captured by a prominent visual artist, Bruce Nauman, in his 1990s installation in a gallery in New York's SoHo neighborhood (at the time, considered the ultimate in artsy downtown cool) titled *World Peace (Projected)*. This installation involved a huge room with many pedestals upon which rested 23-inch TV monitors, each of which had a close-up of a person's face (of varying ethnicities, ages, genders, gender identities, and so on) slowly intoning, "I'll talk, and you'll listen. You'll talk, and I'll listen. We'll talk, and they'll listen. They'll talk, and we'll listen," over and over again. With the Speaker-Listener Technique described as analogous to this famous exhibit (which the couple had seen and loved), they were willing to try it, and it transformed their relationship.

The Plateauing of a Particular Technique's Usefulness

Because all approaches are incomplete, no one approach typically does the job of transforming a last chance couple into a happy, committed one. Pinsof has somewhat humorously described his integrative approach as "failure driven"—when one approach yields incomplete results, switch to another one (Fraenkel & Pinsof, 2001). The therapist must be attentive to notice when a set of techniques provides diminishing returns, and then suggest experimenting with another approach.

In one young unmarried couple that was trying to decide whether they were compatible enough to make a life together, the first three sessions focused on discussing their attitudes about the balance between work and relationship time. His heavy involvement in work—to the occasional neglect of time with her (despite her pleading that he work less)—had led her eventually to have an affair. By the fourth session, it felt like we were going around in circles, having discussed the reasons for and impact of the affair, and having determined that their ideas about work–life balance were more similar than they had believed. I pointed out that we seemed to have reached a place of repetitiveness, they agreed, and I suggested doing some family-of-origin work. This work turned out to be quite important in identifying their different attachment styles—she insecure ambivalent, he more avoidant—and in working on a plan to coordinate time together and time apart that would allow him the space he needed but also decrease her family-of-origin-based anxieties about abandonment.

SUMMARY

The Therapeutic Palette integrative approach is well suited to working with last chance couples. These couples typically present with a mixture of conflictual styles of communicating, little effectiveness in resolving differences, including about partners' respective desired plans for their lives, and intense and frequent expression of negative affect, as well as histories of disruptive and even traumatic events in their relationship, difficult experiences in their families growing up, cultural and social locational differences that result in misunderstandings and a sense of mismatch in their expectations and behaviors, and overall, a lack of closeness/connectedness and vicious cycles of coercion and power discrepancies. They often labor under a negative, problem-saturated narrative about their relationship, have lost a sense of the positive aspects that drew them together and may still peek out between the cracks of the problem story, and cannot envision the details of a preferred future. They also come to therapy with their own theories about the nature of the problems, and preferences for how they wish the therapist to work with them.

Therefore, an integrative approach that addresses the present, past, and future, that can shift from more directive to less directive techniques as the couple gains skills and reduces conflict, that is attuned to the openings or affordances that couples present about their willingness to address themes in the present, past, and future, and that addresses their behaviors, cognitions, emotions, and physiological arousal, is most effective. In Chapters 4 and 5, I provide detailed guidance about how to work with high-conflict couples. Even when couples present issues around value and safety violations (Chapters 6 and 7), differences in their hopes and dreams for the future (Chapter 8), or low passion (Chapter 9), these issues are often accompanied by high conflict. Thus, many of the techniques described in Chapters 4 and 5 will be applicable to couples with these various specific challenges.

However, before we turn to the core techniques and practices to use in an integrative approach to couple therapy with high-conflict and other couples, let's look in Chapter 3 at two intersecting aspects of couple life that usually undergird many of the challenges couples experience, irrespective of their presenting problems and styles of interaction: time and emotion.

CHAPTER 3

TIME AND EMOTION MODULATION

Underlying Patterns of Couple Conflict

COUPLES ARGUE ABOUT MONEY, SEX, in-laws, housework, parenting, and communication, among many other topics. Beneath these topics often lie differences in how each partner relates to time. Temporal "dyssychronies" are often the hidden source of conflict around these common topics. Although some temporal differences are explicit—one partner preferring to be punctual, the other chronically late, one partner wishing to devote more time to the relationship and the other preferring more time devoted to work or other activities— many temporal differences are unrecognized sources of distress but, once named, help partners understand their chronic dissatisfaction. Interestingly, when couples are not aware of the temporal substrate of their differences, these are often represented in global complaints that "we just seem to have different lifestyles."

Partners' differences in life pace (fast- versus slower-paced), punctuality practices (preferring to be on time or early, or disregarding punctuality concerns and being frequently late), time perspective (a focus mostly on the present versus the future versus the past), time orientation (adhering to the clock and calendar versus preferring to forget about these constraints and inhabiting a sense of timelessness), daily and weekly rhythms (early versus late risers, early versus late bedtimes, daily highs and lows in energy, differing work schedules and times for leaving and returning home), differing projected life chronologies (what they want to have in their lives and by when), and in how they prefer to allocate their time among different activities and relationships are often an initial source of attraction. Over time, these differences become polarized and create conflict around the core dimensions of closeness and power (Wood, 1985). The four steps to helping couples address these temporal splits are (1) revealing the differences; (2) revaluing those differences and how they can still provide useful complementarity (a "both-and" about time in which each partner's temporal style is validated and viewed as a useful balancing dialectic and source of checks and balances); (3) revising them so that they are no longer polarized but seen as that healthy dialectic; and (4) rehearsing the revised patterns as they emerge in other issues.

These differences in how partners inhabit time often connect to how each partner recruits the other to modulate their emotions. For instance, the fast-paced partner turns to the slow-paced partner to calm them down, while the slow-paced partner relies on the fast-paced partner to energize them. This recruitment of the other to modulate one's emotions is often unconscious and is part of the initial implicit contract between partners about how they will take care of each other. But like the temporal differences, the very role that one partner recruits the other to play in their emotional life becomes resented, outgrown, and no longer required, and a source of constraint rather than comfort. This chapter provides a guide to identifying and altering the temporal dyssynchronies and differences in emotional experiencing and expression that drive many of the other issues couples disagree on, as well as their overall sense of incompatibility and frustration. Changes at this deeper level must occur for last chance couples to find harmony.

TIME ISSUES IN COUPLES: AN INTEGRATIVE THEORY

The details of this theory and numerous clinical vignettes are described in Fraenkel (1994, 1996, 2001c, 2011, 2018; Fraenkel & Wilson, 2000). The theory was developed and refined over 30 years by synthesizing research from child development, social psychology, anthropology, chronobiology, and music theory (Fraenkel, 1994, 2001c, 2011, 2020). This chapter summarizes the main points and how the theory assists in work with last chance couples.

Time is the ineffable, ever-present factor in all relationships among elements of a system, whether human, animal, botanical, artistic, mechanical, biological, ecological, or cosmic. For the elements of a system to work together to create the "whole that is greater than the sum of its parts" (Steinglass, 1987, p. 31), they must be coordinated in time. The timing of the chambers of the heart as they work in rhythm to pump blood throughout the body is one of the first things a doctor listens to in assessing a patient's health. The temporal coordination within and among the different systems of the body—cardiac/circulatory, respiratory/pulmonary, nervous, gastrointestinal, excretory/urinal, endocrinal/hormonal, integumentary, lymphatic, skeletal, muscular, and reproductive/sexual—is central to the body's functioning.

Guiding all these systems are the chronobiological rhythms that operate in seconds, minutes, and hours (ultradian), and across a day (circadian), and at even longer periodicities (infradian; Moore-Ede et al., 1982; Pittendrigh, 1972). Everyday machines malfunction—for instance, when cylinders get out of sync or the timing belt breaks in your car. On the global ecological level, disruption in the earth's climate has changed yearly temporal patterns of heat and cold, and periods of dryness and wetness, in dramatic ways that affect plant and animal life, gathering, hunting, and production of food, and the safety of communities living in already ecologically precarious environments but to which humans had developed adaptations over many years (e.g., rhythms of planting and harvesting, when to board up and leave homes on the seashore; building homes on stilts that are no longer high or strong enough to avoid powerful tsunamis).

Partners may be separated in space—thousands of miles away from one another when one partner is on a business trip, visiting family abroad, separated by immigration challenges, or by a pandemic that forces them to be apart. But to engage in back-and-forth interaction (rather than monologic communication through texts, emails, or phone messages), they must meet in time. Even these monologic, noninteractive forms of communication include implicit expectations regarding the appropriate length of time within which to respond, although partners' expectations can vary depending on a host of factors, including how each partner wants to be viewed by the other, and the intended effects or "pragmatics" of communication (Watzlawick et al., 1967).

For instance, when meeting someone online for prospective dating, people often manipulate how quickly or slowly they respond to texts from the other to indicate either eagerness or feigned indifference (playing hard to get). In one lesbian couple, Teresa's insecure attachment style translated into demanding that Robin respond within seconds to a text or else risk angry confrontation. In one instance, they had a major conflagration because Robin was getting an MRI and, of course, was locked in the machine for several minutes and could not access her phone when Teresa repeatedly texted her.

However, early writings suggesting that happier couples simply are more temporally coordinated (Cooklin, 1982; Keeney & Cromwell, 1979; Larson et al., 1991) miss the great variety of temporal patterning that may be associated with happiness or distress. Partners may be perfectly coordinated in time but "out of phase" (Moore-Ede et al., 1982), meaning their daily schedules keep them from interacting with one another. For instance, in one distressed couple, Rob woke every day before Alyssa and left the house before she got up, and would go to sleep before she came home, keeping them perfectly, and deliberately, apart in time. Another couple's exactly coordinated rhythms were based on the male partner powering over the female partner. Cynthia complained that Darrel forced her to be home at exactly 6 p.m., to have dinner at exactly 7:30 p.m., and to go to bed together each night at 11 p.m. He also demanded sex four times a week. If she was even five minutes late coming home or was not feeling up to having sex, he would intimidate and berate her. In contrast, some happy couples have largely asynchronous schedules of work and home time during the week but make sure to spend some quality or quantity time together on the weekends.

These examples indicate that there are no simple empirical relationships between temporal patterns in couples and degree of satisfaction or distress. Rather, the therapist must explore with the couple the meaning of temporal patterns and differences, and the respective preferences of each partner, in order to understand how these patterns enter into struggles around power and closeness. Likewise, the causal relationship between temporal patterns and distress is not a simple one: In some cases, distress due to other factors (for instance, shift work in which one partner must work during the day and the other at night; Fraenkel & Capstick, 2012) results in partners' conflicts around time, and in others, the temporal differences partners bring to the relationship erode satisfaction over time.

Furthermore, there are multiple potential influences on how each partner inhabits time and on the temporal splits between them. An integrative, multifactorial approach to assessment is needed, just as in assessing other areas of difference and difficulty. Biologically based temperament, values and attitudes about time-related behavior learned in family and culture of origin and each partner's stance toward what they experienced in those contexts (e.g., to transfer patterns and preferences learned, or to act in contrast to those early learnings and experiences), pressures from the larger contexts of work, medical issues and involvement in medical treatment, and other factors shape how partners relate to time and view relationship time.

For instance, research on temperament (Kagan, 2010) shows that infants demonstrate temperamental styles including speed and intensity of reactivity to unfamiliar stimuli, and these styles tend to be stable into adulthood. Although research has not demonstrated the link between biological temperament and one's overall tempo or pace of behavior, it can be hypothesized that such a relationship exists, especially given that when people's pace is pointed out to them, they often remark that they've always been fast or slower paced, and their pace tends to be the same across different forms of activity—at work, in preferences for how to spend leisure time, in talking and walking, and even in thinking through problems (Kahneman, 2011).

People acquire beliefs about how to relate to time in their families of origin, and some of these beliefs have a quasi-moral quality: For instance, they may be taught such temporal values as the importance of punctuality, adherence to the clock and calendar, and a future-focused planning perspective (as a sign of respect, responsibility, and an achievement orientation). Or, in contrast, they may be taught to reject these traditionally Eurocentric attitudes and values about time, and that they should be more relaxed about punctuality and more immersed in the present moment. The fascination with Buddhist thinking and practice, especially mindful meditation, over the last few decades in Western societies demonstrates how many of us attempt to free ourselves from the traditional Western adherence to clock, calendar, and future planning (Kabat-Zinn, 2005; Nhat Hanh, 1990, 2015; Tolle, 2004).

Culture also may greatly affect our beliefs and behavior around time. Social psychologist Robert Levine (1997) did extensive cross-cultural research on the concepts and behaviors around pace and punctuality. When exploring each partner's cultures of origin, it is always crucial to include questions about how their cultural backgrounds influence their approach to time.

In line with the findings of chronobiology, time issues can occur within different temporal periods: micro (seconds to minutes), molar (within a day), and macro (days, weeks, months, years) (Fraenkel, 1994). For instance, dyssynchronies in conversation occur at the micro level, wherein speech rhythms are discordant, such as when one partner dominates the conversation and, as soon as the other speaks, interrupts that partner and continues on, or one partner speaks and the other takes a long time to respond, raising anxiety and frustration in the waiting partner, and a sense that the silence is being used to control them and the exchange; or one partner speaks quickly and the other slowly (pace). At the molar level, partners may be out of sync in their pace of getting ready to leave the home, in completing household chores, or in their timeliness in getting to a long-scheduled and anticipated concert. At the macro level, partners may argue about which family of origin to spend time with on yearly holidays, or when to take a vacation, and on long-term planning around when to have a child, when to reach a certain level of financial status, or when to move from an apartment to a house.

Events can be either recursive (repetitive) or nonrecursive (one-time events), and recursive events can occur regularly (rhythms) or irregularly. For instance, each time a couple attempts to make love, they may conflict about the pace of the act (he approaches sex like a fast-paced heavy metal tune; she prefers a slower and more languorous groove). Their sexual relationship is recursive—it occurs repeatedly but irregularly (nonrhythmically), and only after one partner complains about their lack of physical intimacy—and they also argue about whether to create a regular rhythm of weekly time for sex—she thinks they should; he wants more spontaneity.

There are five temporal aspects or elements in all behaviors: location (when it occurs in clock and/or calendar time), duration, pace, frequency, and sequence. Couples' conflicts can center on one or more of these elements. For instance, couples may argue about when to go to bed and wake up (Larson et al., 1991), have sex, eat dinner, or walk the dog (temporal location); for how long to sleep, make love, eat dinner, or walk the dog (duration); how quickly or slowly to eat dinner, do the housework, make love, or walk the dog (pace); how often to share meals together, do the housework, make love, or walk the dog (frequency); and which activity should precede or follow another— make love on the weekend before doing chores, versus do chores and then relax into making love . . . and then, of course, walk the dog (sequence).

In the following sections, I give examples of how couples get out of sync around the six major temporal attributes of human thinking and behavior: pace, punctuality, time orientation, time perspective, rhythms, and time allocation.

Pace or Tempo

Differences in partners' paces was the first temporal pattern I noticed as I started doing couple therapy as a clinical psychology intern at

NYU Medical Center back in the late 1980s. I have been a drummer since the age of 10, studying at the Berklee College of Music in high school, and later, with a plan to be a full-time professional musician, went to college at New England Conservatory of Music. As a drummer, my responsibility is to hold down the tempo for the rest of the band, and so I am acutely aware when a fellow band mate is dragging or rushing. We drummers have little rhythmic tricks to get the errant band member back in line tempo-wise (musician note: For some reason, guitarists are the most likely to rush, and I often have to pull them back to the groove!).

As I sat with one of my first couples, it struck me that each was trying to force the other into their respective tempo of speech. Audrey was a 36-year-old Wall Street executive, and Clyde was a 39-year-old ropes course instructor in an outdoors adventure company that catered to companies that sought to improve employee cohesion through recreational activities. In keeping with their respective occupations, Audrey was dressed in a smart gray suit, a string of pearls, and fashionable black pumps. She sat eagerly on the edge of the sofa, while Clyde, dressed in a flannel shirt, jeans, and hiking boots, rested with his back against the couch, with one arm cast across the top. They'd met when Audrey's company did a weekend adventure retreat. Audrey spoke quickly and intensely, whereas Clyde spoke in a strikingly slow, languorous style.

Asked what brought them to therapy, Audrey jumped right in and fired off her assessment in a rapid tempo: "Clyde and I get along pretty well, but when Clyde's son Tim comes for the weekend, we don't have much time together, and we end up fighting about that." I asked Clyde for his opinion; he took a few seconds to even start to speak, then said, "Well . . . [pause] . . . I think that [pause] . . . " and Audrey jumped in and said, "And this is the other issue! He never wants to talk about our issues!" Clyde looked flustered and said, again in his molasses way, "Yes I *do*, and I'm *trying* to talk, but you don't give me a chance!" Although relatively early in the relationship, they were both wondering if they could be compatible in the long run. The couple glared at me, imploringly.

A therapist could readily apply the concept of "pursuer-withdrawer" to this interaction—certainly, this was Audrey's take on their manner of communication—but I sensed something different at work: Each seemed to operate from a different temperament, which translated into a fast-paced agitated style for Audrey and a laid-back, slow-paced style for Clyde. I asked what was it that attracted each to the other: Audrey smiled and said she loved Clyde's laid-back style, and that it helped her calm down, while Clyde found Audrey's high energy and drive inspiring and exciting. Yet over the three years they'd been together, they'd come to feel annoyed by each other's style, without having a name for the underlying issue: differences in life pace. I offered my observation about their differences in tempo, and they both responded as if a light bulb had gone on: "Yes, that's exactly it!" said Audrey, and Clyde nodded (silently). Audrey laughed as she recounted how, growing up in a wealthy town in Connecticut, her parents often tried to slow her down, saying that she talked, walked, and ate too quickly starting at an early age. Clyde recalled the opposite— his parents were always "tryin' to light a fire under [his] ass," as he tended to move and do things slowly—even by Southern standards (he grew up in South Carolina). "I was on the slow side!" I noted that life pace appears to be linked to basic, inborn biological temperament, and while it can be modified somewhat, it cannot be completely altered.

With this pace difference now revealed, I moved to revaluing the difference. I noted that it seemed part of their initial attraction to one another centered on this difference in tempo: Audrey initially felt soothed by Clyde's slowness, and she found it sexy, while Clyde found Audrey exciting. I noted that both paces were useful at different times and wondered if they could try to accommodate those initially attractive differences (revising). Back to the problematic weekends with Clyde's son Tim, they decided to have one "fast and furious" day where they took him to the zoo, the park, roller-skating, and other faster activities, with the other being a "slacker day" where Clyde and Tim could play video games and Audrey could take some time for herself. In a later session, I also taught them the Speaker-Listener Technique, which, among other things, equalizes the amount of talk time each partner gets, and suggested that it would help them "come to the middle" in their pace of talking about issues, mindful that they would never completely change their respective paces. As they came to revalue their pace differences and find ways to compromise or revise their pace patterns, the couple became convinced that they could make a life together. With practice of these compromises (rehearsing), they gained the observable evidence they needed to commit to a future with one another.

Punctuality

Whereas couples are often unaware of the role that differences in life pace play in their discord, differences in how much each partner values and adheres to being on time are usually an explicit irritant. Sam was a 65-year-old businessman and Sheila was a 63-year-old home-maker and artist. Married for 35 years, they were on the brink of divorce after years of conflict, much of it centered on power struggles that manifested around punctuality. Sam was highly punctual, and saw being on time as a sign of respectfulness, reliability, and responsible adulthood. He was never late to a business appointment, and became enraged when Sheila was frequently late in being ready to leave their city apartment for their country house, or for the reverse commute. Sam always wanted to "beat the traffic," but because Sheila often was more than an hour delayed in being ready to leave, they typically got stuck on the highway.

Sheila acknowledged that Sam was right about the need for punctuality, at least when it came to the commute, but resented being "pushed around and insulted by Sam" about her lateness. He retorted that he resented having to "be on [her] ass about it." He noted that their two sons also complained about her in this regard; she felt it was unfair that he recruited their perspective to make his case. Sheila noted that she had struggled her entire life with being organized and, although never formally diagnosed, said she believed she probably suffered from ADHD. Her intensive chemotherapy for cancer a few years earlier had made focusing even harder. She noted that she often found herself "putzing around" the house fixing and arranging things to feel ready to leave and said that she tended to lose track of time despite her intent to accede to Sam's requests about when to leave.

I noted that her attempts to leave their homes perfectly in order likely was a way she was compensating for her loss of focus, about which she felt quite anxious. She agreed, and said she felt understood for the first time. Sam's attitude also softened with this interpretation. Sam offered to remind her to get ready two hours before they were slated to leave, and she appreciated this help. The problem was resolved quickly (with some further guidance to Sheila about ways to get organized—see below), and both partners remarked that they wished they'd understood and "had the words" for this basic temporal difference much earlier in their marriage.

Time Orientation

Interestingly, like many couples, Sheila and Sam's struggles around punctuality also seemed to be infused by their different time orientations. Sam, who was prone to irritation and anxiety, structured his life carefully by the clock and calendar, in part to avoid these emotions; this time orientation was also essential to his business success. In contrast, Sheila was happiest when released from chronological time structure, when she could immerse herself deeply in creating her quite extraordinary artwork.

The ancient Greeks had three concepts of time: *chronos*, or clock and calendar time; *aeon*, or a sense of time standing still, a sense of timelessness; and *kairos*, which they defined as the "opportune moment," often accompanied by a heightened sense of engagement and emotional experience. I explained this interesting piece of temporal history to the couple and suggested that they seemed to differ markedly in which form of time they preferred. They found this interesting and readily agreed with my sense of their differences around time. I noted the link to their differences in punctuality. In part, I brought this perspective to help Sheila feel less pathologized by her own self-diagnosis of ADHD and the effects of her cancer treatment on her ability to focus, about which she worried and felt ashamed. We then came up with some ways for her to handle household tasks in a more organized fashion, so that she could meet Sam's request for leaving on time (which, as noted, she agreed would be good to do). Sam also agreed to help out more with household tasks, taking some of the burden off Sheila. Sam also said he was deeply proud of Sheila's artistic productions, and reflected for the first time that her predilection for entering a zone of timelessness was something he could learn from her, as it could help him relax a bit more, given that he described himself as generally driven and "Type A." Sam decided to begin a meditation practice to foster more of this sense of release from the clock.

Time Perspective

People often differ in terms of their dominant time perspective—being future, present, or past focused. These different time perspectives organize much of their approach to their lives. Louise and Charlie were a couple in their mid-30s, and many of their conflicts seemed driven by a fundamental difference in time perspective.

Charlie was co-owner of an automotive shop, and his work involved intense focus on the present moment's challenges in repairing cars. Louise was an occupational therapist; in her work, she designed her patients' treatment in a careful stepwise fashion. Despite a strong attraction to one another, they'd had a tumultuous relationship for three years and had broken up once for several months. They came back together and sought therapy to decide whether they could resolve a number of issues and stay together.

Charlie was somewhat impulsive. He'd used alcohol and drugs since his teenage years, and had now been sober for five months. He would occasionally say quite insulting things to Louise when irritated by her "pushiness." Louise felt she had to monitor Charlie's behavior and was still on guard about his propensity for alcohol overuse. She also complained that he never seemed willing to plan anything with her. Although she initially enjoyed his spontaneous nature, she had grown tired of trying to get him to think ahead in terms of trips and their social life. Charlie resented her "nagging."

Although I praised him for taking charge of his drinking and drugging, I suggested that Charlie might benefit from the support of a 12-Step program, especially because in the past he tended to respond to feeling upset by bingeing on alcohol. He eventually joined a 12-Step group, and liked that there were other somewhat impulsive people in the program who had learned to address their addictions "one day at a time." He liked what one member said in a meeting: Quoting the venerable Vietnamese Buddhist monk Thich Nhat Hanh, if he took care of the present moment, he would automatically take care of the future. Although his automotive shop was fairly successful, he acknowledged that a bit more future planning would benefit the business as well. In this respect, he admired Louise's forward planning approach to her life and treatment of patients.

Charlie said, "I'm the kind of person who wears my heart on my sleeve," meaning that he would express how he felt without thinking about the possible long-term impact of his words. He couldn't understand why Louise would "hold on" to his occasional hurtful outbursts, and noted that in his family, members would express themselves this way and then "get over it and move on." Louise countered that because she was emotionally sensitive, tended to brood about negative experiences, and assumed others did so as well, she was always careful to think about what she expressed, as "what we say in the moment will shape how others feel for a long time," and she wished Charlie would "be considerate" and think about his impact on her. Charlie came to understand Louise's perspective on how the present shapes the future, and also agreed to work with her about how to plan their lives a bit more. I suggested that they could combine their time perspectives— use Louise's future focus to plan activities, but once in them, go with Charlie's capacity to immerse completely and be more spontaneous, which required Louise to relax more into the present moment.

Daily and Weekly Rhythms

Many distressed couples differ in their preferred daily and weekly rhythms. One partner may be a "lark"—up early, with lots of energy in the morning, and preferring an early bedtime—and the other an "owl," up later and preferring a later bedtime (Larson et al., 1991). This difference, which may be linked to biological differences in the set points of their circadian rhythms, has many ramifications for couples, including when partners prefer to have sex and engage in other intimacy and leisure activities, occupational choices and schedules, and child-rearing (the owl will resist taking the morning shift with babies and young kids, while the lark will resist taking the evening shift with teens, who generally prefer later bedtimes).

Partners' work schedules and rhythms of leaving and coming home—sometimes dictated by their employer and sometimes controlled by themselves—may diverge, leaving partners out of sync, with little time for connection. Preferences and/or ability to set boundaries between work time and couple time may differ—one partner may be constantly checking their texts and emails, and responding to the needs of work colleagues, whether by choice or by the employer's requirements, whereas the other sets a firm boundary on access to themselves by clients and colleagues (Fraenkel, 2001a, 2011, especially Chapters 7 and 8; Fraenkel & Capstick, 2012). Indeed, a person's choice of profession typically centers in large part around the required work hours, with some gravitating to a 24/7 type of job (sometimes due to promised financial rewards, sometimes for excitement and the need to be needed), and others to a profession that ensures a firmer work-life boundary.

Partners often differ around their desired frequency and regularity of sex, leisure time, housework, visits with in-laws, and other aspects of a life together. In a couple mentioned briefly earlier, Robert, an Italian American physician, and Maria, an Italian American elementary school teacher, grew up in the same homogenous working-class Italian neighborhood and culture in Brooklyn (Bensonhurst), where regular contact with family is the norm. Maria wished to sustain this strong connection to her family, insisting on weekly Sunday visits, whereas Robert was repelled by the "claustrophobic and boring" tradition of regular contact with in-laws. They eventually divorced because they could not agree on their preferred rhythms of time with family.

The transition to parenthood often results in a decrease in couple satisfaction (Cowan & Cowan, 2000, 2012). One common reason is that partners do not establish regular rhythms of relationship—time to talk and to be intimate. Especially when both partners have demanding jobs, work, childcare, and housework often takes precedence over regular time for intimacy and problem discussions (Fraenkel & Capstick, 2012). Marcus and Destiny were an African American couple in their late thirties, with a 2-year-old son and 4-year-old daughter. Marcus had a demanding job in finance, and Destiny had an equally demanding job running a women's healthcare clinic, although one that allowed her to be home by 5 p.m. Although their daughter had been a good sleeper from birth, their son often woke up crying a few times at night. They took turns helping their son settle down, and both partners were exhausted.

In addition, Marcus had received a promotion a year earlier, which although financially lucrative, often required him unpredictably to stay later at the office or entertain clients at dinners. Destiny understood that Marcus could not control his schedule entirely, but tension nevertheless ensued between them about the last-minute changes about his arrival time home. Destiny also resented Marcus for not doing his "fair share" of the housework; Marcus felt unjustly criticized, pointing out that he always throws out the garbage and cleans the dishes—the two tasks Destiny had assigned to him—to which Destiny countered, "Not always! I really need to have a clean sink in the morning when I'm running around trying to feed the kids and get ready for work before the nanny comes; and you seem to only throw out the garbage when it's overflowing!" Marcus sighed and shrugged, saying "Look, I'm stressed out, too!" The couple sank into angry silence.

When Destiny and Marcus met six years earlier, they had an active social life and enjoyed going out to dinner and to hear music. But ever since their first child was born, they had felt so overwhelmed with their responsibilities and so tired that they neglected to carve out reliable time to enjoy each other. Each resented the other for not initiating sex or even time to watch a movie together. Marcus said that their sex life had always been so "spontaneous," and now when he tried to initiate sex with Destiny, she was usually too tired. Destiny countered that she felt the same thing happened when she was in the mood—Marcus would often be exhausted, or anxiously emailing a colleague. They both felt that they'd lost the passion that characterized their early years, and with all the bickering between them, were considering separation.

My first intervention was to normalize their challenges. I briefly summarized the research on the transition to parenthood, and on the challenges faced by dual-earner couples. I noted that for many couples, the first thing that gets lost in the "time shuffle" is time for each other. Rather than seeing the cause of their distress as largely due to these multiple responsibilities, partners end up attributing the problems to one another's lack of desire for intimacy. I also asked them whether as African Americans, they each felt any extra pressure to perform well at their jobs, given that many African Americans experience such pressures. They both strongly concurred that they felt this way. Marcus shared that he was one of the few Black men in the company, and one of the first to become a vice president, and said, "I often feel that all eyes are on me." Destiny noted that she sometimes had difficulty managing some of the white doctors and nurses, and at times felt that this might be due to them having "difficulty taking direction from a Black woman." I reflected that these concerns likely led to even more exhaustion for each of them—all the more reason that we should think about how to create some regular rhythms of relationship that would allow them to decompress at the end of the day, offer each other some soothing, and share moments of pleasure.

We then discussed how to experiment with some new daily and weekly rhythms. Marcus agreed to do the dishes and throw out the garbage each night so that Destiny would not have to go to bed worrying that in the morning she might find a pile of dishes and baby bottles in the sink and an overflowing bin. He also offered to take over doing the laundry on the weekend—a task he'd done and enjoyed growing up—which greatly surprised and pleased Destiny. Marcus laughed and said he'd get their daughter to help him with folding and putting clothes away, and that this would give him and his daughter some good "quality time." The couple agreed to having a 20-minute decompression period at the end of the day (at least on those evenings when Marcus wasn't home quite late after client dinners, and when he was out, to have at least a short decompression phone call). They agreed to alternate weekend mornings where one could sleep in while the other took the kids. They also decided to make Sunday night a movie night (after each had been able to catch up on sleep), order in some great takeout or even cook together . . . and possibly, forgo the movie and restart their flagging sexual relationship.

Two weeks later, the couple returned in much better spirits, holding hands and smiling at one another. They also noted that they'd arranged for Marcus's mother to come up next weekend from Philadelphia to take care of the kids while they went out on the town. I expressed delight at these developments and highlighted the remarkable rapidity of this positive shift—further evidence of how powerful the various temporal and other pressures were in leading them to consider separation. With just a few new rhythms of connection, they were able to restore their affection for one another and confidence in their future together.

Time Allocation

Closely related to issues around rhythms is another area of frequent conflict: each partner's different desires about how to spend their time on a daily, weekly, monthly, and yearly basis. Partners often differ on how much time they want to spend on various relationships—with each other, with each other and friends or family, with their kids (if they have kids), separately with friends or family, and alone. They argue about the balance of work time and nonwork time.

Geetika, a second-generation Bengali American physician who grew up in a homogeneous Bengali community in New York, liked to spend a full day each weekend with her family, whereas Aadesh, a first-generation Bengali American who grew up in Birmingham, England, found time with her family boring, uncomfortable, and exhausting. He said he required hours after these visits to be alone and "recharge [his] batteries," resulting in Geetika and her family feeling rejected by him.

When I first met Geetika and Aadesh, it was clear that the future of their relationship centered on whether they could find compromises between their preferences around all the ways of spending time. We spent weeks developing, testing, and refining a "time pie" that would allow Geetika enough time with her family (with Aadesh uncomfortably in tow) and with her friends (whom Aadesh found largely uninteresting intellectually and too chatty, which Geetika found somewhat insulting), time together in activities, and the large amount of alone time Aadesh needed after social engagements. One form of time together that had not occurred to either of them until I suggested it was silent time together on the couch, each immersed in their own reading—perhaps with legs entangled. This form of time greatly reduced Aadesh's need to honor his "deep introversion" (as he called it)—he could be alone in his mind and yet together physically with Geetika. You will learn much more about this couple and the multiple layers of their time differences in Chapters 4 and 5, as they are the featured vignette.

The Five Myths About Couple Time

In some couples, one partner presses for regular rhythms of activities and managing household, financial, and other responsibilities, whereas the other advocates for spontaneity or an "as needed" approach for engaging in these activities. I generally suggest that regular rhythms are important when it comes to sex, leisure time, and handling household and financial chores. Partners are often so overbooked with other work-related commitments and kids that unless rhythms are created and preserved for couple activities, they often don't occur, and do so only when one partner complains to the other about the neglect or absence of these activities. Partners who adhere to the fantasy of having sex only "when the spirit moves them" are under the sway of what I've called the Myth of Spontaneity (Fraenkel, 2011), because the spirit often doesn't move both busy partners at the same moment. However, within the time set aside regularly for such activities as sex and other intimate encounters, there can be a great deal of spontaneity.

Importantly, the term *rhythm* for regularly occurring intimacy is much more palatable to couples than the term *schedule*, which came to prominence during the Industrial Revolution as managers strove to regularize workers' time and get more production out of less and less time. The Scottish poet John Burnside (2020) notes that over the millennia, the experience of the passage of time has changed due to how it is tracked, marked, and divided, from "looking up to the sun and the moon" to early devices that relied on the "flow of water in a clepsydra, the movement of a shadow across the face of a sundial, sand trickling steadily through the neck of an hour glass" to mechanical clocks that led to "the intense regulation of day-to-day life that the *measurement*—and eventually, the industrialisation—of time imposed" (p. 7, emphasis in original). He notes:

> . . . we came to inhabit a world of infinite temporal subdivision, a lifetime of shift-work and comfort breaks, of upload times and nanoseconds. Now, for too many, the daily round is a long monotone dictated by the mobile phone and the online schedule, a condition of voluntary servitude that allows us, by "checking in" continuously, to verify the validity of our existence. (p. 8)

As a result of the link between work and scheduled time, no couple finds the notion of "scheduling" sex or date night very romantic. Likewise, the word *routine* has a double meaning—regularly occurring activities, but also connoting boring and predictable in a negative way (as in, "Yeah, we had kinda routine sex the other night"). Although some in the field have used the term *ritual* rather broadly to denote the importance of regular mealtimes and other daily activities, the real meaning of *ritual* is an event of heightened emotional and symbolic meaning that typically marks a transition from one form of identity (for instance, the transition from a boy or girl to a man or woman, or dating versus married, or from life to death), or that occurs on a regular, repetitive basis, as in daily, weekly, or yearly religious rituals.

These important, often culturally based transitions signify a heightened sense of meaning and connection to higher values and sense of identity (Fiese, 2006; Fiese et al., 2002; Imber-Black et al., 2003) rather than just regular daily activities of a more mundane (in the sense of earthly and secular versus spiritual) but still pleasurable sort. Yet couples can get onboard with establishing rhythms, a word that connotes music, dance, and the beating of the heart. As I noted in Chapter 1, the language and metaphors we use to suggest new ideas and practices are crucial to our intervention's impact, its "transportability" and salience for couples as they leave our sessions and reimmerse in their daily lives.

Another myth—that housework and other chores should not be combined with intimacy—gets in the way of couples making use of the naturally occurring life maintenance rhythms (cooking, cleaning, laundry folding, yard work, even finances) as a time for connection. Couples can talk about events of the week, their dreams, and other topics while taking care of life business and chores, and can experience a sense of satisfaction in teamwork. Doing so also greatly reduces a major source of conflict in many couples around who does the most housework (in cisgender heterosexual couples, usually the woman; Fraenkel & Capstick, 2012). Increasing this sense of teamwork and fair distribution of mundane life-supporting tasks increases women's sense of the fairness of the relationship (Coltrane, 2000). For women, the degree of experienced fairness of a relationship is highly and positively correlated with marital satisfaction (Coltrane, 2000) and inversely correlated with women's rates of depression (Piña & Bengtson, 1994). Not surprisingly, given the few hours most men devote to housework, their perceptions of the fairness of housework distribution are unrelated either to their own or their wives' degree of unhappiness or marital distress (Robinson & Spitze, 1992).

On the other hand, one or both partners may labor under three other related myths: the Myth of Perfection, the Myth of Total Control, and the Myth of Quality Time—which, when combined, result in a fantasy of being able to perfectly manage one's time. The Myth of Perfection is that, with enough careful scheduling, one can fit into one's life all the activities one wants, and with the regularity or rhythmicity one desires.

For instance, some couples believe that despite having two young children, they should be able to maintain the active social life and outside dining routines that characterized their prechildren phase.

Unless they have live-in childcare and household help, this is unrealistic and leaves partners chronically frustrated because they cannot make the complex schedule work. Instead, couples need to prioritize which activities are most important and doable in different phases of their lives. This does not necessitate completely dropping desired activities. Rather than bemoaning that they can "never" go out, or have to give up a previously time-consuming avocational interest like playing music with others, or golf, instead they need to recalibrate the rhythm or periodicity/frequency with which these activities can occur. For instance, couples with young children can decide to go out once every two weeks or even once a month on a regular basis. This allows going out together to remain a part of their ongoing shared narrative, rather than dropping this important part of their connection entirely.

The Myth of Total Control is based on the larger sociocultural Euro-American "heroic rugged individualist" story—the notion that we are totally in charge of our lives and our destinies, no matter how embedded we are in workplace demands, family demands, health issues, and other constraints on how we spend our energy and organize our time. In one couple, Rob was the founder and president of a company that provided light, sound, and other technical support to outdoor theater and musical events. Denise was a nurse who had elected to leave her job to be a full-time mom with their one-and-a-half-year-old son, Mark. When I met them, Rob was deep into organizing the staging of a major outdoor music festival. With a small staff who turned to him for guidance constantly on all manner of details, he was working 16-hour days. Denise was on the one hand sympathetic about his stress levels, but on the other held the naive belief that because he was president of the company, he should be able to control his schedule and be home regularly for dinner. Try as he might to be home on time, he frequently called to say he'd be an hour (or more) late, even though he very much wanted to take a break from work and be with his family.

I noted that, as much as he wanted to exert control over it, Rob's daily schedule was not up to him entirely, and that this position is not uncommon for people higher up in an organization. On the other hand, I sympathized with Denise's dilemma—she felt unable to control her own evening schedule because she was "yoked" to Rob's, which in turn was tied to the music festival organizers' demands. The issue was resolved, albeit imperfectly, by Rob calling each afternoon to provide a two-hour window within which he would be home, or to say that he really didn't think he'd make it for dinner and Mark's bedtime. Rob made a commitment to taking on less demanding contracts after this one, so as to better balance their time together as a family with his need to build the business and support his wife and child.

The Myth of Quality Time feeds into both the Myth of Perfection and the Myth of Total Control. It received a lot of play during the 1990s, just as did another time-saving myth promoted by managers, which became prominent in that decade, called multitasking. Careful cognitive psychology studies have found it virtually impossible and actually counterproductive: The average amount of time it takes to shift back fully into one task from another is 20 minutes. Promoted as a solution for busy parents overwhelmed with the increasing demands of the 24/7 work culture (or sometimes, their ambivalence about making the transition to parenthood), the Quality Time myth claimed that as long as a parent was fully focused on their child when together—in other words, engaging in high-quality time—the ever-diminishing amounts of time parents were spending with their children (for working fathers, an average of seven minutes a day!) could continue, and both parent and child would be satisfied.

However, children are simply not as goal-directed as adults and need time that is unstructured within which pleasurable activities can then organically emerge. Brief bits of highly structured playtime does not make sufficient space for the valuable psychological aspects of play. As psychoanalytic psychologist Donald Winnicott (1971) wrote, "It is in playing and only in playing that the individual child or adult is able to be creative and to use the whole personality, and it is only in being creative that the individual discovers the self" (p. 54). To sit down with one's five-year-old for a seven-minute (and no longer) Lego building session, or a seven-minute joint video game, or even a playful and humorous conversation, is bound to result in frustration—the Lego airplane or truck will not be built, the video game will not be won, and the conversation will feel more like a check-in with a colleague or boss at work.

Summary of Time and Couples

In sum, a variety of temporal dyssynchronies and misguided myths about time can underlie a couple's conflicts around other more common themes, and may operate below the awareness of the partners. Time issues can also represent a major explicit issue about which couples are acutely aware and that threaten to break them apart. The couple therapist can use the guide presented above to assess the presence of these temporal differences and introduce them as part of the therapeutic dialogue. My repeated experience is that naming these differences when they are implicit acts as a powerful frame for understanding why partners feel so disconnected, and why they experience power struggles. Casting these as long-term aspects of personality that are affected by biological temperament, family- and culture-of-origin experiences and learnings, and their involvement in larger systems like the workplace reduces the mutual blaming that characterizes so many last chance couples, and helps partners learn to accept and even revalue their differences and put them to work in a modified, less polarized manner. All ways of relating to time have their place and purpose; the key for couples seeking harmony is to see the positive contribution each partner's ways of inhabiting time can make to their own lives and to their more flexible, resourceful functioning as a unit.

A THEORY OF TIME AND MUTUAL EMOTION REGULATION OR MODULATION

As the vignettes presented above illustrate, the ways in which partners differ in how they prefer to inhabit time are linked to how they handle their emotions. And how partners handle their emotions represents another major, and often unconscious, aspect of partners' initial attraction to one another, transformed in distressed couples to a source of conflict over time. This section outlines a theory of how partners come to rely on one another to regulate, or "modulate" (Jurist, 2018), each other's emotions. A great deal has been written about partners' "coregulation" of emotion (Fishbane, 2013, 2015; Johnson, 2019, 2020; Solomon & Tatkin, 2011). John Gottman's prospective research on variables that predict better or worse outcomes for newlyweds over time (Driver et al., 2012; Gottman, 2011; Gottman & Gottman, 2018) affirms the importance of partners engaging in mutual regulation and soothing, and emotional attunement more generally. These applications of the concept of couple emotion regulation draw heavily on the basic science of ER conducted with individuals (Gross, 2015) and on findings in the field of interpersonal neurobiology (Siegel, 2012).

A Critique of Adult Attachment and Emotion Regulation Theory

These theories and supporting research examine mostly one aspect of emotion regulation, known as downregulating or calming/soothing the partner. As noted briefly in Chapter 2, the capacity to self-regulate and to regulate one's partner is believed by some theorists to be associated with the degree to which each partner is securely or insecurely attached, as the capacity for self-soothing has been assumed to begin in the parent-child bond during infancy (Johnson, 2019; Solomon & Tatkin, 2011). Partners who are insecurely attached have more difficulty with self-regulation and with offering calming and soothing to their partners. Gottman's research is not based on attachment theory but, rather, simply on observation of couple interactional patterns and physiological assessment (blood pressure, pulse, galvanic skin response, shifting in the seat) along with self-reports of experienced affect in happy versus unhappy couples during problem discussions (Levenson & Gottman, 1983, 1985).

A large number of publications argue that there is a strong link between adult attachment styles based on childhood attachment, the quality and stability of adults' intimate relationships, and associated capacities for emotion regulation and coregulation. However, there are a number of serious problems with these assumptions.

First, there are no studies that conclusively indicate that the majority of childhood attachment styles remain stable into adulthood, or that there is a substantial correlation between mothers' degree of responsive caretaking with their infants and toddlers and those children's attachment styles as adults. Even Hazan and Shaver (1987, 1994), the acknowledged founders of the exploration of the link between attachment styles and romantic relationship quality, have questioned the assumption held by some (Hendrick & Hendrick, 1994) that "early caregiving experiences should be fully or largely responsible for individual differences in attachment style" (Fraley et al., 2013, p. 829). Indeed, in summarizing the results of the only large sample prospective study conducted to date from infancy through late teenage–early adulthood years, Fraley and colleagues wrote that:

> Although the present findings suggest that individual differences in adult attachment may have their origins, in part, in developmental experiences, it is important to note that, in absolute terms, the associations we report were relatively small. Collectively, the antecedents we examined explained, at most, 29% of the variation in global avoidance, for example. Thus it is certainly not the case that individual differences in adult attachment are largely a result of early caregiving experiences, at least with respect to factors investigated in the present report. (Fraley et al., 2013, p. 828)

This research indicated that a number of factors shape attachment attitudes and behavior in an ongoing, developmental fashion, including social competence, quality of childhood friendships, and changes in levels of maternal depression and father absence from the home. The reasons for father absence were not examined, but it is likely due in part to marital conflict (possibly resulting in divorce) between parents, and marital conflict has been shown to negatively affect children's emotional and behavioral functioning (Repetti et al., 2002). Increases in maternal depression may also be related to father absence through the mediating variable of marital conflict, as depression in married women is strongly associated with marital conflict (Whisman & Beach, 2015). Thus, mother's depression and father's absence may be marker variables (indicators of other underlying processes not examined) for the impact of marital conflict on children, which might affect their degree of security in adult relationships and may disrupt their emotion regulatory capacities from childhood into adulthood.

Importantly, Fraley et al. (2013) demonstrated that maternal sensitivity was unrelated to anxious attachment, but only to avoidant attachment: When children experienced lower maternal sensitivity, they were more likely as adults to be avoidant in attachment style. However, once again, the association is not strong, and social competence as rated by parents and teachers had a stronger relationship to avoidant attachment than did maternal responsiveness. Likewise, children's' ratings of the degree to which they had a close friendship were more strongly associated with attachment-related avoidance at age 18 than was maternal sensitivity during the child's early years. This suggests that if therapy is to take a retrospective approach, the better focus would be on what sorts of difficulties adult partners had in forming and maintaining friendships, rather than on the partners' experiences as infants and toddlers with their parents (which are difficult for most adults to recall), especially as a sense of friendship with one's partner is found to be a major factor in successful long-term relationships (Gottman & Gottman, 2018).

Second, research suggests that most children and adults do not neatly fit into one of the four categorical attachment styles (secure, insecure/anxious-ambivalent, insecure-avoidant, and insecure-disorganized). A dimensional approach to assessing attachment style has garnered more empirical support than the categorical approach (Fraley et al., 2015). Yet the categorical approach continues to be propagated in work by Johnson (2019, 2020), Solomon and Tatkin (2011), and others. A dimensional conception of attachment opens the possibility of examining how "individual differences in attachment partly reflect the ongoing experiences that people have in their interpersonal relationships" (Fraley et al., 2013, p. 829), as the sense of adult attachment security may be more dependent on what is going on in the adult intimate relationship than mostly on early childhood experiences. For instance, disruption in the sense of trust between partners—due to communication problems, a lack of mutual empathy, or violation of values and expectations, such as happens when a partner has an affair—can lead to a sense of insecurity (Gottman, 2011), even when partners enter the relationship with a predilection for forming secure attachments based on childhood experiences.

In contrast, a categorical conception of attachment assumes stability across time and relational context in attachment security, thereby discouraging investigators and clinicians from formulating hypotheses about how the features of a couple's relationship might influence their degree of attachment, irrespective of their childhood-based attachment security. Research by Pierce and Lydon (2001) and La Guardia and colleagues (2000) supports this latter, more fluid and contextually driven understanding of partners' level of security in their relationships.

Third, there are no prospective/longitudinal studies that have assessed newlyweds' attachment styles and followed these newlyweds over time to see if their attachment styles remain stable even as marital quality either declines or remains positive. Publications on the link between attachment styles and marital quality and particular patterns of emotion regulation—such as those described by Solomon and Tatkin (2011; high-arousal couples, low-arousal couples, and biphasic couples in which one tends toward high and the other toward low arousal)—are based on cross-sectional evaluation of partners once they are already distressed.

These studies and clinical anecdotal descriptions confuse correlation with causation, based not on prospective evaluation of couples but, rather, on retrospective construction of each partner's reported early relationship quality with their parenting figures. Yet neuroscience indicates that the hippocampus, an organ within the limbic system largely responsible for creating memories, does not come online until age two. As a result, even memories from later early childhood (ages three to five), prior to the development of fluent language—which assists in encoding memories through narratives—can be considered questionable in their veracity. This critique of the questionable accuracy of retrospective accounts of early childhood has long been a central criticism of psychodynamic theory and practice, and yet attachment-based couple therapy theorists and clinicians seem to have forgotten or overlooked this concern.

Fourth, there is an obvious logical problem with these cross-sectional assessments of the relationship between current attachment security and relationship quality in distressed couples, in that it can be assumed that newlyweds are relatively happy and demonstrate some degree of mutual care, attunement, and empathy initially, albeit as shown in Gottman's research, with some variability across couples (Driver et al., 2012). Given that attachment theory assumes that partners come to the relationship with their attachment styles in place, one would assume that the problematic patterns associated with insecure attachment would be evident immediately in all their intensity, and might lead partners to choose not to marry in the first place. Even with last chance couples, it is relatively rare to encounter a couple that described an absence of care, security, and connection even during dating and the early years of the committed relationship.

Numerous studies reviewed by Fraley et al. (2013) as well as their own findings indicate that there is greater variability within us in attachment styles than between us (p. 829), and attachment security is influenced more by "proximate causes" (p. 830) than by variations in the early parent-child bond. Clinical anecdotes support these findings: It is common for one or both partners to indicate that they felt secure with each other initially and that this sense of security changed as a result of changes in partners' level of attention to one another during such life cycle changes as the transition to parenthood, noted earlier to be well documented as a cause of decline in marital satisfaction (Belsky & Rovine, 1990; Cowan & Cowan, 1988; Trillingsgaard et al., 2014). When a couple has their first child, the primary parent, usually the mother in cisgender heterosexual couples, often becomes more emotionally connected to the infant than to the male partner, leaving the male partner to feel excluded.

In addition, as noted earlier, given that women most often take the role of attending to and attempting to enhance the quality of the couple's connection, when her attention and energy are diverted (understandably) to the infant, the man must take over the role of relationship enhancement and support, but often fails to do so effectively. Additionally, social class may affect the degree of decline in a couple's relationship following the birth of a child: Research documents that low-income fathers often struggle to provide adequate financial and other support to their families and withdraw or leave the partner altogether (Cowan et al., 2009).

As noted earlier, other proximate causes that can reduce attachment security are an affair on the part of one partner, persistent alcohol or drug use, decrements in sexual and other forms of intimacy due to work and child-rearing pressures, high levels of conflict (in some cases including intimidation and violence) and poor communication (and the accompanying high rates of negative affect), or simply due to boredom with one another. Partners often describe their sense of unpleasant surprise at how the quality of their connection has dissolved over time, will sometimes note that in previous relationships (which ended for reasons other than attachment issues), they never felt this level of insecurity, and will also often describe having felt securely loved by their parents. When reflecting on their previous histories, they express genuine puzzlement about why they feel so shaky in their present connection to their partners, and generally attribute these feelings to conflict and lack of sufficient loving attention in the relationship.

Johnson (2020) and Solomon and Tatkin (2011) suggest that the common pursuer-distancer pattern—in cisgender heterosexual couples, with women more likely to pursue and men more likely to distance and withdraw (Christensen & Heavey, 1990)—is due to differences in attachment style. However, whereas this assessment might be supported in the case of couples in which the female partner clearly demonstrates a history (prior to the current relationship) of anxious-ambivalent attachment and the male partner demonstrates a history of avoidant attachment, there are other research-supported reasons why men may be more likely to withdraw and women to pursue.

For instance, research shows that boys are less encouraged by parents to share their vulnerable feelings than are girls, or are even discouraged (Parker et al., 2012; Thomassin et al., 2019). As a result, in marital conflicts, men may be less skilled and less inclined to share their feelings of hurt, fear, loneliness, or other less "strong" or assertive emotions, resulting in them feeling incompetent and more emotionally or physiologically flooded than women, and withdrawing to avoid extending the conflict. Indeed, Levenson and Gottman's (1983, 1985) early physiological studies on marital conflict found that men become more negatively aroused relative to their resting baseline than do women, and stay negatively aroused significantly longer after a conflict than do women, even though men engage in significantly more stonewalling (freezing the musculature of the face, flattening voice tone), a behavior that the female partner often assumes signals a lack of emotional engagement, leading her to pursue even more vigorously in an attempt to engage her male partner.

Moreover, many feminist scholars have noted the larger social scripts about gender and relationships that encourage women to be the caretakers of intimate and other relationships more than men (Goldner, 1985; Hare-Mustin, 1978; Knudson-Martin, 1997; Knudson-Martin & Huenergardt, 2010; Walters et al., 1988), even when women are in abusive relationships (Goldner, 1998). Attributing women's tendency to pursue in order to take care of the relationship (at all costs) to their childhood-based attachment insecurity—a historically based, intrapsychic cause, rather than a proximal, socioculturally informed aspect of the current relationship—obscures this feminist understanding of power and care dynamics in cisgender heterosexual relationships, with potentially destructive consequences. Guided by attachment theory, a therapist might encourage a woman staying in an abusive relationship to view her behavior as mostly due to her upbringing and need for connection, rather than all the reasons (intimidation, violence, financial dependency, threats of taking the children, and more enacted by the abusive partner) that are well-documented reasons women stay in these relationships (Fraenkel et al., 2022; Stith et al., 2011).

Although the capacity for self- and mutual soothing, and its relationship to a partner's meta-emotions (beliefs about emotion; Gottman, 2011; Gottman & Gottman, 2018) and attachment style are important findings, in the present theory, I suggest that the processes of mutual emotion regulation are more complex than is described in existing theory and research. As I'll describe, mutual emotion regulation includes both soothing and activation of general arousal by one partner with the other. In addition, certain specific emotions—anger, sadness, and others—are often felt and expressed by one partner for the benefit of the other. I find clinically that attachment style is not the sole or even the major determinant of how and to what degree partners engage in regulating each other's emotions. Instead, mutual emotion regulation seems to be based on an unconscious contract or agreement that partners make with one another—a kind of quid pro quo.

A New Theory of Couple Emotion Regulation/ Modulation: The True Meaning of the Marital Quid Pro Quo

In 1965, family systems pioneer Don Jackson published a seminal article titled "Family Rules: Marital Quid Pro Quo" in the *Archives of General Psychiatry*. Jackson wrote:

> When two people get together, they immediately exchange clues as to how they are defining the nature of the relationship; this set of behavioral tactics is modified by the other person by the manner in which he responds. . . . Quid pro quo, then is a descriptive metaphor for a relationship based on differences, and

expression of the redundancies which one observes in marital interaction. (p. 591)

Like most of the early theorists in the emerging field of family systems theory and practice, Jackson was initially trained as a psychoanalyst. I believe that what he meant to capture in this concept of the quid pro quo was the largely unconscious manner in which people provide emotional and behavioral information to one another—often expressed nonverbally, through voice tone and speech pace, speed of response to one another's expression of affect, and facial and other bodily gestures and posture—about the degree to which they experience psychophysiological arousal (excitable versus calm), their tendencies toward positive versus negative affect, and their level of comfort experiencing and expressing specific emotions.

People become attracted either to someone who shares their affective style or, perhaps more frequently, to someone who represents a different affective style that can help them modulate their own emotions in a complementary fashion. One partner is more excitable and easily aroused, and is attracted to someone who is calmer, steadier affectively, and slow to arouse. In turn, the calmer person finds the more energetic one exciting and enlivening. Or one partner is cheerful and upbeat and finds the other's more critical perspective, shown through gentle sarcasm and nihilistic attitudes, sexy, appealing, or even suggestive of greater well-worn worldliness compared to their own seemingly youthful, innocent, cheerful naivete. Or one partner is generally anxious and has difficulty asserting himself or herself, and is drawn to a person who has more aggressive fantasies and is better at being assertive. In turn, the more aggressive/assertive partner experiences the other's more tentative stance toward the world as a corrective to their own intense approach to the world—and maybe even finds that being around this person helps them make space for their own unacceptable anxiety. Partners become intrigued with each other's emotional differences just as partners often get intrigued with a partner who comes from a different cultural background or a different way of inhabiting their own culture.

Sadly, I believe that Jackson's fascinating observation and theoretical intent was lost as the theory and practice of couple therapy developed. Couple therapy theorists, especially behavioral couple therapists steeped in Thibault and Kelly's (1959) social exchange theory applications to marriage ("I'll do this for you if you do this for me") interpreted Jackson as commenting on how partners divide up roles and responsibilities in a marriage. This led to a major therapeutic focus on how partners distribute responsibilities for earning income, doing housework, and raising children, and to attributing the source of conflict to couples' failure to do so fairly. Although many couple conflicts certainly do center on these more explicit distributions of tasks (Fraenkel & Capstick, 2012), there is a more profound relational arrangement that centers on how partners recruit one another to modulate or regulate their emotions.

Certainly, in the early days and weeks of a relationship, it can be assumed that new partners rarely have explicit discussions about how they will divide up responsibilities should they move on to a committed, cohabiting relationship. Rather, the experience of falling in love is more about feeling one has met one's soul mate, one's match, that one fits together with one's new lover like a hand in a glove or two puzzle pieces. Although partners discovering their shared values, shared sources of enjoyment, shared aesthetics, and other aspects of conscious selfhood play a role in this powerful coming together of minds and hearts, the present theory suggests that the sense of one partner completing the other has even more to do with emotional compatibility and fulfillment of emotional needs—what you do for me emotionally, how you "complete me."

The Temporal Basis of Mutual Emotion Regulation

The vignettes presented earlier on couples out of sync on one or more aspect of how they think about and inhabit time illustrate the link between temporal patterning and mutual emotional regulation. Life pace differences between partners are the most obvious example of how temporal styles are linked to emotions and mutual emotion regulation, as one's life pace is often associated with varying levels of emotional/physiological arousal or activation. Audrey was fast-paced and was drawn to Clyde's slow pace because it relaxed and calmed her after a long day of Wall Street trading. In turn, Clyde was drawn to Audrey's fast pace as it brought exciting energy into his life and nervous system.

The large body of research on interpersonal neurobiology and its implications for couple functioning—summarized elegantly by my colleague Mona Fishbane (2013, 2015)—provides a possible explanation for how this largely subliminal and automatic process of mutual emotion regulation occurs. Research indicates that the brains of humans (and of other species such as chimps) have mirror neurons, which lead us to respond to behavior, including emotional displays, as if we are doing or feeling what the observed person is doing and feeling. Mirror neurons make possible the crucial process of emotional attunement and empathy. Therefore, it can be hypothesized that when one partner observes the other's behavior that is linked to their level of arousal (high or low), the observing partner's level of arousal is modulated to match (to some degree) the observed partner's arousal level.

Adding to this important research on mirror neurons are studies that demonstrate how our brains respond in a mirroring fashion to sound, especially music, and the connection between music, emotion, and communication. I mentioned some of this research in Chapter 2 to make the case for integrating music into couple therapy (see also Fraenkel, 2020). Lee and Schögler (2009) write that "something in the pattern of flow in the movement of music, dance or gesture communicates directly and elicits emotion and, sometimes, sympathetic movement" (p. 83). They also reference a number of studies that support the link between time and emotion: "Ultimately, perception and cognition have inherent relationships to the generation of motivated psychological time, the time of moving and experiencing that is regulated emotionally . . . which is the key to social communication in all animals" (p. 84).

Their neuroscientific research has explored the question, "how does an expression or gesture pass from the mind of a musician into the body of a dancer through the medium of sound?" (Lee and Schögler, 2009, p. 84). Numerous studies of the musical, nonverbal aspects of mother-infant communication—voice tone, rhythm, and pitch—repeatedly demonstrate that babies respond emotionally and physically to the mother's communicative music, and that some degree of synchronicity between mother's voice and baby's vocal rhythms (albeit with important moments of disconnection that invite repair and resynchronization) is associated with secure attachment (see review in Panksepp & Trevarthan, 2009).

It can be hypothesized that in adult intimate relationships, people respond similarly on an emotional or neuropsychological level to the musical aspects of their partner's emotional expressions. Some research has shown that people alter their voices (to a lower pitch) when speaking with a more attractive person than when speaking with someone not viewed as attractive and as a prospective mate (Hughes et al., 2010). However, no research has explored how what is experienced as an attractive voice may differ depending on one's emotion regulatory needs. For instance, although lower voices are found to be more attractive generally—perhaps signaling an associated state of calmness and groundedness, and the greater parasympathetic arousal central to sexual arousal—it may be that someone looking for a partner who will upregulate or activate them is more drawn to a higher-pitched voice and a more rapid pace of speech. Otherwise, it might be that faster-talking people with higher vocal pitches would never find a mate, and that is clearly not the case.

Jed and Julia were one such couple. Jed had a laid-back style and a low melodic voice, whereas Julia had a high-pitched, somewhat scratchy voice tone. Although I as the therapist found Julia hard to listen to at times, especially when she got emotionally agitated, Jed loved her and even spoke about loving her voice. Julia enjoyed Jed's low voice tones, although at times they triggered her anxiety that he was slipping back into being a "stoner"—he'd had a history of drug and alcohol use that led to a breakup months before they came to therapy to see if they could be compatible and commit to each other.

Back to Audrey the Wall Street executive and Clyde the outdoors adventure instructor: In a period in which they are not distressed and are getting along well, when Audrey comes home hyperaroused and moving fast and sees calm Clyde laid out on the sofa in a relaxed, low-arousal state, her mirror neurons are activated and trigger a process in her of calming down. Likewise, Clyde may become a bit more aroused physiologically in seeing Audrey in her highly aroused state. But if the couple has come to agree that time after work is time to unwind, Audrey will allow herself to be more influenced by Clyde's relaxed vibe and join him in his low-arousal state. On a weekend when the couple has planned to get up and out to explore the city or for some other activity, Clyde may allow himself to join Audrey in her higher state of arousal—indeed, he relies on her to upregulate or energize him.

Fast forward to their current state of distress: Audrey comes home from work, sees Clyde lounging on the couch, and, rather than sliding down with him into his low-arousal state, resists the signals from her mirror neurons so as to maintain her higher level of activation, and asks him "to get up and do something around the house for a change!" Clyde responds by attempting to defend his arousal state, rejecting the messages from his mirror neurons' response to seeing Audrey's high energy, and telling her to "chill out!" Thus, the couple engages in a power struggle over what was originally a powerful aspect of their coupling—how each inducted the other into a different and desired arousal state. Each is irritated by the other, not only because of the conflict that ensues, but because of the internal conflict between their existing arousal state and that presented by the partner. Over time, couples like Audrey and Clyde come to resent the very tendencies toward fast and slow pace and accompanying high and low arousal states that initially acted as a major source of their attraction.

To buttress their respective emotional/arousal stances and attempt to commandeer the other into their level of arousal, a couple in this physiological/emotional tango may recruit beliefs and attitudes from their relationship to their respective families and cultures of origin— and may weaponize what they know about their partner's family history and culture. For instance, in one painful fight about their respective paces, Audrey declared that it was high time Clyde start getting more energized himself without her needing to prod him, noting, "You're not in the sleepy South and in your family of couch potatoes, Clyde. You should be glad you're with a woman from an ambitious Connecticut family!" To which Clyde shrugged dismissively and fired back, "Right, glad to be with a representative of uptight self-centered pushy Northerners who have no manners and no gentility! You need to live where I came from to learn some Southern manners!"

Although pace differences between partners are the most obvious potential links between time and mutual emotion regulation, other differences in how partners inhabit time also often serve this function and provide an initial, although sometimes counterintuitive, source of attraction. For instance, Allen, a highly anxious 56-year-old Jewish American New Yorker (he reminded me a lot of Woody Allen) and Claudia, a laid-back 54-year-old Brazilian American, were on the brink of divorce around differences in attitudes and practices around punctuality. Allen was extremely punctual in all his affairs and, in fact, often arrived quite early for work meetings. Claudia was frequently late, not only for activities with Allen, but in her work life. Allen saw Claudia's chronic lateness as a sign of enormous inconsiderateness and disrespect, whereas Claudia viewed Allen's "obsession with punctuality" as a means of controlling other people, including her, and as a manifestation of his neurotic character. In this latter assessment she was not far off, as research has linked high degrees of punctuality to neuroticism, a personality trait associated with a generally negative view of the world (Back et al., 2006).

However, upon exploration of how they met and what attracted each to the other, Allen acknowledged that in the early days, he was intrigued by Claudia's devil-may-care approach to timeliness, as a part of him wished he could be "less uptight" about time. He longed to be relaxed like Claudia, but then his anxiety would kick in and return him to his punctiliousness. In later sessions, Allen revealed that his father had been severely bipolar, and Allen had been charged with monitoring the father's wake times so that he would get to work on time. For her part, Claudia acknowledged that she admired Allen's responsibleness, and felt that his punctuality provided her a secure base from which to deviate as she wished.

In later sessions focused on her family of origin and mixed cultural background, she came to realize that her attitude and behavior about punctuality developed as a teen rebellion against her punctual parents. The parents had immigrated from Germany as young liberal anti-Nazis to escape persecution, yet often criticized Brazilians for being lazy and irresponsible about time, although they loved most other aspects of their adopted homeland. Claudia identified strongly as Brazilian and differentiated herself from her parents and her German roots around their attitude about punctuality. We came to see that she was attracted to Allen partly because it provided her another opportunity to work through and master her unresolved feelings about independence from her parents.

Likewise, Charlie the present-oriented partner and Louise the future-focused partner, described earlier, each credited the other's time perspective as part of their initial attraction, once I had introduced this concept to explain their current struggles. Charlie aspired to be a better planner and thought being around Louise would help him learn how. He imagined that a bit more emotional restraint toward sustaining business relationships would improve his prospects. Louise, for all her criticism of Charlie's impulsiveness, acknowledged that there was "something sexy and exciting" about his ability to be impulsive in the present moment. She recognized that her careful planning for the future often meant deferring spending money and having fun in the present to finance future goals. In their good times, like on vacation, Louise was able to emulate Charlie's relaxed, in-the-moment passions.

Nontemporal Forms of Mutual Emotion Regulation

Partners often differ in emotional styles in ways that have nothing to do with the ways they inhabit and behave in time. For instance, in one last chance Modern Orthodox Jewish couple I worked with, Talia had a somewhat agitated, irritable temperament for which she never received adequate soothing responses from her parents. Her role as her mother's confidant about her mother's unhappiness with her father only accentuated Talia's tendency to focus largely on problems and express negative affects—she had learned to value these as a form of connection to others through her coalition with her mother. Moishe had an easygoing, relaxed temperament, but had difficulty making space for negative affect—when he allowed himself to fully recognize problematic issues, he tended to become extremely anxious, almost to the level of panic, and so he had developed a perspective that "your reality is based on what feelings you walk around with—a bag of coal, or a bag of feathers."

Although Talia was initially attracted to the calming effects of being around upbeat Moishe, and Moishe relied on Talia to name problems and negative affect, over time, their differences became polarized. In one powerfully illuminating session in which I identified this emotional polarity and how they had come to rely on one another too much to "raise the flag" for either negative or positive assessments of their life together, Talia angrily said to Moishe, "I know you have negative feelings, but you put them in my person! So get your own so that I can have space for more positive feelings." In a remarkable way, she had named the process of projective identification, described in Chapter 2.

I supported Talia's wish, and Moishe's response to me was, "So you're asking me to be less positive?" I replied, "Not less positive, just allowing more negative feelings to exist side by side with the positive, so that Talia can feel free of the burden of holding and expressing negative feelings for you and can become the more positive person you want her to be, and that she also wants to be. . . . You're each doing too much emotional work in one area."

Another frequent emotional polarization presents as one partner being rational and unemotional in general, and the other being the one to express emotions for both partners. As this difference is often divided in cisgender heterosexual couples, with men being more inclined toward relentless rationality and women left needing to voice emotions, many publications have incorrectly attributed these differences to biologically based tendencies between men and women, rather than gender socialization (Hare-Mustin, 1978; Jackson, 1965). It is interesting to note that in his 1965 article on the quid pro quo, Jackson presaged the later feminist critique of the widely accepted theory of men as biologically determined to be instrumental and women to be emotional:

All manner of behaviors quite removed from primary sexual differences can be brought into the framework of male-female differences, which framework then becomes an explanatory model of marriage. This view pervades our popular mythology of sexual stereotypes, it influences marriage manuals and similar advisory accouterments and it certainly guides our scientific study of the marital relationship, no matter how inconsistent or unspecific this theory proves to be. (p. 589)

SUMMARY

In sum, it is essential to assess a couple's underlying temporal struggles, how in a less-polarized version of these temporal differences were a powerful, usually unnamed (but felt) source of attraction, and how these temporal differences are often linked to each partner's unconscious recruitment of the other to modulate or regulate their emotions and arousal levels. By identifying these patterns and their source in partners' personal "temporal temperament" and family and culture of origin, and by teaching partners better self and mutual emotion regulation strategies such as couple mindfulness practices (Adair et al., 2018; Atkinson, 2013; Wachs & Cordova, 2007) and overt skills in mutual soothing, empathic listening, and emotional attunement (Fishbane, 2013, 2015; Gottman, 2011; Johnson, 2020; Solomon & Tatkin, 2011), partners can end the temporal and emotional tug-of-war that provides a frequent source of friction and threatens to end their relationship. Patterns of the unconscious quid pro quo of emotion regulation not linked to temporal differences must also be identified and transformed, so that partners no longer rely so heavily on one another for positive or negative affect, for being rational or emotional in general, or for experiencing or expressing specific emotions. Likewise, whether linked to mutual emotion regulation processes or not, revealing, revaluing, revising, and rehearsing new, less polarized patterns of how partners inhabit time separately and together are essential to improving the functioning of couples and strengthening their chances of going forward together—in time.

CHAPTER 4

HIGH-CONFLICT COUPLES

Action-Oriented Techniques

THIS CHAPTER PRESENTS ACTION-ORIENTED TECHNIQUES that apply to work with most last chance couples. These techniques target problematic patterns of interaction. Although for some the major issue leading partners to consider ending the relationship is persistent high-conflict forms of interaction and polarizations (scenario 1), couples in other last chance scenarios—those in which one or both partners have violated values or safety (scenario 2), those with mismatched projected life chronologies (scenario 3), and those with low passion and connection (scenario 4)—also usually engage in high conflict. In the case of couples with low passion and connection, they are often burned to a crisp by years of high conflict and have settled into a pattern of extreme disconnection and avoidance, for fear that reconnecting will lead to restarting high conflict. Therefore, consider this chapter a general guide and toolbox of action-oriented techniques for working with all last chance couples. Chapter 5 continues discussion of working with high-conflict couples, but introduces insight-oriented techniques as well. Subsequent chapters on last chance scenarios 2–4 are briefer; they draw on the techniques in this chapter and Chapter 5, but focus more on the additional techniques needed to address these specific scenarios.

ELIMINATING DESTRUCTIVE COMMUNICATION AND BUILDING PROTECTIVE RELATIONAL PRACTICES: A SCIENCE-BASED APPROACH

Many therapists feel most daunted by the prospect of working with high-conflict couples and may avoid doing couple therapy entirely for fear that seemingly unmanageable high conflict will erupt. Partners that launch critical, contemptuous, defensive diatribes, interrupt one another, roll their eyes, shake their heads, and then glare at the therapist imploringly for a judgment of who's right and who's wrong can indeed be intimidating at first, and exhausting until a significant change starts to occur. Goldner (2014) writes:

> In the face of that raw intensity, one's ordinary working state cycles between hot and defensively cold, between anxious, hyperattentive caregiving (regulating, soothing, comforting, all hard-wired responses to distress in those we love), and the private abdication of that caregiving ("I've had it with you two"). The heat, the threat, the confusion, and finally the sheer clinical exhaustion can ignite a defensive withdrawal in even the most devoted clinician. Instead of allowing oneself to receive, contain, and ultimately metabolize the couples' traumatic states, the therapist thinks ironic thoughts. One of my favorite phrases from the heyday of family therapy captures this mind set: "The Situation is Desperate, but not Serious." (p. 403)

But of the four types of last chance couple scenarios, those whose primary issue is high conflict are usually the easiest to treat successfully. The other types of last chance couples present significantly greater challenges. Almost all last chance couples benefit from psychoeducation about the empirically supported communication skill alternatives to their destructive patterns.

I draw largely from the research conducted and techniques developed by the creators of PREP (Prevention and Relationship Enhancement Program; Markman, Rhoades, et al., 2010; Markman, Stanley, et al., 2010) and related psychoeducational programs (Halford, 2011; Leuchtmann et al., 2018) designed to prevent destructive conflict and enhance positive, protective factors. Although PREP was designed as a primary prevention program for happy, premarital or early-marriage couples, even with high-conflict last chance couples, the focus should be on equipping the couple to prevent further conflict. The theory, ideas, and techniques introduced are of course similar to cognitive–behavioral couple therapy (Baucom et al., 2015; Dattilio, 2010), but I find that emphasizing how all couples, at any stage of the relationship and level of happiness, need to adopt a firm determination to prevent destructive conflict, and can do so with a few simple skills, immediately helps couples feel a bit less hopeless and unique in their "dysfunction" (Fraenkel & Markman, 2002). In other words, along with teaching these skills, we are also encouraging a new commitment to protect the We through distress prevention and relationship protection and enhancement practices.

Along with these skills, couples need what Fishbane (2013) has termed "neuroeducation"—understanding what happens in partners' brains and their overall autonomic nervous systems when they detect or anticipate (accurately or not) signs of disdain and criticism from their partners, and how to engage mindfulness practices to self-soothe. Writing from the theoretical perspective of dialectical behavior therapy, Fruzzetti (2006) has also stipulated the importance of teaching mindful, self-soothing practices in work with high-conflict couples. A large literature has emerged on the effectiveness of these skills (including not only mindful meditation, but also mindful movement approaches such as Tai Chi and Qigong) on individual mental and physical health (Baer, 2003; Jahnke et al., 2010; Kabat-Zinn, 2003, 2005; Osypiuk et al., 2018) as well as on couple emotion regulation and promotion of positive, empathic, secure connection (Adair et al., 2018; Atkinson, 2013; Khaddouma et al., 2017). Without such calming practices, couples are not able to engage new communication skills.

High-conflict couples also benefit from ideas and skills, based on John Gottman's (Driver et al., 2012; Gottman, 1994; Gottman & Gottman, 2018) groundbreaking research, that foster repair after a relational rupture; learning to take influence from one another and leveling the power playing field; reorienting their attention to one another (responding to bids for attention) and away from distractions like their phones; and other practices that strengthen mutual admiration and respect, friendship, and pleasure. As described in Chapter 2, although I draw upon some techniques developed by others that are supported by outcome research pretty much as they were originally presented, in other instances I use the science of couple relationships as a base to create individualized suggestions for a particular couple that connects with metaphors that make sense knowing their culture and meaning system and their unique backgrounds.

The Therapeutic Palette integrative approach recognizes that underlying these skills are relational values usually not named in the original cognitive–behavioral sources of the techniques—the values of fairness, equity in power and voice, nonaggressiveness, and an ethic of care, and therefore represents social justice as applied to the couple context. Feminism's (Gilligan, 1982; Goldner, 1985; Hare-Mustin, 1978; Knudson-Martin, 2012, 2013, 2015; Knudson-Martin & Huenergardt, 2010; Knudson-Martin & Mahoney, 2009) emphasis on these values in relationships provides the guiding framework and rationale. Although feminism began with a focus on cisgender heterosexual relationships and how patriarchal sociocultural beliefs structure relationships between men and women, the ethics of equity between partners has been applied to same-sex and other Queer relationships (Richards et al., 2015).

Learning these communication and problem-solving skills often results in challenging inequitable power arrangements between partners, leading to important conversations about fairness and decisions about whether partners wish to transform these power arrangements, not only in the domain of communication but more broadly in terms of their roles in the couple and family around domestic labor and childcare, entitlement to time alone for decompressing after work, and other daily activities (Fraenkel & Capstick, 2012). Not infrequently, a partner who has assumed power privilege in the relationship balks at engaging in these skills, as they lead to equalizing partners' power and voice. This reluctance to engaging in fair and equitable communication opens up important conversations about assumed and exerted power and the sources of these "power over" attitudes and behaviors in larger social narratives about gender, race, ethnicity, class, and other social locations (Knudson-Martin & Huenergardt, 2010).

Once couples have an actual, observable experience demonstrating that they can communicate without conflict, the therapy can better explore each partner's family- and culture-of-origin sources of emotional sensitivity and vulnerability (Scheinkman & Fishbane, 2004) and the models of communication they witnessed growing up. As described in Chapters 1 and 2, openings or affordances often are presented spontaneously by partners during training in communication skills, as they reflect on how different these skills are from what they saw growing up, or from what their cultural backgrounds taught them about who gets to speak, have opinions, and proffer solutions to problems in a relationship. Rather than waiting until partners have achieved some measure of competence in these skills over weeks, the therapist can briefly pause the skills training and explore these family and cultural beliefs when partners raise them, and then return to fostering mastery of the skills. In later sessions, a fuller exploration of each partner's past and cultural references can occur. This represents the productive shifting of time frames from present to past and back again to the present described by the Therapeutic Palette approach.

In sum, although these communication and problem-solving skills are drawn from cognitive–behavioral couple therapy and CBT-based distress prevention programs, from the integrative, multiperspectival vantage point of the Therapeutic Palette, they achieve goals suggested as important by other approaches to working with couples. From a structural couple therapy point of view, they provide a prepackaged guide for an enactment of a better way to resolve problems, eliminate vicious cycles of distancing and pursuing, overfunctioning and underfunctioning, or blaming and placating, and can bring partners closer. From a feminist perspective, they equalize power and voice between partners. From an intergenerational couple therapy perspective, they help partners differentiate from their respective families of origin. From a sociocultural and multicultural perspective, they help partners examine their often-implicit beliefs about power in relation to gender, ethnicity, class, and educational background, and about who knows the right way to talk about issues, the appropriateness of expressing vulnerable versus more aggressive feelings, who is most entitled to "have the last word," and about how to view and address intimate conflicts.

Learning skills of respectful turn-taking may even prompt reflection about cultural traditions that embody similar practices of peaceful, respectful talking and listening (for instance, in Native American cultures, passing an eagle feather to signify whose turn it is to talk, or in the Maasai culture of Kenya, passing a talking stick). From a social constructionist and narrative therapy perspective, these skills provide a slowed-down, emotionally safer opportunity for partners to hear their often quite divergent stories of what happened, provide a method for addressing future conflicts so that they quickly arrive at a shared story, and help shift the couple's identity from dysfunctional or hopeless to competent, compassionate, and skilled. From a solution-focused perspective, they provide tools to actualize hopes for improved communication that typically emerge in response to the miracle question.

Vignette: Geetika and Aadesh

I use the following case to illustrate how to teach couples these skills. Geetika was a 30-year-old cardiologist and Aadesh was a 32-year-old lawyer. Both were Bengali Americans. They met online and were immediately attracted to one another physically, intellectually, and by their shared cultural heritage. However, almost from the beginning, they engaged in high-conflict arguments. Aadesh pronounced them to be a "really dysfunctional couple," and Geetika agreed. The content of their arguments centered largely on different desires about how to spend time. Geetika was highly social and extremely close to her family, who lived nearby and who often invited the couple to spend weekends with them. Aadesh described himself as "highly introverted" and tended to be a bit curt and emotionally restrained in social situations. He found himself quickly "getting to zero" in energy reserves after a weekend with her family, too many other social occasions one after another, or extended periods of intimate conversation with Geetika. Aadesh would desperately request some "alone time to recharge," which led Geetika to feel unloved and rejected, hearing in Aadesh's declarations of exhaustion that he found time with her depleting rather than enlivening and pleasurable.

Each partner was offended by the other's emotional style during their conflicts and worried about what the other's styles indicated about their personality and, therefore, whether each could change. Aadesh felt Geetika was too sensitive, often bursting into tears and needing a lot of reassurance when he behaved diffidently with her or others, and Geetika felt Aadesh was rude and mean when he got angry and withdrew.

After two years of almost constant fighting, they broke up, but got back together seven months later, hoping to make it work. They tried some couple therapy, but the therapist did not help them change their interaction patterns, focusing only on each partner trying to understand the other's feelings. They read some self-help books with general information about communication, but not specific enough to equip them with skills. As Aadesh said, "We have very different styles of communication; we agree on 90% of the substance of our lives, but it takes a lot to get there, if at all." Referred to me by another former last chance couple in the South Asian American community, they stated they did not "want to waste time with each other if things couldn't improve, because of [their] age." Close to calling off the relationship, they initially requested several double (two-hour) sessions per week.

Like all high-conflict couples, Geetika and Aadesh initially required a present-focused, interaction-focused, and highly directive approach. They felt great urgency to see if their communication style could become more compatible, and firmly noted they did not want to repeat the exploratory approach that the previous therapist had taken. With my having heard enough about their issues in the initial 30-minute Zoom consultation to determine a useful first step in working with them, they agreed to have me teach them in the first session research-based information about the typical problem patterns couples engage in, and communication and problem-solving skills that would avoid these patterns. I essentially conduct a private psychoeducational workshop with couples on this material. In what follows, I trace Geetika and Aadesh's progress and reactions in learning these skills as I describe each component of the workshop.

Steps and Script for Teaching Communication and Problem-Solving Skills

The skills and ideas couples need to communicate and solve problems, and to identify their expectations and the larger issues in their relationships, can be taught across four sessions. Here's the breakdown of sessions and topics, assuming sessions are 60 minutes long:

1. Session 1. Research on typical problem patterns; Speaker-Listener Technique and XYZ statement; coaching the skills on a low-intensity topic
2. Session 2. Review of home-based practice of skills; Problem-Solving Technique; Speaker-Listener Technique and XYZ statement on a higher-intensity topic followed by problem-solving on the issue
3. Session 3. Review of home-based practice; techniques for identifying expectations and hidden (broader) issues of closeness and caring, control and power, respect and recognition, integrity and safety, commitment, trust, and acceptance; Speaker-Listener Technique and XYZ statement that includes naming hidden issues and expectations
4. Session 4. Using all the skills to address a high-intensity topic

Although many therapists are somewhat familiar with CBT-based communication and problem-solving skills, and the skills seem straightforward and easy to understand in the abstract, over 30 years of teaching these skills to beginning and experienced couple therapists, I've realized that many therapists don't have a clear sense of how to teach them to couples most effectively. Cognitive–behavioral therapy skills are not just an assemblage of techniques to foist on clients in a cookbook fashion—they require all the aspects of building and maintaining a therapeutic alliance discussed in Chapter 1 and many nuances in motivating and guiding people to try new relational movement. I've seen experienced couple therapists show videos at conferences in which they demonstrated how they introduce these skills, and, with all due respect, they make serious errors—for instance, failing to set the stage and build motivation for using these admittedly awkward and unnaturally structured skills by summarizing the research on the problem patterns the skills are designed to avoid before teaching them. In one demonstration, the therapist repeatedly interrupted the couple to point out these problem patterns (which she had not fully explained beforehand), and finally, the couple turned on the therapist angrily and said, "This isn't working—we're already mad at each other and now you're pissing us off!"

I've also added some important "neuroeducation" (Fishbane, 2013) to help couples understand what happens in their brains and autonomic nervous systems during conflict, which usually starts even before the conflict as partners get ready to hear criticisms and defend themselves. Knowing what happens in our "conflict brains" encourages couples to engage in mindfulness practices before and during problem discussions—crucial acts of emotional self-regulation to avoid escalation and other dysfunctional patterns of communication.

The steps, general script, and approximate duration for each step in a 60-minute session are described below. If possible, an initial 90-minute or 120-minute session is preferable for introducing the skills, but it can be done in 60 minutes. Consider this a detailed manual for how to introduce and engage couples in these core communication and problem-solving skills. The "script" (what to say to couples) is in quotation marks. Sentences without quotations are instructions to you, the therapist.

SESSION 1: RESEARCH ON TYPICAL PROBLEM PATTERNS, THE SPEAKER-LISTENER TECHNIQUE, AND THE XYZ STATEMENT

1. 5 minutes. Brief description of the history of research on couple conflict

"In the early 1970s, research on couples shifted from questionnaire studies and attempts to identify personality styles associated with better or worse outcomes in marriage to detailed observational studies in which couples talked about a 'hot topic' for 20 minutes and tried to solve it. These conversations were videotaped and then coded for partners' verbal and nonverbal behaviors. Good news! Aside from one personality style, personality is not associated with better or worse chances of having a happy marriage. The one personality style associated with poorer outcomes is 'neuroticism,' which basically refers to a person who takes a negative view of events, a kind of 'glass half empty' approach to life. It's not surprising that this would be related to unhappy relationships, because a person high on neuroticism is more likely to engage in the problematic forms of thinking and interaction I'll describe in a moment. Instead, research with many different groups of couples in many different studies in several countries has found that there are a few problematic patterns of communication that distinguish happy from unhappy couples, and that also predict, from groups of newlywed couples, which will end up unhappy over time. Point being that even couples who are initially happy may engage in these problematic forms of communication, and over time, these interactions degrade the quality of the relationship. Furthermore, the skills I will teach you can override and correct for problematic personality styles or other individual psychological difficulties (depression, anxiety, and so on), because sometimes, feelings of depression and anxiety are largely due to a sense of fear, upset, and hopelessness about how communication goes between oneself and one's partner."

2. 20 minutes. Describe the four major problem patterns and a few subflavors of escalation

Believe it or not, you can go through this script or your own version in 20 minutes—I've done it hundreds of times. Note that I take a break between explaining escalation and the remaining four major problems patterns—withdrawal, invalidation, and negative interpretations—to explain the time-out rule, to do some neuroeducation and training in mindfulness techniques, and to describe the three problematic expressed emotions or affects of criticism, contempt, and defensiveness.

Escalation

"There are four major problem patterns that research has found characterize distressed couples' communication, and that predict from groups of newlywed couples which ones will head toward distress and divorce: escalation, withdrawal, invalidation, and negative interpretations. Escalation is a pattern in which one partner speaks with negative affect or expressed emotion, the other expresses themselves with negative affect, Partner A responds again with negative affect, and on it goes, in a kind of painful volleyball match of negativity. Happier couples may start an escalation but quickly exit it—by one partner saying, 'Wow, we got off to bad start,' and the other agreeing; or a partner may apologize for their tone, explain that they are a bit stressed out, or even may make a self-effacing critical comment ('Well, I'm certainly being a jerk. Sorry, honey'). So the first technique I want to teach you is what we call the 'time-out' or 'stop-action' rule: If you see that you are getting into an escalation—or any of the other patterns I'll describe today—the best thing you can do is stop and take a break. These patterns have an almost magnetic pull, and they lead nowhere good fast. So to protect yourselves individually and the relationship, agree that if one person calls the time-out, the other will respect it and not insist on talking further at that moment. However, in order not to slip into the second major problem pattern—withdrawal, where one partner pulls out of the conversation—it's important that you decide on how long a break you will take, and schedule a time to come back to the conversation. That can be within a few minutes after you've had a chance to cool down, or it might be that the conversation came up at an inopportune time when one of you has to get to work, or is too tired, or the baby needs tending, so schedule a time within the next 24 hours.

"I encourage couples to come up with their own code word or verbal flag to signal a time-out—I've had couples call it Red Balloon, Code Red, Chill Time, Volcano, and others. One couple even used the words 'Tuna Fish' so that their little girl wouldn't suspect what was happening and ask about it! Can you think of a term that would work for you, and maybe even one with a sense of humor to lighten the moment?" Brainstorm with the couple a personalized verbal signal for a time-out.

Neuroeducation and teaching mindfulness techniques. "Now when you take the time-out or whatever term you agreed on, what you *don't* want to do is to be like boxers retreating to their separate corners of the ring to think about what they will do when the bell rings and they start fighting again. Instead, it's best to spend the time calming your nervous system. One thing important to know is how the brain operates during relationship conflict. As you may know, the autonomic nervous system has a sympathetic branch and a parasympathetic branch. The sympathetic branch readies us to deal with perceived danger, putting us into fight-or-flight mode. What's happening is that a small organ called the amygdala within the limbic system—

the emotion center of the brain—senses possible danger and sets off a cascade of events: cortisol and adrenaline coursing through your veins, activating the neurotransmitter norepinephrine, all designed to help us protect ourselves. Essentially, the limbic system hijacks our higher cortical functions, the centers that allow us to be reasonable and reflective. You may still be using words, but you're likely not making a lot of sense, or you're saying things that you will later regret. Importantly, when we know we are about to have a problem discussion, we often already are moving into fight-or-flight mode—we anticipate that we will hear things from our partners that will be hurtful, that will make us angry, or about which we might feel some guilt or shame. The amygdala doesn't differentiate between danger signals from outside and those from inside—our expectations and feelings." Often, partners will interject that they've seen this happen, and regret what they've said during fights, or can't even remember a day later what the fight was about—all they can remember is how they felt and the hurtful things said.

Ask the partners what they already do when they are stressed and need to calm down. Many people will respond that they have no reliable method for dealing with stress in the moment, or need to do things that take more time, like watching TV or exercising. In a subsequent session, or sometimes at this moment if a partner brings it up, it might be appropriate to briefly explore each partner's family-of-origin history of receiving soothing. Sadly, many people report that they rarely received soothing from parents or others in the parenting role (grandparents). Suggest that you teach the couple a simple mindful breathing practice that works quite rapidly (see the website Coherent Breathing, https://coherentbreathing.com).

"So, I'd like to teach you a mindful breathing technique that has been found in many studies to significantly reduce stress, anxiety, depression, and other psychological issues, like trauma symptoms. What we're going to do is breathe in through the nostrils to a count of five, hold the breath for one second, and then breathe out through the nose to a count of five and hold the 'empty' for one second. When you breathe in, notice the coolness of the breath coming in through the nostrils, and when you breathe out, notice the warmth of the air going out. This is a good kinesthetic focusing technique to help you move away from ruminative thoughts and upset feelings. In addition, you can say in your mind's voice, 'I know I'm breathing in' as you breathe in, and as you breathe out, 'I know I'm breathing out.' You can close your eyes or keep them open as you breathe, but if you keep them open, try to look at something pleasant—a nice stone, a flower, anything nice (but not your phone, unless you have a photo of such an object on it!). Don't expect to fully relax or forget about your upset, but if this helps you calm down a bit, it will put you in a better place to resume the conversation, but with the help of the communication skills I'll be teaching you soon. Shall we try it?"

Lead the couple through three to five repetitions of breathing in and out. Then ask them if they notice any change in their arousal levels or how they feel. Inevitably, partners will report that this led them to feel calmer, and they are often surprised at how quickly the technique works. I even found this to be true with one couple who was irritated that I was 10 minutes late to our session—I had a good reason, believe me!—and the husband was a self-described "rage-aholic," yet with three mindful breaths, he was remarkably calmer, and noted that this would help him at work as well, where he occasionally burst into angry tirades, to the consternation of his colleagues.

I also invite couples to let me teach them a few Qigong moves. Qigong is an ancient Chinese internal martial art quite similar to Tai Chi but less complicated. It involves pairing slow breathing with slow movements of the hands, arms, torso, and legs, a kind of movement meditation. I find that my peripatetic New York clients often have difficulty doing sitting meditation and prefer Qigong. I've studied it for 30 years, but anyone can easily learn some moves (on YouTube you can find videos of Qigong masters, including Lee Holden and my teacher William Kaplanidis, demonstrating these moves). There is a large body of research demonstrating the effectiveness of Qigong and Tai Chi on physical and emotional health (Jahnke et al., 2010; Osypiuk et al., 2018).

I have the couple do three Qigong moves with me, and again, they inevitably like them. I've also had some interesting moments with highly distressed couples when I've taught them the moves and they've burst into laughter, commenting that they never expected they'd be doing these sorts of things in couple therapy. One partner, who had been highly reluctant to come to therapy, liked it so much that when contacting me for future appointments, he'd write, "Can we do tree swaying next Wednesday at 6?" ("Tree swaying" is one of the Qigong moves.) I suggest that couple partners practice three mindful breaths and three Qigong moves five times a day—in the morning when they wake up, midday, somewhere in the afternoon when most of us experience a biorhythmic slump of fatigue, at the end of the work day, and before bed. My experience is that five short practice sessions of these mindfulness activities across the day works better for maintaining a sense of relative calm than one long sitting meditation in the morning, which many clients have tried and found doesn't protect them from the inevitable stressors encountered during the day. I suggest that if possible, it's lovely for couples to do the morning and bedtime practice together, as a way to start to create a "climate of calmness and compassion." If they are working at home (as many couples did during and following the COVID-19 pandemic), they potentially can do all five practice sessions together.

The three problematic affects or expressed emotions. After teaching couples these mindfulness practices, continue with a more nuanced definition of what researchers mean by *negative affect*, as follows: "So, let me go back to what we mean by *negative affect*. I should say that I find the term *negative emotions* problematic, because these emotions, although unpleasant, are important to feel and to express. Feelings like sadness, loneliness, fear, anxiety, boredom, anger, and so on are certainly not pleasant, but are inevitable and very important to recognize in ourselves and share with our partners. But guess what? Research has even discovered that the expression of frustration and anger—without being colored by the problematic affects I'll describe in a minute—is healthy and actually a predictor of positive relationships over time, as long as the anger is expressed in a modulated way that is not overwhelming, aggressive, or intimidating. This finding shows how research is important, because for decades there have been books on 'anger as the dangerous emotion.' But it's inevitable that we get irritated, frustrated, and angry at our partners sometimes, and it's important to express those feelings.

"What research by John Gottman and others has found is that there are three really problematic negative affects: criticism, contempt, and defensiveness or belligerence. Criticism is putting down your partner's point of view ('That's what you think happened? You've got to be kidding!'), their ideas about a situation ('That's a really stupid idea. That will never work and you know it!'), their feelings ('How can you possibly be upset about that?'), their behavior and attempts to contribute to mutual well-being ('You call this cleaning a kitchen? You didn't do anything! It's still a mess!'), or their whole personhood in what we call a character assassination—like, instead of saying, 'I'm irritated when you leave your socks around the bed and I have to pick them up,' it's 'You're a slob!' or 'You're so inconsiderate!'

"Contempt adds a whole other flavor of disgust, sarcasm, or even revulsion to the communication. It's expressed in nonverbal ways—like eye rolling, grimacing, mocking voice tone, deep hostile sighs and snorts, and in words like, 'You're sooo pathetic,' or with hostile humor, like, 'Oh I *see*. You think you don't need to clean your own dishes because you were born a prince [or princess]—so sorry, I forgot! Couldn't see the invisible crown!' Yuck! Cringeworthy!

"Defensiveness or belligerence is when a partner responds to a reasonable suggestion or request with an outsized angry response, a kind of blowback: 'Are you for real? You expect me to take out the garbage when I work 14-hour days to support this family?!' Criticism, contempt, and defensiveness are the truly destructive expressed emotions—avoid them! With the skills I'll teach you, I think you'll be less tempted to attack each other in these ways and will be able to express normal anger and frustration constructively."

Withdrawal

"Withdrawal is the second major problem pattern. It's when one partner gives verbal or nonverbal signals that they are pulling out and turning away from the conversation. It can be as subtle as a momentary glance away while the other partner is talking, a sigh, rolling eyes and raising eyebrows, or more obvious through turning away or shaking one's head, or turning away the entire body, suddenly folding arms, or shrugging one's shoulders, as well as by statements, such as repeatedly saying 'I don't know' in answer to a partner's questions, saying 'I don't want to talk about it,' or literally getting up and ending the conversation. The most extreme version of withdrawal is a facial expression John Gottman named 'stonewalling'—freezing the musculature of one's face, kind of the Arnold Schwarzenegger as the Terminator, or Sylvester Stallone as Rocky or Rambo, or Dwayne 'The Rock' Johnson in any of his tough-guy roles' style of communicating [I then imitate one of these characters and their blank face, narrowed eyes, and brief utterances, which draws a laugh]. When one partner withdraws, guess what the other does?" Couples always offer the answer, and often smile knowingly: "Goes after the partner, pursues." "Right! And then you get into the classic circular pattern or vicious spiral of withdrawing and pursuing, which can itself escalate."

With cisgender heterosexual couples, I then add, "Interestingly, research shows that men do two to four times as much withdrawing as do women. Now, that may be different for the two of you." Invite the couple to talk about how this pattern occurs in their relationship. Sometimes it's the woman who withdraws more, but often it is the man. When it's the man, continue as follows: "Gottman's later research in the '80s with his colleague Robert Levenson had couple partners hooked up to five different measures of physiological arousal: galvanic skin response, which is the conductivity of electricity across the skin—the higher it is, the more sympathetically distressed the person is—as well as pulse, blood pressure, and even shifting in the seat. They found that compared to their baseline level of arousal before the problem discussion, men get on average four to five times more negatively physiologically aroused than do women, and stay aroused four to five times longer than do women.

"Remember, research is always about averages, so this may be different for the two of you. But what's interesting about this is that men in most societies are taught not to express vulnerable emotions—the only feelings acceptable to express are so-called strong feelings like anger. Therefore, being in a conversation with your partner when you are feeling anxious, ashamed, guilty, sad, and so on becomes difficult, because these more vulnerable feelings are viewed as not acceptable, and men don't have a lot of practice expressing them, and sometimes, not even practice feeling or naming them. So it's no wonder that they get so negatively aroused—they're being asked to do something that they are not skilled at, and also something seen as 'not masculine,' which threatens part of their identity. And at the same time, they are doing more of the stonewalling, and the other partner is wondering if they're still alive and have a pulse! (Again, generating a moment of laughter.) The skills I'll teach you today will help both of you feel more comfortable expressing vulnerable emotions, as well as anger and frustration, but in a more modulated way."

Invalidation

"The third major problem pattern is invalidation, and it has two forms, an active and a passive form. The active form is two of the problematic expressed emotions I already mentioned—criticism and contempt, putting down your partner's views ('How can you possibly think that?' 'What planet are you on? That didn't happen at all!'), putting down your partner's suggestions about how to solve a problem ('That's a ridiculous idea, you know that won't work!'), and putting down their feelings ('I can't believe you feel that way. You're so sensitive/crazy, etc.')."

In describing the passive form of invalidation—an underresponse to a partner's upset—I use the moment to describe a few other important findings from Gottman's research on responding to bids for attention and the importance of mutual soothing.

Responding to partners' bids for attention. "The passive form of invalidation is a kind of underresponse to a partner's upset. For instance, one of you comes home from work and talks about having a terrible day at work, or an upsetting conversation with an in-law or friend, and the other one is like, "Uh huh, right. . . . Hey, what's for dinner?" while looking away or at your phone, totally disinterested or distracted. Or it might even be your attempt to make the other feel better, but it feels invalidating, as in, 'Oh, honey, you know you *always* have bad days at work,' or 'Don't you think you're making too much of that?' but it feels like a put-down, like your partner's feelings are unreasonable and don't matter. John Gottman found that one of the best predictors of whether newlywed couples remain happy and together over the years is how partners respond to what he called each other's 'bids for attention'—do you 'turn toward' your partner, meaning you look at them when they speak, show interest, and do what I call 'empathic murmurings,' like, 'Oh, really? That happened? And then what? Sounds rough, sorry to hear that happened, honey,' and so on? Or do you 'turn away,' meaning avoiding eye contact, having a flat voice tone, seemingly showing disinterest even if it's just being distracted by your phone or what have you?"

Responding effectively to a partner's concerns: Listening versus solutions. "A partner can sometimes also feel invalidated when the other makes 'unrequested suggestions' for how to solve the problem, when all they're really asking for is that you listen and empathize. Usually, they already know how to handle the problem, so if you suggest something, they may feel you don't think they are competent. Or they may sense that you are impatient with their complaints, especially if the situation has happened before." Again, with cisgender heterosexual couples, I'll add, "It's often men trying to provide solutions and women feeling insulted by that, even if you [the guy] don't mean it that way." This typically gets an affirmative response from the woman—"Yeah, that happens a lot!" For all couples, I say, "I suggest that if you have an idea for how your partner might solve their issue at work or with someone else, you can say, 'I have some ideas for how you can deal with that, if you want to hear them . . . '—in other words, ask for an invitation to share your ideas. But be ready for your partner to say, 'No, that won't really work, because . . . ' or, 'Yeah, I tried that already.' In other words, just because you have an idea, it may not seem useful to your partner, but at least you tried."

Frequently, the partner who is repeatedly being asked to listen to the complaints from the other will say something to the effect of, "The problem is that she seems to have an endless need to talk about her problems at work" or "with her family," or whatever. The other partner will then typically say, "Yeah, well, that's because you don't really listen!" or "Yeah, but that's because you're always offering solutions, but I don't need your advice!" I say to the partner being asked to listen, "I think what she's saying is she just wants you to listen. If you're offering solutions, you're working too hard. Just do those 'empathic murmurings' next time and see what happens. From my experience with couples, I think she might be less needy than you think, because what's happening is you're not listening in the way she needs you to, so she keeps going, hoping to get your full attention." This usually gets a strong affirmative response from the partner who wants the other just to listen more fully.

The importance of mutual soothing. At this juncture I will also share Gottman's findings that mutual physiological soothing between partners is also a strong predictor of relationship success. I'll ask partners whether and how they soothe each other when they're upset about something other than the relationship. Often, partners have not engaged in such soothing, or one wants it and the other doesn't ask for it, even if they may want it, or one may believe that individuals need to calm themselves down, sometimes stating, as one husband did, "You can't really help someone with their feelings about what they're going through. They have to figure it out for themselves." I will challenge this idea with Gottman's research, and suggest à la the PREP program that the skills I'll be teaching them can be used for "friendship talks," in which they have what I've called a daily 15–20-minute "decompression" conversation at the end of the day. I call this the "How was your day, dear?" conversation, in which they focus fully on one another and provide soothing empathic remarks and even physical soothing like holding the other's hand or offering a hug. I ask the couple if they've ever engaged in such talks or physical soothing— if yes, "Do more of that!" If not, I suggest they try it. With last chance partners who are angry at each other, this can seem challenging, but I recommend it as yet another experiment in possibility to see if it softens their attitude and stance toward each other, as part of determining whether the relationship can become more satisfying.

Negative Interpretations

"The last of the big four problem patterns is negative interpretations, and the behavior associated with it is negative mind reading. This is where we develop what I call a 'theory of mal-intent' about our partner's behavior. For instance, with a partner who's frequently late, at some point we might decide that they're late because they don't love us or don't want to spend time with us, or are trying to show that their time is more important than our time, or they're trying to show they don't respect us. Same thing with a partner who frequently forgets to clean up after themselves: 'Your behavior is telling me that you think it's my job to do all the cleaning, or to pick up after you.' Research shows that over time, distressed couples develop these negative theories, what researchers call 'negative attributions.' And once we have this theory, we don't think like good social scientists, trying to collect data that might *disprove* our hypothesis. Instead, we behave more like a litigator and start scanning our partner's behavior to collect supporting evidence for our theory. These theories are hard to disprove just with words, which is why it's important to discuss the issue and make a plan to change behavior to provide evidence that they're not true. The changed behavior can be both by the partner being accused of doing (or not doing) something and, also, changes in the complaining partner in which they start to notice that the partner is behaving in ways that they hope for.

"Usually, these theories center on what the PREP researchers call 'hidden issues,' which are sometimes not so hidden, but represent broader themes that pop up in specific complaints. In a later session I'll teach you a way to identify and work on these bigger issues. They include feeling unloved or uncared about by one's partner or, on the other end of the spectrum, that your partner seems to require too much affection or reassurance; feeling controlled or pushed around by your partner or, on the other end of the spectrum, like you have too much responsibility and power in the relationship to handle things; feeling disrespected or not recognized for your efforts, your challenges with work or childcare, or even disrespected as a whole person, expressed as a character assassination—as in, 'You are a_____'—fill in the blank: 'unloving, irresponsible, unkind person, slob, loser, brute,' what have you.

"Then there's the issue of integrity and safety, feeling your partner is asking you to do something that violates your values, or they are behaving in ways that violate your values or sense of emotional or physical safety; feeling your partner is not committed to the relationship or to trying to improve it; feeling that you can't trust your partner; and the biggest underlying issue is acceptance—not feeling basically accepted for who you are as a person. I should note that I do not agree with an old idea from the 1960s, that we should have unconditional acceptance for our partner. This is an idea that came from client-centered therapy, and was more about a therapist having 'unconditional positive regard' for their client. But it doesn't really apply to relationships, because we do have conditions for the relationship—we don't want to feel pushed around or controlled, or unloved, or disrespected, or unsafe, or that we can't trust our partner."

Having described the four major problem patterns, I ask couples at this point if any of these patterns sound familiar. This is often the first time in a session when partners look knowingly at one another and a bit more softly—and with less mutual blame—and agree that all or at least some of these patterns are quite familiar; and they will spontaneously describe a few instances in which these patterns occurred. I then provide reassurance by saying, "Well, the good news is that with the skills I'll teach you, you can avoid all of them—if you use the skills consistently! It's just behavior, and we can change our behavior."

Subflavors of Escalation

"Before we get into the skills, I want to briefly describe a few subflavors of escalation. They're kind of the Ben and Jerry's of pain, the Häagen-Dazs of hurt [this often elicits a smile]. Summarizing self syndrome is when one partner states her point of view, the other states his point of view, Partner A responds again with her point of view, Partner B with his. . . . It's essentially a standoff. A version of that is 'Yes, but'—'I know you think we watch too much TV, but I feel like I need to keep up with that series because everyone at the office talks about it.' Other partner: 'Yeah, but it's too much—we need to find other ways of spending time together.' 'Yeah, but . . . '

"Cross-complaining is when one partner brings up an issue in one domain of life—'You didn't clean the kitchen like you said you would!'—and the other, rather than addressing that issue, brings up an issue in a totally other domain: 'Well, you didn't call my mother to wish her a happy birthday, so we're even!' In the method I'll teach you, you pick one topic to discuss, and each of you offers your opinions and feelings about it.

"Another pattern is called 'kitchen-sinking'—as in the old expression, 'everything but the kitchen sink.' I think of it as the deli salad bar approach: Just as we fill up our plate with a bit of all the many offerings on the salad bar, here you're piling the plate with every complaint you have about your partner, all at once: 'Okay, we have to talk. You never clean up after yourself; you don't greet me nicely when I come home; you're not sensitive to my sexual needs; you're not nice to my mother . . . ' and on and on. All the other partner can do is feel like a total jerk. Instead, with this method you'll pick one issue to talk about and stick with that.

"Finally, there are three versions of what I call 'globalizing' from specific complaints to general statements. One is character assassination, which we discussed already. Another is 'always/never' statements: 'You never pick up after yourself. I always have to do it.' 'You never greet me when you come home. You're always distracted by your phone.' And finally, there's blaming: 'It's all your fault that we're having these problems, that we can't get along, that we have no friends,' and so on. And that's it! It's a pretty exhaustive list gathered from studies with thousands of couples in various countries. Any of these sound familiar?" Once again, couples typically report that they engage in many if not all of these patterns.

The reasons for spending time describing the research on couple problems and the specific patterns before teaching the skills are as follows:

a. Couples usually experience conflict as a kind of undifferentiated gray mass and get quickly overwhelmed. Providing them a language for identifying specific patterns helps them discern the specific patterns so that they can more quickly call a time-out.
b. The therapist and the therapy process itself gains credibility by showing couples that you already are well versed in the types of problems they are experiencing, and as I discussed in Chapter 1, the credibility of the therapy and therapist are essential to building a strong therapeutic alliance.
c. Hearing from you that many couples get into these patterns—even newlywed, happy couples—helps couples feel less alone in their problems, and reduces the sense of shame and stigma or sense that they are a hopeless, dysfunctional couple.
d. The communication and problem-solving skills you will teach them admittedly feel artificial at first, and to motivate the couple to practice them, it's important that they know what they will be able to avoid if they use them.
e. Providing the information on typical problem patterns before teaching the skills allows you to refer back to that information if the couple gets into one of the patterns, as in, "Umm, that sounds a bit like what I talked about earlier, negative mind reading. . . . Can you rephrase that so that it's clear you don't know for sure that that's what Jim thinks and feels, but maybe that sometimes you wonder if he still loves you?" Or, "Okay, that was kind of a

criticism, let's try it again, and this time, drop out the critical stuff and just say how you feel when Sally does that." Or, to the listening partner, "Reggie, you seemed to be withdrawing a bit there while Janessa was talking when you were shaking your head and rolling your eyes. Let's have her say that again, and this time, no matter what you're feeling, remember at this point, you're just trying to hear what she's saying and show her that you are listening, even if you completely disagree. You'll get a chance to speak pretty soon."

What does not work well is to teach couples new skills and then point out when they are interacting in these problematic ways without having first told them about the general findings about how many couples interact in these ways. Remember that when couples are trying something we're suggesting and teaching to them, they will have the normal level of anxiety that anyone experiences about learning to do anything new, and they want to show you (and themselves) that they can do it. This is especially true for last chance couples, who come to therapy in a great deal of pain and confusion about the destructiveness of their communications, and often feel shame and a sense of failure. To then interrupt their attempts to learn a new way to communicate and point out their problematic tone or words will compound their anxiety and sense of failure.

3. 20 minutes. Communication skills: the Speaker-Listener Technique and the XYZ statement

Explain the skills as follows: "The Speaker-Listener Technique is the main communication skill. One of you will be the speaker at any one time, and the other will be the listener. This avoids talking over one another and makes sure that the listener hears and understands what the speaker is saying. The speaker speaks for 10 to 15 seconds at most, using 'I' statements—meaning, 'I feel that . . . , it seems to me that . . . , I think that . . . '—not mind-reading statements like, 'You feel, you believe,' and so on. If you want to say something about what you think your partner feels and thinks, you can say something like, 'Sometimes I wonder if you don't love me' or 'Sometimes it seems you're trying to control me,' or 'I sometimes feel that you don't respect me.' In other words, you're stating your belief or impressions about what they think, feel, or intend toward you. Putting it in terms of your perceptions is completely different than stating that you definitely know how your partner feels or thinks, or what their intentions are behind their behavior. Does that make sense?"

Make sure the partners understand this distinction. Then go on: "The listener should repeat back what they heard, as accurately as possible, which is why we keep the speaker's statements brief. Don't try to paraphrase or put what the speaker said in your own words at this point. One you get comfortable with the skill, you'll be able to take slightly longer turns as the speaker, and the listener can then paraphrase the gist of what the speaker said, but for now, I want to make sure you get the basic process of speaking and listening and really hear exactly what each other is saying.

"When the listener repeats what they heard, the speaker should then say, 'Uh huh' or 'Yeah, you got it,' to let the listener know they repeated it correctly, and then go on to another statement on the same topic—remember, we're avoiding the 'salad bar' style and staying on one topic. If the listener didn't get it quite right, the speaker should say, 'Not exactly,' and then repeat the part the listener didn't get correctly. Once the listener gets it completely, the speaker goes on to another statement on the same topic. As the speaker, you get up to four or five turns on the same topic, each time with the listener repeating back correctly. Then the floor goes to the listener, who becomes the speaker, on the same topic, because we want to avoid cross-complaining.

"As the listener, you have the hardest job because you need to put aside your reactions, rebuttals, and so on, and just focus on understanding what the speaker is saying. Remember that in repeating back what the speaker said, you are in no way saying you agree—you're just trying to show that you hear each other and are trying to understand your partner's point of view and feelings. When you get the floor, you may say that you have a totally different memory of an event or sense about the topic."

Ask the couple if they have any questions. Once these are addressed, go on to explain the XYZ statement: "A subtechnique of speaker-listener is the XYZ statement. This is designed to avoid those three forms of 'globalizing' from specific things you're upset about to general statements like character assassinations, always/never statements, and blaming. It is a kind of 'communication algebra'—'When you do X behavior (fill in the blank) in situation Y (fill in the blank), I feel Z specific emotion (fill in the blank).' For instance, 'When you don't greet me when you come home, I feel hurt.' 'When you leave your socks all around the bedroom, I feel frustrated.' You can switch the order of the terms: 'I feel embarrassed (Z) when you get drunk (X) at parties (Y).' Or, 'When we're visiting my mom (Y) and you go after her about her political views (X), I feel angry (Z) and like I need to protect her from you.'

"One more thing: It's really important that for the Z term, you tell your partner what specific emotion you're feeling—sad, hurt, upset, disappointed, angry, frustrated, and so on. We sometimes use the word *feeling* to indicate an opinion, like, 'I feel we'll never get along,' or to express a desire, as in, 'I feel like running away.' Here, you really need to say how you are feeling emotionally, because your emotions are the window into empathy for the listener. Also, the XYZ statement is just to state your complaint or concern clearly at the beginning of your turn as speaker—you don't need to stick to it with each subsequent statement. Instead, you might give an example, or talk about how what your partner does triggers old feelings from your family growing up, or just explain why you feel as you do."

One other note on expressing anger: As was noted earlier, Gottman's early longitudinal research on predictors of happiness and stability for newlywed couples showed that the expression of anger without criticism, contempt, or defensiveness was not a predictor of problems over time (Gottman et al., 1998). Although it is important for couples to know that they can express the inevitable anger and frustration that occurs in relationships, high-conflict last chance couples often are so rageful and reactive to one another's anger that they need help identifying their underlying hurt, fear, disappointment, or other vulnerable feelings. This process is central to emotionally focused couple therapy, and is known as "softening" (Johnson, 2019, 2020). I describe to couples the research on anger, indicating that it is a secondary emotion, a reaction (often quite rapid, within milliseconds) to those primary, vulnerable feelings.

I also use a metaphor to distinguish anger from the initial vulnerable feelings. "Anger is like the breaking whitecaps on an ocean wave, while feelings of hurt, fear, disappointment, and so on are the 'roiling currents' unseen beneath the whitecaps." I encourage couples to "'speak your anger' rather than 'do or demonstrate your anger.' It's fine to have distress in your voice tone, to sound angry or frustrated if you are—although try to modulate your voice tone, because loud, aggressive anger tends to result in the other partner 'turning down the speakers or receptors' in their own mind, as a form of self-protection. Don't use your speech in this moment to cause further hurt."

Coaching the Couple in Communication Skills

Ask the couple if they have any questions, and once those are answered, suggest that they try the techniques with you coaching them. Ask them to pick a low-intensity topic and note, "We're not going to try to solve the problem today. We're just using the topic as some content to learn the skills. In fact, I haven't yet taught you the second part of this method, which is problem solving, coming up with an action plan. The speaker-listener part is just for talking about your points of view and feelings. We separate problem discussion from problem solving for a few reasons: first, to make sure each of you has a chance to fully express your perspectives and feelings. Sometimes, the partner receiving a complaint just wants to jump into solving the problem because it's uncomfortable hearing the partner's upset feelings. Separating problem discussion from problem solving makes sure that both partners get a chance to share their points of view and feelings. Second, when couples move too quickly to solutions, they may not be solving the real problem but something more on the surface. Third, I'd estimate that about 80 to 90% of problems don't need a whole action-planning process—it's often obvious what to do about solving the problem once both partners have had a chance to share their views."

Sometimes last chance couples have difficulty identifying a low-intensity topic, but encourage them to find one. This is often a useful exercise in itself, as it helps the couple see that not everything is a 10 on a 10-point scale of seriousness.

When one partner comes up with a low-intensity topic, have them state it to make sure the other partner agrees that it is low intensity. Once they agree, ask who would like to start as the speaker (it will usually be the partner who came up with the topic). Have the speaker start with an XYZ statement. Your role now is to guide the couple to use the technique. Remember the basic behavioral principle of "shaping"—reinforcing approximations to the goal.

After the speaker speaks and the listener repeats, ask the speaker if the listener got it right. If the speaker says the listener said it correctly, remind the speaker to affirm to the listener that they repeated correctly by saying, "Yeah, you got it" or "Uh huh," and then ask the speaker to go on to another statement on the same topic. You should also positively reinforce the listener and the speaker by saying, "Yes, good listening, and good speaking, too!" You'll be surprised by how even your most intellectually sophisticated couples appreciate a little positive reinforcement. I sometimes play with this a little, especially when the couple has young kids, by saying, "A star for you [to the listener] and a star for you, too [to the speaker]!" This reinforcement of both partners encourages them to keep trying. If the speaker says, "No, she/he didn't get it," ask the speaker to say it again, until the listener repeats it correctly. Then administer reinforcement.

On the other hand, if the speaker says it was a good repeat, but you remember something that seemed important that the listener missed, say, "Oh, well, I think I remember you also saying that . . . " (restate what you heard). Usually, the speaker will then remember and can then restate that part and let the listener repeat it again until they say it correctly. Often, what the listener missed is the speaker's feelings about the issue, so make sure that the listener repeats the feelings. It's also common that the speaker will not have stated their emotions in doing an XYZ statement, or will express an opinion or desire rather than a feeling, so have them state how they feel, and remind them why this is important.

At first, when partners take the role of speaker, they may make a statement that includes one of the problem patterns you've described and suggested they avoid—a mind-reading statement, an always/never statement, even a critical or contemptuous statement. As a coach, you need to focus initially on the basic rhythm of the technique, helping the couple take turns (e.g., stay in the speaker and listener roles), keeping the speaker's turn to 10–15 seconds or so, and helping the listener repeat back accurately without interjecting their own point of view. If the speaker uses an always/never statement, or a mild blaming statement (e.g., "It's because you don't clean up that the house is a mess," or a mild mind-reading statement ("Since you don't like to go out with other people, we have practically no friends"), you can overlook it in the moment the first time around in favor of reinforcing that the basic communication rhythm is happening.

After the speaker has made such a statement and the listener has repeated it, then point out the always/never, blaming, or mind-reading statement, and have the speaker say their piece without those problematic types of statements, and have the listener repeat it. Then go on to the speaker's next turn/statement. For instance, "Tanya, I noticed that you said Jill 'never' cleans the kitchen well—can you say it again, but drop the 'never'?" Or, "Lawrence, I think I heard you use a blaming statement when you told Richard that the money problems are 'all your fault.' See if you can stick with an XYZ statement like, "Richard, I get really upset when I see you've taken $500 from our account when we've agreed not to spend that kind of money unless we discuss it first."

However, no matter what stage of learning the couple is in, stop the speaker if they make a character assassination (e.g., "You're just a stupid jerk"), use an obviously contemptuous or critical tone, or make a more intense mind-reading statement (e.g., "You just don't care about me," "You obviously don't want to take any responsibility"). Point out the problematic statement and refer back to the research showing that these are destructive, and ask the speaker to use an XYZ statement that avoids these forms of expression.

Likewise, sometimes the listener will dutifully repeat back what they heard, but in a flat, disinterested tone—a kind of parroting of the speaker, as if to communicate, "That's what you think, but I don't agree" or signaling a lack of interest in the other's point of view and feelings. Sometimes the speaker will comment on this, other times not. In either case, you should note it, ask the listener to try again, and remind them that they don't have to agree with what their partner is saying, that they will get a chance to state their point of view, and that the goal right now is to show the speaker that they take their partner's feelings and perspective seriously, and to try to understand them, even if they don't agree with them.

Remember that, especially at first, the speaker's statements should be kept short—approximately 10–15 seconds maximum. The listener's difficulty remembering what the speaker is saying can be due to a host of factors: disinterest, emotional arousal about the topic, even receptive language difficulties and attentional issues. You can briefly explore what's getting in the way of the listener repeating back what they heard, and if they are truly trying their best but are still having difficulty, have the speaker cut the statement in half, or at some logical point of the statement (e.g., up to the comma, where they would take a breath before going on). Emphasize that the technique is not a memory test; the statements should be manageable for the listener, so that the listener can repeat the statement accurately and come to understand the speaker's point of view.

The speaker may offer a general wish about solutions, such as, "I wish there was more affection between us," or "I really want to share the household responsibilities more." This is fine. But if the speaker then launches into specifics about how they envision solving the problem, stop them and remind the couple that we separate problem discussion from problem solving, and that in the next session, you will introduce them to the technique for coming up with action plans.

4. 5 minutes. Discuss the couple's experience with the new skills and give homework

Ask the couple how they experienced using these techniques as an alternative to their usual ways of talking about problems. Couples will inevitably say that these techniques are much better than how they usually argue, but will also usually comment that the techniques feel artificial. Validate this experience, noting that the feeling of awkwardness and artificiality shows that they are doing something new, and say that with practice, the techniques will feel more natural. I often ask them about their experiences learning any new behavior, in sports (a new way of swinging a tennis racket or golf club, throwing a basketball), music (playing a new figure on an instrument), or getting used to a new software package, phone, or computer, and whether these new actions felt awkward and artificial at first—the answer is always, "Yes," of course.

I also remind them of one of the principles of the Creative Relational Movement approach to change, described in Chapter 1—that any change they experiment with will inevitably feel awkward and artificial initially, but with practice, they will find it more natural. You can also mention that when we are learning new habits, we are literally rewiring our brains based on neuroplasticity, creating new neural pathways that with repetition become automatic, and that with practice will override the old, problematic patterns (Fishbane, 2013).

I suggest that couples practice the technique two times for 20 minutes each time before the next appointment, on a low-intensity topic. I also suggest that the couple set aside one hour a week for relationship care. Most last chance couples have never established a regular time for talking about ongoing issues or issues that came up during the week that they did not have time to fully discuss. As a result, problem discussions end up infiltrating the relationship at inopportune moments: during an attempt at having a romantic dinner, while taking care of kids, just before bed, before or after sex, first thing in the morning when one or both need to prepare for the day, and other ill-timed moments. Ask the couple to decide on a regular rhythm of relationship care. Note that in their work lives, they likely have staff meetings to address issues and work on projects; relationships also need regular time set aside for discussing and solving problems. They can practice the technique at least once during that time.

Vignette: Geetika and Aadesh

As I noted earlier, couples often spontaneously reflect on how these ways of communicating and taking care of the relationship are quite different from what they witnessed in their families growing up. Geetika noted that her parents were constantly fighting in private, although in public they tried to show that they had a happy marriage. Aadesh grew up in Birmingham, England, and his parents aspired to a more upper-class "British" style of handling conflict, which meant never discussing difficulties in front of the children. Aadesh knew from talking with each of his parents that there was much tension between them, but he never witnessed them successfully discussing their differences or finding resolution. Rather, they took the stance of agreeing to disagree, even though this meant a gradual decline in their marital satisfaction. Geetika and Aadesh both expressed enthusiasm for these new skills, and said they finally had a sense of hope that they could now have a life together. In later sessions, I explored their respective families of origin and the problematic models of relationship they witnessed enacted by their respective parents.

SESSION 2: REVIEW HOME-BASED PRACTICE, TEACH PROBLEM-SOLVING TECHNIQUE, AND COACHING ON A HIGHER-INTENSITY ISSUE FROM PROBLEM DISCUSSION THROUGH PROBLEM SOLVING

1. Review of home-based practice

Ask the couple how their week went, and if they feel prepared to continue learning the skills as planned. If something urgent has come up, you need to address it and may need to forgo proceeding with teaching the skills. If what's come up is mostly continued ruminations about whether to stay in the relationship or dissolve it, remind them that you're suggesting they give the therapy a few weeks if possible to experiment with possibilities for improvement to make a better decision about whether to stay together or not. If the couple has kids, remind them that they will still be coparents even if they divorce, and that the skills you are teaching them will be important to reduce conflict and to avoid triangulating the children. If another issue has arisen that really can't be put aside, address that issue.

Otherwise, ask the couple how it went with practicing the skills. Address any problems they had with the skills, or questions about how to use them. A frequently reported issue is that the skills are difficult to use when they are quite upset. Validate that experience and remind them about the time-out rule to use when they are too negatively aroused to use the skills, and ask if they came up with a personalized verbal flag to signal the need for a time-out. Remind them about the neurobiology of couple conflict and that they need to calm down enough to engage the skills, using the mindfulness techniques you taught them. I often tell couples, "Respect your nervous system! It's sending you important signals that you need to calm down before talking." Review those techniques and have them engage in some mindful breathing and Qigong as further practice.

2. Problem-solving technique

Remind the couple about why we separate problem discussion from problem solving (see above). Then explain: "The Problem-Solving Technique is captured by four letters on the other side of the alphabet from XYZ: the ABCs plus F. A is for setting the agenda. You may have had a discussion about needing to redistribute household tasks: Now you want to pick one task and work to come up with a plan, whether that's who takes out the garbage, washing and putting away dishes, cleaning the counters, and so on. Or you may have discussed not having sufficient time for each other—during the week, on the weekends, or that you haven't had a vacation in years.

"Now you will pick one of those issues and come up with a plan. B is for brainstorming. You should come up with any ideas, even ones that seem initially improbable, and write them down. Don't censor or criticize any ideas because you think they won't work—just let them flow. Even humorous ideas can sometimes be transformed into realistic solutions. There are three Cs: combining, compromising, and contracting. Combining means taking the best of your respective ideas and trying to come up with a plan that honors them both. One of the assets of being in a couple is that you each may have different ideas about how to address problems. Although couples often bemoan their differences, these can become one of your greatest strengths if you can harness them."

Before continuing with the rest of the script, let's take a moment to discuss the importance of the strategy of combining in problem solving, as it is not described in the original materials from PREP (Markman, Stanley, et al., 2010). Assuming that in a first session you inquired about how the partners met and what it was that attracted each to the other, you've likely heard that each was in part attracted to ways in which their partner was different from themselves. Remind the couple of that conversation and note that research shows that neither the sayings "birds of a feather flock together" nor "opposites attract" tell the whole story of why people connect. Rather, all couples have a combination of differences and similarities. I usually also describe family systems theory founder Gregory Bateson's (1979) notion of "double description" as applied to couples—that, at their best, couples have a kind of "binocular vision," with each partner perceiving a situation differently. Just as our two eyes pick up slightly different images of an object and those images are combined in the brain to create depth perception, partners' different points of view and desires can be combined to create a deeper, more usefully complex, resourceful solution to problems.

One example around parenting: One parent might be inclined to reward a young child for doing his homework when he's had difficulty doing so; the other is more inclined to punish the child for not doing the homework. Developmental psychologists and parenting experts suggest that it's always best to start with a positive reinforcement approach—it helps shape the child's behavior and avoids the negative feelings and parent-child stress that occur with punishment. But if that approach fails, then move to taking away privileges. Both approaches can also be used simultaneously—rewarding the child for doing his homework, and taking away privileges if he doesn't.

Another example is about how to spend leisure time. As discussed in Chapter 3, many couple partners differ in their overall pace, and this typically manifests in different preferences for how to spend leisure time—one preferring faster-paced exciting activities, the other preferring slower-paced more relaxing time together. Partners are initially attracted to one another by these differences, and then get polarized around them, but they can be framed as equally valid and combinable in an overall plan for spending pleasurable time together.

I also often use a bit of humor to make a memorable point about the preferability of differences in relationships. Having been raised in the Boston area, I adopt an authentic heavy Boston accent and say, "After all, if you wanted to be with someone just like yourself, you could go to Target, 'cause they have a sale on full-length mirrors, $19.99 plus tax! Then you can just talk to yourself and watch yourself say the same words you're saying, simultaneously!"

Or I sometimes use the analogy of harmony in music to support the value of differences: "Musical harmony requires at least two notes played together. Without two different notes, what do we get? Monotony—the same note played by two different instruments. And of course, another meaning of the word *monotony* is *boredom*." Interestingly, as I learned when lecturing many times in Hong Kong, many popular books about couple and family relationships in the more collectivistic Chinese culture hold that harmony is a central value and goal in intimate relationships. Our more individualistic Western cultures tend to promote self-sufficiency, personal freedom, autonomy, and independence above all, leading to more struggle for couples around combining and compromising.

Vignette: Geetika and Aadesh

Presenting this material frequently elicits a conversation about how troubled last chance couples are by their differences. With Geetika and Aadesh, her more extroverted social tendencies contrasted greatly with his more introverted need for alone time and discomfort with extended periods of socializing. In addition, by their own description and as demonstrated in their interactions, Geetika tended to be more sensitive emotionally, easily hurt and prone to tears, whereas Aadesh could be a bit gruff, taciturn, and seemingly emotionally hard to upset, although his more sensitive side was revealed through their speaker-listener conversations. At one point, I teased Geetika that, as a physician, she knew that the skin is the largest and most exposed organ of the body (she had initially considered dermatology as a specialty, and remained interested in it), and perhaps her greater sensitivity related to her career choice, which made her laugh. Likewise, I noted that although Aadesh turned out to be quite sensitive under his gruff exterior, he could, as Geetika said, sometimes be "quite rude" when feeling overwhelmed, and behaved at those times like a "bull in a china shop" in responding to Geetika's upset, which elicited in him a confirming smile.

Exploring what attracted each to the other initially, Geetika said she was drawn to his "coolness," strength, and apparent unflappability, and Aadesh acknowledged that he loved that Geetika was "emotionally available and expressive," something he had not experienced in his family.

In problem solving about their differences in preference for social time and alone time, the couple used the principle of combining to devise a detailed daily and weekly schedule of time spent in one-on-one intimate activities, time spent silently "in their own heads" but together—for instance, on the couch reading, with legs entwined— time alone, primarily to catch up on the last work emails at the end of the day; and time with family and friends. Aadesh practically pleaded to be allowed some alone time or "silent together" time after social activities to help him recharge, and Geetika assented, now understanding better how desperately he needed to pull into himself after these events and no longer taking it as a rejection by him.

The couple found that the Speaker-Listener Technique itself represented a structured way to combine their different levels of comfort expressing vulnerable feelings. They also adopted the nightly practice of a "decompression chamber" in which they would first greet each other at the end of the workday (at the time I worked with them, Aadesh was working at home due to the coronavirus pandemic, and Geetika was still seeing patients in the hospital) and talk about their respective days and feelings for 20 minutes. Aadesh would then spend 20 minutes engaging in solitary activities that helped him calm down and "reboot" while Geetika called family or friends. They then would reconvene for dinner and go on with the rest of their evening together.

Now back to the script for teaching problem solving: "Compromise is the second C. Compromise is inevitable in relationships, yet is often the hardest thing for partners to do. Hearing how important something is for your partner helps. I generally take the 'lowest common denominator' approach—if possible, the person who has the greatest emotional or practical investment in a certain solution should have their way, or more of their way. Over time, when the partner who compromised more feels very strongly about something else, it's likely the other will return the favor. If not, that becomes an issue for you to talk about—that is, when one partner ends up compromising more than the other. But struggling over finding the perfect 50-50 fair and equitable compromise is often a painful waste of time.

"Commitment researcher Scott Stanley, one of the creators of PREP, notes that some degree of sacrifice is necessary for couples to sustain a relationship [Stanley et al., 2006]—giving up a bit or sometimes a lot of what you want or need in order to please your partner and establish the We, a sense of joint identity as a couple." It is often useful at this point to hear partners' responses to these ideas about compromise, to hear their history of difficulty achieving it, and to learn about what they witnessed in their families of origin around compromise.

"The final C of the three Cs is contracting. This means deciding exactly who is going to do what by when, where, and how. You've already established the 'why' for trying a solution (the 'what')—now you need to pull out your phones, to-do lists, and calendars and make some notes about what you will each do to achieve the goal. It may seem obvious and unnecessary, but I've seen couples come up with a great plan and then not get specific about the who, when, and how of what they need to do, and in the busyness of life, the plan gets forgotten.

"The final letter in the Problem-Solving Technique is F, for follow-up. You need to set a time to follow up with each other to see whether the proposed solution worked. This also provides a motivating deadline to get it done. You can use your one-hour-per-week relationship care meeting as the time to review the success of or impediments to enacting the solution. Keep in mind that, just like our work together, everything new that you try is an experiment, and there may be unanticipated circumstances that block getting the solution in motion. You can then tweak the plan and try again, or devise an entirely new one as needed.

"If you get stuck at any place in the problem-solving sequence—difficulty setting the agenda, brainstorming, combining, compromising, or contracting—that means you need to go back to the Speaker-Listener Technique and discuss the issue further. Oftentimes, it may signal the presence of a hidden or broader issue around power and control, closeness and caring, respect and recognition, integrity or safety, trust, or commitment. I'll be teaching you a method for identifying these broader themes in our next session."

Ask the couple if they have any questions about the Problem-Solving Technique. If not, suggest that they do a short speaker-listener discussion about a higher-intensity issue, or use the one already discussed in the previous session, or one that they talked about during the week, and then have them try out problem solving. Your role as always is to keep them on task and to encourage them when they seem to hit a roadblock. Homework for the coming week should be doing a problem discussion and problem solving on another issue.

SESSION 3: REVIEW OF HOME-BASED PRACTICE, TEACH EXPLORING EXPECTATIONS AND HIDDEN ISSUES

In this session, make sure the couple is still up for continuing to learn the skills. If a pressing issue emerged during the week, ask them if they feel they can use it to learn the next set of skills, or whether they need to talk more freely with you about it. Check in with the couple on how they did with discussing and solving another problem, and address any issues they had in using the techniques.

Explain the role of expectations as follows: "All partners come to relationships with expectations and hopes of various sorts, about virtually all aspects of life together. Partners bring expectations about the division of household, financial, childcare, and other responsibilities; sex (how often, for how long, what they prefer in terms of sexual engagement) and other forms of intimacy; how to spend leisure time; relationships with in-laws and friends; the balance of work versus relationship time; religious or spiritual practices, cultural practices, and more. According to the PREP researchers, there are three types of expectations: those we are aware of ourselves but haven't expressed to our partners, sometimes because we fear that they may disagree or critique us about them; those we were not even initially aware of ourselves but that emerge when we sense that our partner has different expectations about something we simply took for granted; and those that are unreasonable, at least in relation to our partner's needs and capacities."

By this time, the couple has likely discussed their different expectations about one thing or another, and you can point out what you've heard as a different expectation or hope about some aspect of their lives together. Note that the Speaker-Listener and Problem-Solving Techniques are designed to help partners address these different expectations and suggest that in a future session you might work with them on one or more such expectations.

Next, describe a method for addressing hidden issues. "PREP researchers identified what they called hidden issues, broader themes in the relationship that pop up and fuel conflicts in specific areas like money, sex, child-rearing, domestic chores, and so on. I briefly described these earlier when I talked about the typical sorts of negative interpretations or 'theories of mal-intent' partners hold. There are six of these:

1. Caring and closeness: Feeling unloved or uncared about by your partner—or, on the other end of the spectrum, feeling that your partner's needs for expression of affection and love are excessive and overwhelming.
2. Power and control: Feeling pushed around or controlled by your partner—or, on the other end of the spectrum, feeling that you have too much control, too much responsibility.
3. Respect and recognition: Feeling your partner doesn't respect your ideas about how to solve problems, your beliefs, your feelings, the work that you do; or feeling that your partner doesn't recognize your efforts to improve the relationship or to contribute to a good life for you two [and if the couple has kids, you can add, 'for the family').
4. Integrity and safety: Feeling that your partner is doing something or asking you to do something that violates your values or your sense of comfort and safety.
5. Commitment: Feeling that your partner is not committed to the relationship.
6. Trust: Feeling that you can't trust your partner, that they are not honest.

"The 'mother' or 'father' of all hidden issues is acceptance—feeling that your partner just doesn't accept you for who you are, with your faults, even if you're working to correct some of those faults. I should note again that the need for acceptance does not mean 'unconditional acceptance.' The popular notion that we should accept our partner no matter what they do is problematic, because it goes against all those other hidden issues that are important: We expect to be loved and cared about, not to be pushed around, not to be made to feel unsafe or that our partner is doing something that violates our values, and so on. There are conditions for all relationships. But there's also the need to realize our partners have their challenges and imperfections, and that we also may have differences that are not entirely resolvable but can be lived with."

Here are the steps for helping couples identify the hidden issues or broader themes that fuel conflict.

1. Pick an issue that the couple has discussed with the Speaker-Listener Technique. Ask one partner to identify the hidden issue(s) (there may be more than one) that they sense are associated with that specific issue about money, housework, time together, and so on. If they get stuck, you can suggest what you've sensed are the hidden issue(s). Ask the other partner to do the same: What is (are) the hidden issue(s) underlying that specific issue?

2. Ask one of the partners to use a modified form of the XYZ statement that now includes the hidden issue: "When you do X behavior, in situation Y, I feel H [hidden issue] and Z emotion." For instance, "When you spend a lot of money (X) on downloadable music (Y), I feel I have no control over where our money goes (H), and that frightens me (Z)." Or another partner: "When you come home (Y) and don't greet me (X), I feel unloved (H), and hurt (Z)." Have the listener repeat what the speaker said.

3. Now ask the speaker to think about other issues that trigger that hidden issue for them. For instance, "I also feel controlled by you and powerless (H) when you insist on your desires (X) for how we should spend our weekends (Y), and that makes me feel silenced and frustrated (Z)." Or, "I also feel unloved and abandoned by you (H) when we go to a party (Y) and you quickly disappear and spend the evening talking with other people (X)—I feel sad and lonely when that happens (Z)." Have the listener repeat what the speaker said. The speaker should name up to three issues where the hidden issue seems relevant.

4. Now have the listener become the speaker. The new speaker

should go back to the original issue the first speaker discussed and name the hidden issue(s) underlying it: "When you criticize me (X) for spending money on downloadable music (Y), I feel unloved (H1) and unrecognized about all the stress I go through at work to support us (H2), especially since I think you know how much music helps me relieve stress; I feel really hurt about that (Z)." This partner has named two hidden issues underlying the conflict about his spending money on music. Have him pick one of those hidden issues and identify other specific issues in which he feels that hidden issue comes up: "I know I should be contributing more to keeping the house tidy, and I'm fine with that (Y), but when you get on my case about not doing my chores right when I come home and am exhausted (X), I feel hurt and insulted (Z) and unseen and unrecognized (H) for all the efforts I've made all day for our family." Once again, the speaker can name up to three issues where the hidden issue seems relevant.

5. Now that each partner has identified the hidden issue(s) underlying several specific areas of conflict, have them pick one of these to do some problem solving. Make the point that one cannot dissolve something as broad as a hidden issue all in one conversation. People can't just abstractly commit to no longer being controlling, unloving, disrespecting, and so on. The couple needs a specific plan for each partner to change their behavior so that the other feels there's some progress in chipping away at the hidden issue. Suggest that their efforts to eliminate the hidden issue in one domain will have multiplicative rather than additive effects. This means that it gets easier to address the presence of the hidden issue in a subsequent problem-solving conversation around a different specific issue.

For instance, if they've addressed how control issues fuel arguments about money and leisure activities, by the time they get ready to take that on in decisions about whose parents to visit over the holidays, they may find there's no longer a control struggle, and that they readily create a fairer balance of spending time with in-laws, because they've already addressed the control issue in other domains and are working toward greater power equity. Remind the couple that you will address the hidden issues each of them has named over subsequent sessions.

Vignette: Geetika and Aadesh

Geetika felt that Aadesh's reluctance to spend time with her family and his need to spend time alone after doing so connected to the broader, hidden issue of feeling unloved. She said, "When you become emotionally removed when we visit my family, and sometimes short and rude with them, I feel unloved and rejected by you, and lonely." Asked to reflect on other moments when she felt unloved, she said, "When I want to talk about my day, and you get distracted by your phone, look impatient, and say nothing, I also feel unloved and hurt." She also noted, "When you criticize me for crying and being 'overly sensitive,' I feel unsupported and unloved, and I get even more upset. She also reflected on her expectation that as a person of Bengali background, she had assumed he knew that Bengali families are very close and expect a great deal of connection with children's partners. She found herself having to explain his behavior to her family and to apologize for his rudeness and emotional distance.

For his part, Aadesh connected most to the hidden issues of control and respect or recognition. He said, "When I tell you I just can't take so much socializing with your family, or with friends, and you insist that we see them and even make plans without asking me, I feel you put me in an emotionally uncomfortable position, and I feel resentful and kind of frantic, because I know I just can't muster the energy to be social for so long. I've told you so many times that I am highly introverted and need a lot of private time in my head, but you still push me out of my comfort zone. I also feel that you don't recognize and respect how different my family is from yours—yes, my family is Bengali, but we don't talk a lot or spend that much time together, and I feel kind of hurt that you seem not to get that."

As to Geetika's feeling unloved when Aadesh criticized her for being too sensitive, he said the same issues of control pervaded these moments with her. He often felt her need for one-on-one intimate conversation was "endless" and felt controlled by her need for talking. Geetika responded, saying that she didn't feel her needs were so extraordinary, but that when she sensed he was pulling away, she would express herself more intensely in the hopes of reengaging him. Aadesh had been reluctant to fully immerse in dialogue about her feelings for fear that this would result in an endless conversation.

Further conversations explored all three of these hidden issues. The detailed plan they created about how to balance time with her family, with friends, time in one-to-one conversation, time alone, and the new category I suggested—time together but spent silently, with each engaged in their own reading—was a first important step toward dissolving their hidden issues. We also addressed Geetika's feeling of being criticized for being emotional and Aadesh feeling overwhelmed, by me pointing out that these moments represented the classic vicious cycle of withdrawing and pursuing—when Aadesh started to feel these conversations were limitless, he'd withdraw, and Geetika would pursue, confirming his worst fears. Setting a regular 20-minute period at the end of the day for talking greatly reduced Aadesh's worry that he'd be overwhelmed, and he experimented with being fully present to her during that time. He immediately saw, to his great surprise, that Geetika was fully satisfied with this amount of full attention from him.

BEGINNING ANEW FOR COUPLES: A MINDFULNESS-BASED APPROACH TO COUPLE COMMUNICATION

The distress prevention techniques of communication, problem solving, and identifying expectations and hidden issues, and related techniques and ideas from cognitive–behavioral couple therapy, have been shown to be effective (Baucom et al., 2015; Markman & Rhoades, 2012). However, with high-conflict last chance couples enveloped in strong negative affect and set in their negative views about one another, the Speaker-Listener Technique can sometimes result in a more civil, but still unempathic form of summarizing self syndrome, with each partner repeating their point of view and failing to gain compassion for the other's perspective and feelings.

To address these impasses, and to help couples more fully engage self-regulation techniques prior to talking, I've developed a mindfulness-based approach to couple communication that blends a tradition of conflict resolution used in Buddhist monasteries (yes, even monks and nuns have conflicts living together!) with the research-supported tools of cognitive–behavioral couple therapy. The Buddhist approach is called "Beginning Anew" (Khong, 2014), and the original format involves five steps, after a short period of silent, joint mindful breathing before speaking:

1. Flower watering: Giving the other a compliment or other statement of appreciation. This step aligns well with Gottman's (2011; Gottman & Gottman, 2018) finding that couples in which partners

make regular statements of admiration and appreciation do better over the years than those where such comments are absent.

2. Expressing regret: Sharing one or more things one regrets doing and apologizing for it.

3. Checking in: Asking for more information; asking the other partner if one has hurt them in some way.

4. Expressing hurt or disagreement: Naming a hurt that one feels the other has caused or an area of conflict. Particularly useful in this approach is that the person introduces the hurt felt at the hands of the other by saying, "I need your help with something." Gottman's (2011; Gottman & Gottman, 2018) research shows that couple conversations go better when partners engage in "soft startup"— gently raising an issue—as opposed to "hard startup," raising it with anger and resentment. His research indirectly supports this Buddhist-based method.

5. Hugging meditation: Even in the original format, this is an optional step; many highly distressed couples are not ready for physical contact, but eventually if things improve, it is, as Sister Chan Khong writes, "a wonderful way to end a session of Beginning Anew" (2014, p. 31). She notes further, "be sure to do it only when it feels right to you" (p. 31).

Whereas in the original Buddhist version the speaker can speak for as long as they desire while the other person listens quietly, the listener in a distressed couple cannot process that much information at once. Amending this approach by adding the rhythm of 10–15 seconds of speech from the speaker followed by the listener repeating it allows the listener to check in with the speaker to make sure the speaker was heard correctly. In addition, I've found that with couples, it works better to blend Step 3 (asking for more information) into Step 4, so that the speaker first describes what they found hurtful, and then asks the listener if there was something the speaker did that led to that hurtful behavior. When the listener gets the floor, they can comment on what has felt like hurtful behavior by the partner.

Here are the steps of this mindfulness-based approach to couple communication, which is integrated with the communication and problem-solving skills from PREP. I introduce this approach only after first teaching couples the basic Speaker-Listener and Problem-Solving Techniques. Highly distressed couples are generally not ready immediately to be authentically empathic, to express the hurts underneath their anger, or even to take much responsibility for their part in conflict. Once partners experience a more productive approach to expressing their anger and resentment, they are ready to take the next step toward empathy and apologies that are the core of this mindfulness-based approach.

Explain why you are introducing this approach to them: "You've done a great job learning the techniques I've taught you thus far. I'd like to introduce you to a mindfulness-based version of the Speaker-Listener and Problem-Solving Techniques, because I've found this can take you to the next step in developing more empathy for one another and becoming more of a team in dealing with conflicts that arise. It's designed to help you develop more calmness and compassion for one another before trying to solve a problem. Although it's based in part on a conflict resolution technique used in Buddhist monasteries, you don't need to be a Buddhist to do it! And remember what I told you about all the research that supports the effectiveness of mindful breathing and other mindfulness activities on anxiety, depression, and trauma."

1. Mindful breathing together: "I'd like you first to do 5 minutes of mindful breathing. You can use a beautiful stone, flower, or other object as something lovely to focus on." Show them a stone or flower as an example—I have several of these ready in my office.
2. Flower watering: Ask one partner to start. "This is a chance to share your appreciation and admiration for your partner. You should mention specific instances when your partner said or did something that you appreciated or admired. This is an opportunity to shine light on your partner's strengths and contributions, and to encourage the growth of your partner's positive qualities. When we practice flower watering, we support the development of good qualities in each other, and at the same time, we help to weaken problematic cognitive, emotional, and behavioral tendencies in each other. As in a garden, when we water the flowers of loving kindness and compassion in each other, we also take energy away from the weeds of intense anger, resentment, other upsetting emotions, and misperceptions."

    After the speaker has finished, just as in the regular technique, the listening partner should repeat back what they heard. If it's not exactly accurate, the speaker should repeat it until the listener gets it correctly. The speaker should try to keep their statement brief—speak only for about 15 seconds, then let the listener repeat, and continue the rhythm of speaking and repeating until the speaker has finished saying what they want to say.
3. Sharing regrets: Say to the speaker, "Now, apologize for something

you've done that you regret and feel sorry about. It doesn't have to be related to the thing you're upset about that your partner did. By offering an apology before naming the behavior you hope your partner will apologize for, you model the very thing you hope your partner will do, and you show that you realize they are not the only one in the relationship that has caused hurt. This has the effect of lowering your partner's potential defensiveness upon hearing about something they did or said that hurt you."

After the speaker has finished, the listening partner should repeat back what they heard. If it's not exactly accurate, the speaker should repeat it until the listener gets it correctly. Again, the speaker should try to keep the statement brief—speak only for about 15 seconds, then let the listener repeat, and continue the rhythm of speaking and repeating until the speaker has finished saying what they want to say.

4. Expressing a hurt: Say to the speaker, "Now you can tell your partner what it was that upset you, hurt your feelings, scared you, angered you, or other feelings—although remember, as we discussed, anger and frustration are secondary reactions to first feeling hurt, upset, insulted, scared, and other vulnerable feelings, so try to stick to or at least include one or more of those more vulnerable primary feelings. Start by saying something to the effect of, 'Honey/my dear, I need to ask for your help with something that happened between us.' Share how you felt with your partner due to their actions, including their speech. You can use the XYZ statement format. If you're going to include anger, remember to 'speak your anger' rather than 'do your anger'—it's fine to have a bit of distress in your voice tone, to sound angry if you are, but don't use your speech in this moment to cause further hurt. Just speak openly and clearly about your feelings. Modulate your anger so that your partner can hear you.

"After the speaker speaks, just as before, the listener should repeat back what was said. Now we're basically back to the Speaker-Listener Technique as you've already learned it. The speaker will get four to five turns to talk about their feelings about what happened. As part of that, you could explain how what your partner did reminds you of painful experiences you had in your family growing up, or in previous intimate relationships, and that these memories contribute to making what the partner did even a bit more painful. Be clear that, of course, these previous experiences are not your partner's fault—but that they do amplify the suffering you experience when your partner does or did hurtful things. Hopefully, when your partner hears about these experiences, it provides further motivation to change and to avoid hurting you again in these ways. In the original Buddhist/mindfulness version of Beginning Anew, talking about how an experience with your partner triggers old feelings and memories from the past is known as 'sharing a long-term difficulty and asking for support.'

"Finally, I'd suggest that you as the speaker ask if there was anything you did that might have led your partner to behave as they did. In other words, show that you are curious and concerned about how you might have done something that led to their reaction. This is in the spirit of that second step, expressing regret, and recognizing that you each usually play a role in the hurtful interactions that have happened. You can say something like, 'When you get to speak, I'd like to hear if there's something I did that upset you and led you to act as you did,' or you could say, 'I wonder if there's something I did that upset you, too.' In the original Beginning Anew format, this is called checking in, or asking for more information."

As you guide the speaker, encourage them to mention if what happened between the partners reminded them of a painful experience from the past, including in their family growing up. Don't push on this, just raise it. And if they forget to ask whether there was something they did that contributed to the other partner behaving as they did, remind them to do so.

Once the speaker has had up to four or five turns on this part of the process, the listener will get the floor, but this time, rather than immediately sharing their feelings and point of view on the topic, ask the new speaker to start with flower watering—saying something appreciative or admiring about the partner (as before, with the listening partner repeating what they heard, in this and subsequent steps). Then have the speaker go to sharing a regret. The regret can be about the topic the partner already raised as a hurt, or about something else. After those two steps, the new speaker should go back to the issue the other partner (first speaker) raised and talk about their perspective and feelings about it.

After both partners feel they've said all they need to say about the topic, have them go on to problem solving if it isn't immediately clear how to resolve the issue. Remind the partner that the next time they use Beginning Anew, the partner who was initially the listener in this conversation can start as the speaker and raise an issue that they "need help with."

Vignette: Geetika and Aadesh

Sensing that they could benefit from further developing a "climate of calmness and compassion" after mastering the Speaker-Listener Technique, I introduced Geetika and Aadesh to the Beginning Anew approach. Aadesh took the role of speaker first and "watered Geetika's flower" by noting that he loved her liveliness and gentleness, and admired her ability to express emotions, even though he had often felt overwhelmed by them. He acknowledged that he hadn't learned to express vulnerable feelings in his family of origin, where the parents discouraged emotional displays. He expressed regret that at times his need to "withdraw and refuel" led him to be terse and rude, including to her family and friends. He asked in a vulnerable, heartfelt manner for her help in making sure they would stick with the plan for how to divide their time, so that he could avoid this experience of being depleted.

For her part, Geetika watered Aadesh's flower by saying she admired his strength, intelligence, ability to be organized, honesty, and forthrightness, even though at times this came across as rude. Now more fully understanding his sense of emotional and energic depletion after social interactions as his area of vulnerability, and his need to take care of himself not as a rejection of her or her family, she apologized for not taking him seriously and pushing him for more time with her family. She, too, said she sought his help to stick with their new plan for "different types of time" and to make sure their nightly "decompression time conversations" happened.

REPAIRING RUPTURES AND MUTUAL SOOTHING

Gottman (2011; Gottman et al., 2015; Gottman & Gottman, 2018) found that couples in which partners repair effectively after conflict do better over time than couples that remain in a state of simmering resentment. Effective repair occurred when partners addressed the rupture quickly; when partners addressed each other's feelings rather than focusing on their different perceptions of the problematic moment or offering solutions; when partners took responsibility for their part; when they disclosed their own feelings but softened their anger, empathized with and validated their partner's feelings, and even complimented their partner; when they used humor; when they provided reassurance to the partner and about the state of the relationship ("We're OK"; Gottman & Gottman, 2018, p. 81); and at the end of the conversation, celebrated their success in repairing their connection by focusing on their teamwork in addressing their conflict. In contrast, partners who did not repair well engaged in rational problem-solving prematurely, criticized each other's suggestions, promised to change their behavior prior to hearing their partner's feelings, and became defensive by providing excuses for their behavior or by referring to times when the partner had upset them.

Gottman et al.'s (2015) research findings centered on newlywed couples just setting off on their journey together, and yet even in this group found those who already had difficulty with repair. Thus it is no surprise that high-conflict last chance couples typically have little sense of how to repair after conflict. The Speaker-Listener Technique provides a ready-made tool for repair. But a few more suggestions are useful to help couples respond to ruptures in the moment, potentially reducing the number of times they need to engage in a full speaker-listener and problem-solving conversation.

1. Easy apologies. To avoid defensiveness, suggest to couples that they apologize for the *impact* of their behavior, even when they had no *intention* of hurting or otherwise offending their partner. Falconier and colleagues (2015) note that an intimate relationship inevitably involves "daily hassles"—moments of irritation with one's partner, of feeling misunderstood, not heard, taken aback, and inconvenienced. I call these "sandpaper moments"—when in the rush to get to work, to handle the kids, or other daily responsibilities, we "rub up against one another" in unpleasant ways. High-conflict couple partners have "practiced" their negative attributions about one another (Bradbury & Fincham, 1990) for so long that they immediately assume negative intent when their partner's behavior may simply have been due to being stressed themselves, not paying full attention, or forgetting something the partner asked them to do or be mindful of. From a psychoanalytic perspective, negative attributions result from a rupture in connection which leads to an incapacity to "mentalize" (Asen & Fonagy, 2012)—to hold the partner's mind in mind and construe the motivations behind their behavior in a more compassionate fashion.

Correspondingly, partners are often highly motivated to demonstrate to each other that they are not the evil, thoughtless, self-centered people their partner believes them to be, and so may become defensive when the other complains about their behavior. Normalizing these sandpaper moments helps partners stop feeling they must walk on eggshells with one another—after all, eggshells crack with just the slightest bit of applied pressure, so it's futile to try to avoid these moments. Instead, suggest to couples that they get more comfortable accepting that they can't be perfect with each other, recognize that they will inevitably irritate or even offend their partners on a fairly regular basis, and be ready to offer an easy apology—one that is given even when one had no negative intentions to be hurtful. After apologizing in a genuine, caring tone for the impact of one's behavior (not resentfully, as in, "Well, I'm *sorry*, okay? Geesh!"), it's fine to add reassurance that one had no intention to cause upset. Partners can even explain what was going on in their head—"I was distracted, I forgot," and so on. But they should avoid a defensive stance and long explanation.

2. Neuroeducation and discussion of shame and guilt. Some further neuroeducation and discussion about the emotions experienced when a partner is upset with the other can help partners handle ruptures effectively. Ask them how they feel when their partner tells them they hurt the partner's feelings, insulted them, or upset them in some other way. Partners will usually describe feelings of shame or guilt, and resentment at being "made to feel that way when I didn't mean anything by it." Remind the couple what you taught them in an earlier session about how the sympathetic nervous system (fight or flight) gets activated when we perceive possible danger or threat. When a partner feels insulted or hurt, the natural reaction is to either withdraw or attack. Validate the experience that even if a partner simply voices in a nonconfrontational manner that something the other did hurt them, the partner hearing this complaint may experience it as an attack on their sense of self as a good person, and experience shame ("I've been bad") or guilt ("I did something wrong to someone"). If they didn't intend to hurt the partner, they may then feel unjustly criticized, resentful, and defensive.

Adopting the attitude that, try as one might not to offend one's partner, we inevitably will do something irritating or hurtful accidentally can reduce the intensity of shame or guilt. However, some level of shame or guilt is inevitable, and can be viewed as a good sign—that as angry as someone may generally feel toward their partner, part of them still cares enough about the partner to feel badly about hurting their feelings. Or even if they are so angry at their partner that they don't care much about them, the feelings of shame or guilt at least indicate that they are invested in being a good person—in psychoanalytic terms, they have a conscience or superego. Suggest that in these moments of being told they hurt their partner, accepting, sitting with, and breathing through those feelings of shame or guilt for a few seconds is a good first step before responding. Then offer the easy apology.

However, they must also realize that it takes a little time for the hurt partner's nervous system to settle down. As a result, apologizing doesn't usually lead the partner immediately to feel better. They may even repeat their complaint because they're still upset, and the best thing to do is just to calmly apologize again, rather than say something like, "Why are you still upset? I *apologized* already!"

3. Mutual soothing. This is a good moment also to discuss the importance of mutual soothing in couple relationships (Gottman & Gottman, 2018). Ask each partner what they need most from each other when they're upset, either at the partner or about something else. As noted earlier, partners often say they don't know, and may reflect that in their families growing up, they rarely experienced soothing from a parent figure. For instance, because in Aadesh's family, expression of any sign of emotional vulnerability was discouraged—"My parents adopted the white English motto 'Chin up!' whenever I hurt myself on the playground or had a problem with a classmate"—he rarely experienced comforting from his parents.

In another couple discussed more fully below, Talia related that her connection with her mother centered almost entirely around the mother's complaints about the father; Talia felt she couldn't come to her mother for emotional care and was implicitly forbidden by her mother from seeking out her father, as that would demonstrate to the mother that Talia was being disloyal. In yet another couple, Richard was a high-powered lawyer whose parents had disowned him when he decided not to become a doctor like his father. He received little soothing from them: instead, quite the opposite—shaming for selecting a profession based on his career desires.

Ask the couple to imagine what might be helpful. Often, they will say that a quiet, calm voice tone and words showing empathy and compassion for their feelings might help. Sometimes, some form of physical connection—holding hands, a hug, or a warm gaze—is also desired. Have them try this in the session. Have each partner take turns talking about a previous hurt and have the other experiment with an apology, delivered in a warm and soothing tone.

Next, ask the partners each to talk about something that happened outside the relationship that was upsetting—at work, with a friend or family member, or while shopping or traveling—and have the listening partner try soothing the upset partner. Suggest that they avoid giving each other advice about how to solve the problem. As I noted earlier, in cisgender heterosexual relationships, men often try to soothe their partner by offering advice, and women often feel this is patronizing, or at least not what they are looking for: "I know what to do about it. I just wanted to talk about my feelings!" Suggest again that the listening, soothing partner instead simply utter empathic murmurings such as, "Oh, wow, that happened?" "Really? He did that? And then what happened?" or "So you felt [repeat the feeling the partner stated]" or "Sorry to hear that, honey!"

The challenge in doing this work with last chance high-conflict couple partners is to encourage them to try interactions that go against their well-refined antipathy toward one another and their hopelessness about the relationship's potential. Years of misunderstandings, hurts, anger, grievance, and the resulting loneliness have led them to feel that it is emotionally irrational to treat each other with compassion and care. Yet paradoxically, it is the desperate longing for just such care and compassion that has led to bitter resignation. Framing these efforts as experiments in possibility frees them up to see what the new patterns might yield. Suggest that they have nothing to lose by trying, and that if it doesn't yield positive results, this outcome will still be helpful in deciding about the future of the relationship. Often, couples are surprised at how quickly their feelings toward one another change with relatively simple changes in how they relate.

Derek and Julie were in great conflict around Derek's demanding career that had resulted in numerous placements abroad. What was supposed to be an 18-month position in another country led to 14 years moving from one country to another. This resulted in disruption of Julie's career, and she often felt lonely in the new countries, which led her to feel a great deal of resentment. Although Derek initially balked at apologizing for the effects of his work on Julie's career and social comfort—"We're having a pretty good life, with nice homes, help around the house and with the kids, lots of adventures in different countries!"—he eventually recognized that despite these benefits, Julie's feelings had merit. He apologized for the impact of his career on aspects of her life, and this went a long way to helping her feel validated, which led her to take steps to adjust as best she could to their circumstances.

Other issues may interfere with last chance couples taking this relatively simple, commonsense and research-supported advice about repair and mutual soothing. The following case vignette illustrates how a partner's volatile temperament and issues of gender and power initially blocked a couple's attempts at utilizing these practices as well as the communication skills.

Vignette: Bahir and Sarah

Bahir, 39, a second-generation Saudi American and Sarah, 37, a white Anglo-American whose family, originally from Sweden and Norway, had been in the United States for many generations, were considering divorce after six years of frequent explosive fights. Married for three years, they had a 15-month-old daughter. Both partners had highly successful careers, Bahir as an entrepreneur and CEO of his company, Sarah in public relations. Bahir acknowledged often feeling impatient and exhibiting his "intense temper," which would initially overwhelm and silence Sarah, until she'd "had enough" and would fight back.

The partners described quite different models of communication from their respective families of origin: Bahir said that like many Saudi families, feelings were put "right out there" at a high volume, and then the family would simply move on without discussing the issue, only to fight again once the issue arose. He said, "There was a lot of emotion, but nothing ever got solved, and I was the angriest of all of them." Sarah described her family as "classic WASP—there were never any fights, and if you were unhappy with someone, you were expected to raise the issue in a low-key way, if at all." Although their differences in temperament and emotional style were initially a source of attraction—Sarah admired Bahir's ability to assert himself; Bahir loved and admired Sarah's more "genteel" manner—they had become polarized in their emotional styles and felt they could not, in Sarah's words, "untangle ourselves." With the birth of their daughter Samantha, they realized they needed to change, and if they couldn't, would be better off apart.

The couple agreed that a good start would be to learn communication and problem-solving skills along with mindfulness practices to calm down before or during an argument. Bahir was so impressed with these skills that he said he would start using them in his company, where he frequently engaged in outbursts with his staff and colleagues. Sarah was relieved that Bahir found these skills appealing. However, in the following session, they reported difficulty in implementing them, because Bahir's temper would get the best of him.

As we explored his relationship with his own anger, it became clear that Bahir was ambivalent about working to control it. He spoke with some pride about times when getting extremely angry had helped him deal with other men who tried to intimidate him, and said moreover that this was such a lifelong "part of me" that he didn't think he could eliminate it. I said that the goal was not to eliminate his capacity for intense anger, but to get more control over when and with whom he used his "firepower." By coincidence, he was an amateur rock drummer who was thinking about pursuing more formal lessons, and he and Sarah had seen on my website and in chapters from my book on couples and time that I am a professional drummer. I used this connection between us (and frankly, me being the professional and he the aspiring amateur desiring lessons) to suggest that just as a drummer needs to be able to play soft and slow as well as loud and fast depending on the tune and what the rest of the band wanted, he needed to be able to modulate his intensity in different relationships and that, clearly, his expressions of anger were too fast and loud for Sarah. This analogy appealed to Bahir, and he recommitted to working on reducing his expressions of rage.

However, the couple reported that the day after that session, they had the worst fight of their entire marriage and decided they would ask me to help them get divorced, although the despondent look in their eyes and the strong attachment and love for each other that I'd heard about in the first session suggested to me that they were hoping I could help them avert this path. Sarah described the details of the fight: "We woke up to the sound of leaf blowers, which you hear a lot in this suburban neighborhood [the couple had moved a few months earlier from California and were renting a house while looking to purchase one], and Bahir got very annoyed, and yelled about it. We've been looking at a house online that's near a local airport, and we've been trying to get in touch with the realtor, who's slow in answering our emails, to find out about noise from the airport. Bahir got irritated about that, too, and I suggested he drive to the house to check it out. He got really angry with me, yelling and saying, why did I want him to go there? Did I want to get rid of him 'cause he was angry? I said, not at all. I thought it would give him a break from the leaf blowers, and we could check out the house ourselves. He kept yelling, and I finally snapped, and started crying like I always do, but then later, I got really mad and said, 'I hate you!'—which I regretted right away. I don't hate him. I hate what he's like when this other person comes out, and I can't take it anymore. Plus, Samantha was in my lap, getting upset, and later it took me an hour to get her down—I had to have her fall asleep on my chest, and she's never like that. She usually goes to sleep right away. I know you taught us the communication technique, and I've tried to do it with Bahir, but in these moments, it doesn't work."

Bahir concurred with Sarah's description of the fight, but added, "She said some other things too, like, 'You're just a mean person.' I'm just so sick of this always being about me and my anger."

I sensed a challenging moment in sustaining the therapeutic alliance. I risked alienating Bahir if I agreed with Sarah about his problematic rage. I looked at him with a mix of understanding and regret about what I had to say, and said, "Well, I hope this won't be our last session, because what I have to say is likely to make you feel again that we're focusing on your anger. By saying you don't want to have this be all about your anger, I'm feeling a bit like my hands are tied, but I'm gonna take a chance and say it anyway." Bahir grimaced slightly but responded that I could go on, as if he too knew discussing his rage was unavoidable. "I kind of feel like you were doing a bit more 'research' to see if it's possible to keep responding with that level of intense anger with Sarah, and I think the research suggests it won't work. I guess one way to think about it is that this is the moment for you to really take charge of your 'firepower,' and remember, I said in a previous session that I don't think this is about not being able to get that angry sometimes. I'm not suggesting that you have to change entirely as a person and eliminate anger, just that you need to choose when and when not to use it." Bahir's face showed a bit of remorse, but he agreed.

I then concurred with Sarah that the Speaker-Listener Technique can't work when one or both partners are that rageful, and reminded the couple about the time-out rule (they had decided on the term *volcano* as their signal for calling a time-out). I went on to suggest that if they could catch a "flammable or eruptible moment" (when the volcano is about to erupt) quickly enough and do some repair, they might not need to engage in the Speaker-Listener Technique at all. I introduced the notion of rupture and repair as described above, noting that we inevitably irritate or offend our partners inadvertently and unintentionally at times. I suggested, "An easy apology in which we acknowledge that we upset our partner without getting defensive about it often helps the other settle down. However, it sometimes takes one or two more reassuring apologies to get through and have an effect, because the partner's sympathetic nervous system has its own pace for settling down." Sarah said, "Yes, but I really meant to be helpful to Bahir. I had no negative intentions at all—so why should I apologize?" I agreed that it might seem odd to apologize when our behavior was positively intended, but suggested that she view that behavior as a stimulus that evoked a response due to Bahir's over-sensitivity to criticism about his anger, and that an apology for the impact of her behavior would just serve to tell him he was hearing her incorrectly.

Although both partners understood the possible usefulness of repair, Sarah raised a great point—that as a woman in a world where women are often expected to apologize for their well-intentioned behavior that nevertheless challenges a man, she was reluctant to apologize to Bahir when something she said or did led him to become rageful. "I don't want to have to be the one who tries to control his temper!" I found her response extremely important, and as further evidence that the simple, research-based, and seemingly common-sense ideas and practices we offer to couples are often not so simple, as they are filtered through the couple's issues around power and responsibility—in this case, due to gender and the larger patriarchal assumptions in our culture designed to keep women subservient and docile (Knudson-Martin et al., 2015).

I agreed wholeheartedly with Sarah, and said that this was an excellent point. I restated that indeed, Bahir needed to take charge of his anger, and that this was not Sarah's responsibility. At the same time, if he could instead express a lower level of hurt or irritation and she could quickly offer reassurance that she did not mean what he thought she meant, and if he could then calm down, they could avert an escalation. I emphasized that the practice of apologizing went "both ways"—he needed to offer such reassurances to Sarah as well. I reiterated that Bahir needed to become more attuned to his mounting irritation (which started not with Sarah's comment, but with the noise of the leaf blowers) and needed to actively engage in self-soothing. I also concurred with Sarah's concern, which Bahir shared, about the effects on Samantha, and noted that a large amount of research indicates the negative effects of high couple conflict on children (Repetti et al., 2002). I told them about a public service announcement addressing domestic violence that was posted in the New York City subways some years ago—a large photo of a young child with big eyes, with the caption, "This is a highly sensitive recording device." Both partners looked appropriately distressed to hear about this ad, and Bahir more calmly repeated that he would really get to work on modulating his anger.

Sarah raised yet another important point: that because the couple rarely spent time with each other in pleasurable activities—they were either working, taking care of Samantha, house shopping, or attending to other tasks—they didn't have a buffer of positive feelings between them to rely on to bounce back from these conflicts. She said, "Bahir is so loving toward Samantha, but I don't get any of that! I feel like we don't have a cushion, and when we fight like this, it's like we're dropping from a high building and smashing into the sidewalk!" Bahir agreed and suggested that they reinstitute a once-a-week movie night. I also suggested another activity—the 60-second pleasure point practice, described in more detail below—that could strengthen their pleasurable bond even during this time-pressed busy time, and with relatively little effort. The couple laughed as they brainstormed about fun, pleasurable, and even sensual activities that took only a minute or less that they could institute on a daily basis. Sarah suggested, "A foot massage, I'd love a foot massage, or a hand massage!" Bahir laughed and added, "Any kind of short massage, head, shoulders. . . . " Sarah laughed and said, "Or a kiss!" Bahir added, "Or looking into each other's eyes—we never look into each other's eyes anymore!" Both laughed and looked at each other warmly. The session ended on this much more positive note, with the couple equipped with some repair skills, and Bahir finally committed to taking charge of his anger.

In our session the following week, Sarah and Bahir were warm and friendly toward each other, reported they'd had no conflicts, and felt much closer. Bahir had started reading a book I'd recommended on a Zen Buddhist approach to managing anger written by a self-described Type A lawyer (Scheff & Edmiston, 2010), and found it "spoke to" him. The session focused on exploring hidden issues—particularly, Sarah sometimes feeling unloved and uncared about, and Bahir feeling that Sarah sometimes didn't recognize how he was trying to avoid offering advice about how to solve whatever issue she was facing, which he now saw she interpreted as "not caring." We clarified that although she did not want Bahir to try to solve her work issues, she did welcome caring gestures, she said, "like holding my hand or giving me a kiss or a hug" when she was feeling vulnerable.

For instance, during the week she had a painful medical procedure related to fertility treatments that they were beginning in hopes of having a second child; Bahir was in the room with her, but, she said, "He sat behind me and didn't offer me any comfort." Bahir explained that he "wasn't looking at [his] phone or anything!" and was trying to respect her request that he not try to "fix things," so he sat back. Now that Bahir understood the difference between Sarah's desires for him to "just listen" when she talked about her work travails versus wanting comfort when she was sad, anxious, or in pain about personal issues, he felt ready to offer that comfort. For her part, Sarah revised her belief that Bahir didn't see her suffering, but rather, had been trying to respect her need for autonomy, albeit too globally. This exploration of their respective hidden issues helped them repair that moment in the doctor's office.

PRACTICES TO ENHANCE PLEASURE AND MUTUAL ADMIRATION

The intensity of high-conflict last chance couples' discord can easily lead them, and therapists, to focus solely on their destructive interactional style and assume that if they improve their communication and solve their disputes, they will be convinced that it's worth staying together. But it's important to remember that when they met and found each other attractive, partners didn't think to themselves, "Hmm, that seems like someone I could manage challenges and solve problems with!" They were drawn to each other by a mixture of physical attraction, sexual and intellectual compatibility, shared aesthetics, interests, and leisure activities, shared values, an initial sense of mutual compassion and care, and similar visions for their futures. Reducing conflict does not automatically result in couples increasing engagement in pleasurable activities (Fincham & Beach, 2010).

Therefore, as early as possible, therapy needs to encourage couples to experiment with possibilities of restoring and enhancing these sources of pleasurable, positive connection so that partners can better determine whether they want to remain with each other. Couples are more motivated to work on reducing conflict and engaging the admittedly artificial-feeling communication skills if they sense that the relationship will also provide pleasure and positive, loving connection. Research shows that increasing leisure time from 1.7 hours to 4.9 hours per week led to a 50% decrease in the probability of a marriage ending (Hill, 1988). The amount of leisure time couples spend together has been strongly associated with higher relationship satisfaction and lower levels of conflict (Berg et al., 2001; Birchler & Webb, 1977; Birchler et al., 1975; Crawford et al., 2002). In contrast, the degree to which partners pursue independent leisure activities is associated with lower levels of relationship satisfaction (Holman et al., 1984).

Yet high-conflict couples are reluctant to engage in extended potentially pleasurable activities such as the oft-prescribed date night or a full weekend day together centered on enjoyment. They worry, rightly so, that if they sit at a table for a few hours of an attempted reboot of the romantic dinners of the past, that light conversation will devolve into conflict, starting perhaps with disagreements about the quality of the food or service, or the cost of the entrees, leading relentlessly on to criticisms of each other's too-high or too-low standards, on to complaints from one partner that the other has been too devoted to work to make time for dinners (even though they are now there, having dinner); and on from there to all manner of criticisms. Or they will fear that they have little to talk about, given that their conversations for months or years have been solely focused on disagreements and mutual antipathy, and possibly ending the relationship; or even that awkward attempts at an evening together will remind them of how easy it once was, eliciting a discouraging contrast to their current level of disconnect. All not good for digestion!

Instead, initial experiments in pleasurable connection need to be brief and emotionally safe. Below are listed some recommended low-cost, high-yield pleasure and positive connection starters. These activities can be suggested even in a first session as homework to experiment with before the next session.

The Daily Relational Vitamin: Statements of Enjoyment, Appreciation, and Admiration

As noted earlier, Gottman's research indicates that couples in which partners make regular statements of appreciation and admiration do better over time (Gottman & Gottman, 2018). Most high-conflict couple partners complain of feeling unappreciated, disrespected, unseen, and taken for granted. They often bitterly and jealously contrast the sparse attention given them by their partner with how excited their partners get when talking with friends, acquaintances, work colleagues, and family members about their activities, recent achievements, interests, and ideas. They may notice that their partners comment on how great someone else looks in a new set of clothes or with a new hairstyle, but never receive that kind of approving gaze from one another. They may show more pleasure and warmth interacting with their kids—and even their pets—than with one another. It's not uncommon for one partner to comment to another in session, "If you only showed me the same love you give to our cat/dog/pig, I'd be happy!"

Suggest that each morning, partners make one statement of enjoyment, admiration, or appreciation to their partner. Just like taking a multivitamin, such statements start the day with an act of strengthening the couple's bond, which will help them weather ongoing "attacks" on their relationship's "immune system." Appreciating what the partner does for the couple's shared life—even if it's something they do regularly, like working hard to provide support, taking care of the kids, domestic chores—can start to restore a sense of being valued and can correct the sense of being taken for granted.

Even more powerful are statements that center on aspects of the partner that have nothing directly to do with what they do for each other. Partners can compliment one another on how they look today, on a recent work achievement ("I'm proud of you/delighted for you that . . . "), or on small moments of nonverbal behavior that they enjoy and that they may never have commented on, or haven't for some time—how the other laughs, and smiles, and frowns; how they walk purposefully down the street in a determined gait; their voice tone when making a point, being gentle, or when sad; how their eyes light up when telling a story; how they have a distant gauzy look when sitting quietly with a cup of tea and staring out the window. These small observations of one's partner fall into the category of what I call "getting a kick out of you," after the Cole Porter song made famous by Frank Sinatra (Fraenkel, 2001b): We enjoy the very presence of our partner, as "human poetry in motion"—taking pleasure from who they are apart from what they do for us, and apart from what they're accomplishing in the couple's shared life.

The 60-Second Pleasure Point Activity

After validating the partners' trepidation about spending extended time together, tell them that you will offer an activity that makes use of quite small amounts of time to start experimenting with positive connection (Fraenkel, 1998b, 2011). Ask them to brainstorm with you all the fun, pleasurable, or even sensual (but not sexual) activities they can do with one another in which the activity is 60 seconds or less in length—a minute or less of fun, pleasure, or sensual sharing. Even highly distressed couples will offer up, often with a surprising smile, the following sorts of activities: a hug, short massage (hand, foot, shoulder, head), or even a kiss; stroking each other's hair, looking into one another's eyes, looking together out the window at a tree or squirrel or a deer passing through their property while holding hands; a short dance to music; feeding each other a piece of chocolate or a berry; smelling a calming or invigorating scent; or, as one elderly Jewish gentleman from Brooklyn suggested in a gravelly voice during a couple workshop years ago, "stroking your partna wid a velvet mitt!" In another workshop, a young couple attired in punk rock regalia offered, "Dressing the cat!" and explained that they had a small chest of drawers filled with cat-sized clothes with which they would dress the cat and post photos on Instagram.

Next, ask the couple to brainstorm things they can do that take less than 60 seconds when apart. Suggestions have included a loving, erotic, or humorous text; sending a photo of something interesting or humorously mundane that captures how their day is going, or a close-up photo of an object with the tag line, "Guess what it is?"; a short affectionate call; or a suggested plan for the evening when they reunite. Explain that a branch of perceptual psychology known as the Gestalt School (Köhler, 1947) discovered that when subjects are subliminally exposed to a row of dots, they reported they saw a line. You can show them a piece of paper with three dots arranged with one dot at the top, two spread apart at the bottom, and ask them what they see, and they will inevitably say "a triangle." Note that this finding established that the mind automatically "connects the dots" of our experience. Suggest that they do six of these 60-second pleasure points across the day—two in the morning before they depart from one another, two when apart, and two when together again, with each partner initiating one of these pleasure points in each of the three time periods. Suggest that they may find that with just six of these pleasure points a day, they will experience an "arc of connection" that greatly exceeds the amount of time invested.

Some highly distressed couples may balk even at just these six minutes or less of connection; suggest instead that they do four of them, or even just two. Some partners may say that they don't feel highly motivated to engage in pleasure, or that enacting these pleasurable moments feels forced, artificial. Remind them of the second and third principle of the Creative Relational Movement theory of change: Trying something new will inevitably feel awkward and even irrational, given how negatively they've felt about one another (Principle 2). High motivation is not necessary to start the change process and, in fact, when coming out of a long period of conflict and considering divorce, it's normal not to feel strongly or consistently motivated (Principle 3). The hope is that in spite of these attitudes and feelings, engaging in small bits of potential pleasure may evoke a beginning, surprising sense of enjoyable connection, and may even evoke memories of such connection from their more positive past, leading them spontaneously to enact longer periods of shared pleasure time.

The Decompression Chamber

Not surprisingly, research shows that the greatest number of arguments between partners occur after reuniting at the end of the day (Larson & Almeida, 1999). High-conflict couples generally do not engage in daily check-ins at the day's end, or, if they do, these conversations center wholly on discussions of tasks not yet completed, often generating criticism ("You call this cleaning a kitchen? What are you doing all day?"), disagreement ("I didn't say I'd clean the kitchen!" "Yes, you promised!"), and resentment ("I thought *you* were going to clean the kitchen! Why do I have to do it when I've worked all day?"). The vast body of research on the effects of "negative spillover from work"—transmitting stress from the day spent in work outside or inside the home (including childcare) into relationships (Fraenkel & Capstick, 2012) indicates that partners need specific practices for reducing work-related negative arousal and for preparing to reconnect. Yet as Gottman's (Gottman & Gottman, 2018) and Markman, Stanley, and colleagues' (2010) research indicates, people view friendship and mutual support as a major component of an intimate partnership, and the end of the day provides a natural rhythm to foster these elements of a happy relationship.

As noted earlier, partners often lack specific, effective means of self-soothing, or have different needs and expectations about how to decompress and reconnect at the end of the day. One partner may want to spend quiet time alone, exercise, take a long shower, or watch TV before talking, while another wants to launch immediately into conversation, and conflict ensues. One partner—especially the main breadwinner—may assume privilege for attending to their needs, leaving the other feeling their needs are viewed as less important. The decompression chamber activity helps couples equitably reconcile their different needs (Fraenkel, 1998a, 2011).

Ask the partners what they each need to unwind at the end of the day and to reconnect. Explain the concept of negative spillover from work and ask how each of them feels at the end of the day. Introduce the metaphor of the decompression chamber: Just as a deep-sea diver needs to come to the surface slowly after being many meters down, people generally need reliable ways to calm down and release stress at the end of the day. Have them create a detailed sequence of solo and joint activities, with compromises as needed.

For instance, Geetika preferred that she and Aadesh greet each other immediately and talk for an extended period, whereas Aadesh needed some quiet time before engaging. They created a compromise routine in which they would greet each other, chat for 20 minutes about their respective days, and then Aadesh would spend 30 minutes with end-of-day emails, while Geetika read or called family and friends. They would then have dinner together and watch a movie or read their separate books together on the couch.

In another couple, Tim spent three hours commuting to and from work, and was "fried" when he came home. Laura, who had decided to leave work and be a full-time parent until their toddler, James, started kindergarten, was equally exhausted by day's end. Tim usually felt that he would need an entire evening to fully relax, which he never did, because Laura wanted him to take James for an hour while she took a walk, and wanted him also to help with housework, activities which he agreed to in principle, but carried out resentfully. The couple worked out a plan in which they would greet each other warmly, and Tim would get 30 minutes to play his guitar in their bedroom, then take over with James while Laura took a walk or spent time knitting for an hour, followed by dinner. This routine brought both partners great relief. Within a few days, Tim found he could obtain the same level of decompression playing guitar in the living room with James crawling in and out of the guitar case, and Laura often joined them.

The Silent Walk

It's almost a truism and certainly a caricature of professional and popular couple experts' advice columns that couples "need to communicate more" to have greater intimacy. I may be one of the few couple therapists who think that couples often need to talk less and do more, silently yet together. A wonderful song by jazz singer Michael Franks ("Living on the Inside," from the album *Tiger in the Rain*) about a couple's cozy weekend day when one partner practices piano and the other works on saving an endangered species while they share a pot of Tibetan tea provides a different model for intimate time, one without words. Especially with high-conflict couples who readily erupt into arguments, learning to spend time together in silence can open a whole new mode of intimate and nonrisky connection. I suggest couples take a silent walk in nature, or in a neighborhood with which they are unfamiliar, with partners occasionally pointing out to one another (silently) something interesting or beautiful (Fraenkel, 2011).

Engaging the Arts for Deeper Connection

Especially with couples who've been together many years, it's unlikely that they can regularly come up with interesting, entertaining things to talk about without some external stimulus. One or both partners may long for a deeper connection, and yet even when they're getting along fairly well, it's unreasonable to expect partners to share novel feelings about their daily lives, their hopes and dreams, most of which have likely been revealed long ago. Partners may misinterpret each other's difficulty coming up with something to say as an unwillingness to connect, when they're simply at a loss for saying something novel and interesting. When couples are in high conflict and considering divorce, they are understandably reluctant to share their feelings, hopes, and dreams—some of which may be about leaving the relationship.

Instead, couples can listen to music together and then talk about what the music evoked for each of them. Music is often treated as aural wallpaper for other activities such as dinners or housework, rather than the focus of an evening together. Likewise, reading a novel or short story together, or poetry, actually looking at those big coffee table photo or art books, watching a film, and engaging other arts can provide novel stimuli to prompt an enjoyable discussion.

Conjoint Mindfulness Activities: Creating a Culture of Calmness and Compassion

I've already discussed the powerful effects of mindfulness practices and how important it is for couples to utilize them before a problem discussion or during a time-out when things escalate. When couples practice these skills together regularly—meditation, Tai Chi, Qigong, yoga, prayer—it can create a culture of calmness and compassion. Encourage couples to pick a mindfulness-based activity and practice it together daily, or take an in-person, DVD-based, or online class on one of these activities together.

Blending Connection With Chores

As I discussed in Chapter 3, one of the five time myths that keep couples from connecting is the notion that chores should not be combined with pleasure (Fraenkel, 2011). Yet chores provide naturally occurring rhythms of activities that can be utilized for connection. Cooking together, cleaning the kitchen, folding laundry, raking leaves, even doing simple financial activities provide opportunities to talk, tell stories, share humor, and so on. In addition, by promoting chores as opportunities for connection, you will also help partners equalize the amount of domestic labor they engage in, eliminating a significant source of conflict (Fraenkel & Capstick, 2012).

Sensate Focus: Restarting Sex

When couples are ready to reengage sexually but have been literally and figuratively out of touch for a long time, the classic sex therapy activity of sensate focus can provide a safe, unchallenging, beginning reorientation to one another's bodies (Masters & Johnson, 1975). One partner takes the role of giver, and the other is the receiver. Encourage them to decide together on sounds (music, recordings of waves or rain) and smells (incense, candles) that will enhance the experience, and to use massage oil. The giver gives a sensual but not sexual massage—avoiding whatever body parts the receiver says are too erogenous—and experiments with pace (slow to fast), rhythm, and depth of pressure (light to firm) on the receiver's body, with the receiver giving feedback on what feels good and what does not through simple sounds and words—"Mmm, yeah, nice," or "Too fast/too light/too firm," and as the giver adjusts the strokes based on feedback, "Yeah, that's great, mmm. . . " So that it doesn't arouse anxiety, instruct the couple that they are not to have sex as part of this activity. Otherwise, one or both anxious partners may have difficulty enjoying it, for fear that it's leading up to sex, for which they're not ready. If they mutually decide to go on to have sex, that's fine, but at the outset the expectation should be that sex will not follow sensate focus.

Introducing Novelty Into Pleasure Time

Research by Aron and colleagues (2000) and others has established two types of leisure time: core and balance activities. Core activities are those that are easy to arrange, require few resources, and are more commonplace, like dinner at home, watching TV or movies, or taking walks around the neighborhood or in an easily accessible park. Balance activities introduce novelty and usually involve accessing resources outside the home: dance lessons, yoga and pottery classes, hikes or athletic activities in new and more distant settings, vacations in faraway places, going to the theater or a jazz club. Research shows that couples need both sorts of leisure—reliable sources of pleasure and connection as well as novel activities, especially those that provide challenges to learn them that couples can experience together, and which provide opportunities for partners to experience normal levels of anxiety in learning something new, and to reassure one another that they are mastering the requisite skills of the activity (Aron et al., 2000). Novel activities promote a sense of self-expansion (Aron et al., 2000; Dyck & Daly, 2006; Graham, 2008; Strong & Aron, 2006). Oftentimes, couples rely on core activities and neglect introducing novelty, especially as they enter the transition to parenthood, are exhausted, and have difficulty finding reliable babysitters (Claxton & Perry-Jenkins, 2008; Such, 2006). As conflict rises, couples also stop engaging in core activities and drift apart. The relationship and their lives more generally become mundane and boring.

Discuss with couples what have been their reliable sources of connection and pleasure, and when and why these ended. Inquire about the types of more exciting, novel activities they engaged in during the early years of the relationship—a period when they occurred most frequently and likely played a role in their bonding (Such, 2006)—and when and why they stopped inviting novelty into their lives. Ask about what sorts of activities each partner introduced to the other, and what were the effects of entering into each other's sources of pleasure. For many couples, these experiences are highly positive, as they promote a sense of self-expansion and a sense that the partner can lead them into new worlds. However, in some last chance couples, even early on, partners were not excited about each other's sources of pleasure or even expressed reluctance or distaste for those activities, which may have been experienced as a major disappointment to the partner introducing what turns them on, launching the couple on the path of disconnection at a crucial time of bonding and developing a sense of We.

Suggest that they begin reviving core activities, but also that they think about what novel activities they would enjoy at this stage of their lives. As they get more comfortable connecting in pleasure through the relatively unchallenging activities of the 60-second pleasure point, silent walks, and the other smaller bits of connection listed above, encourage them to experiment with some new activity that requires more energy and time.

Creating and Sustaining Rhythms of Relationship

As I described in detail in Chapter 3, last chance couples are usually out of sync in their daily, weekly, monthly, and yearly rhythms of connection. They need to reestablish (or establish for the first time) regular times for pleasure (Fraenkel, 2011). They may labor under the

Myth of Spontaneity, with partners expecting that both will desire pleasurable contact at the same time. This expectation is highly unrealistic, given how busy and exhausted most couples are taking care of all the exigencies of their lives. Research reveals an interesting paradox: Although couple and family time is essential to keeping those relationships pleasurable and well connected, partners often view that time as more flexible and easier to rearrange, and tend to prioritize obligations to other activities that have set demands based on other people's and institutional needs (Marks et al., 2001). They assume that the leftover time will be used for active connection, but without intentional creation of regular times for intimacy, it simply doesn't happen. Instead, one partner who is monitoring the lack of connection time will raise a complaint, often with implied or explicit blame of the partner for how they "never make time for us," leading to conflict, which then taints the pleasurable activities. Repeat that cycle, and eventually couples give up on trying to have fun and intimacy altogether, just to avoid yet another argument.

Therefore, encourage the couple to set aside regular times for pleasure. These pleasure times should be integrated into a broader plan of "rhythmizing" the relationship that also includes regular times to talk about problems, so that problem discussions don't bleed into pleasurable experiences. The language of "establishing rhythms" is more appealing than that of "scheduling sex."

SUMMARY

This chapter provides the core action-oriented techniques for reducing conflict, repairing relationships after ruptures, and enhancing pleasurable connection. In Chapter 5, I introduce a combination of insight- and action-oriented techniques to address long-standing polarizations and the problematic relational scripts as well as the psychological, emotional, and behavioral tendencies and challenges that contribute to conflict and impede positive connection.

HIGH-CONFLICT COUPLES

Insight- and Action-Oriented Techniques
to Address Polarizations and Partners'
Psychological Issues

C HAPTER 4 FOCUSED LARGELY ON teaching couples communication and problem-solving skills, how to identify and address expectations and hidden issues, teaching couples how to repair the relationship after ruptures, and a bevy of practices for increasing pleasure in the relationship. This chapter discusses how to address polarizations and partners' individual psychological issues with a mix of insight-oriented and action-oriented techniques.

ADDRESSING POLARIZATIONS

High-conflict last chance couples are always polarized around one or more differences. These differences become readily apparent in the first session and further revealed as the couple engages in the slowed-down, less emotionally volatile process of communication created by the Speaker-Listener Technique. Therefore, although they can be noted and commented upon even in a first session, polarizations are usually best addressed in more depth after a few sessions in which couples learn these skills and attempt to resolve their differences through the Problem-Solving Technique. By removing the variable of poor communication and problem-solving skills that often dominates high-conflict couples' assessment of their problems, they become better able to see the impact of these polarized differences and more motivated to understand and transform them.

The multiple perspectives encompassed by the Therapeutic Palette integrative approach are necessary for effective work with polarizations. From a strictly systemic perspective such as that described by Watzlawick and other members of the Mental Research Institute (Watzlawick et al., 1974), polarizations are vicious cycles of differing behaviors that problematically reinforce and strengthen one another: The more Partner A behaves in a manner not desired by Partner B, the more Partner B feels the need to correct Partner A's behavior, which leads Partner A to reassert the behavior more intensely, and on and on.

Structural family therapy's (Minuchin, 1974) emphasis on the fundamental dual dimensions of power and closeness in relationships, supported by research on interpersonal relationships more broadly (Smith Benjamin, 2002), sheds further light on these polarized patterns. Partners may struggle in a symmetrical way to assert their influence and power, or their desires for particular forms of closeness (one wanting to engage in shared activities, another wanting to engage in intimate conversation; one wanting more together time, the other wanting more alone time). Or they may engage in an asymmetrical pattern, in which the more one dominates, the more the other cedes power, leaving the more dominating partner eventually resentful of their degree of responsibility (overfunctioning) and the less dominant partner resentful of their eventual lack of influence or seeming incompetence (underfunctioning) (Fraenkel, 1997). Likewise, an asymmetrical vicious cycle may occur in which one partner seeks more intimacy or conversation and the other withdraws, leading to the classic withdrawer-pursuer pattern.

Feminist couple and family therapy's focus on power differences in cisgender heterosexual relationships (Goldner, 1985; Hare-Mustin, 1978; Knudson-Martin, 2013, 2015) adds a critical sociocultural perspective on how these patterns of power and different stated needs for intimacy that become polarized are often due to socially constructed gender roles. These gendered assumptions and roles account for the oft-repeated finding that women do more pursuing or demanding and men do more distancing or withdrawing (Baucom et al., 2010; Christensen & Heavey, 1990; Gottman & Gottman, 2018). Women take on more of the essential work of the couple and family, including childcare and domestic chores, even when they work at full-time jobs (Fraenkel & Capstick, 2012).

As a result of this unequal distribution of tasks, which men often incorrectly assert is desired by women ("She insists on her way of caring for our child"; "She has a particular way that she likes to fold the laundry and doesn't let me help") means it falls on women to bring up issues around parenting, childcare, and household management, and leaves men the option to engage or withdraw. Although men often report that they are controlled and dominated ("nagged") by their female partners, it is men who actually hold more power in this pattern—they feel entitled to respond or not respond to the woman's often increasingly urgent requests for problem-solving or assistance (Baucom et al., 2010). Importantly, when it is the man who feels most strongly about an issue, men pursue and women may withdraw (Christensen & Heavey, 1990).

The pursuer-withdrawer pattern around requests for intimacy (with a woman generally seeking more verbal intimacy than men, including around the desire to receive support, soothing, and validation for upset feelings) is also mediated by socialized gendered beliefs around the appropriateness, acceptability, and worthiness of experiencing and expressing such emotions—what Gottman and Gottman (2018) call "meta-emotions," or feelings and thoughts about feelings. Men tend to be socialized away from these feelings from early on, whereas women are encouraged to experience and express them (Parker et al., 2012; Thomassin et al., 2019). Even the posture used in intimate conversations has been found gendered: Men tend to sit side by side or shoulder to shoulder when talking to each other, whereas women tend to prefer face-to-face interaction (Gottman & Gottman, 2018). This results in "meta-emotion mismatch" (Gottman & Gottman, 2018), with each partner attempting to assert their orientation toward emotions and communication of them.

As I briefly noted in Chapter 2, from a feminist perspective, it seems more correct to label this problematic pattern as distancer/pursuer, or withdraw/demand. Although it is understood that it is a circular pattern involving both partners, naming it "pursuer/distancer" suggests that the first move is made by the pursuer, who is usually a woman, and implies support for the male stance that women are always demanding and nagging. However, in my clinical experience with hundreds of couples, I've found that the couple's narrative reveals that early in their relationship, women initially approach men in a reasonable manner about an issue of importance to both partners—what Gottman and Gottman (2018) call "gentle start-up"—and men then refuse to engage, which leads the woman to intensify her efforts to engage him in an important conversation. Over years of frustration with her husband's withdrawing, the woman may come to initiate conversation in a "hard start-up" fashion, but it is the husband's repeated withdrawing and nonengagement that "recruited" or shaped her over time into this approach.

Power struggles and differences in desired levels and quality of intimacy may also be due to social locations of race and ethnicity (Killian, 2013), within same-sex couples around whether a partner is out or not (Greenan & Tunnel, 2002; Richards et al., 2015), gender identities (Linville et al., 2012; Subirana-Malaret et al., 2019), and differences in social class (Walsh, 2019), as well as through the intersectional combinations of various locations, such as race and gender (Watson, 2013) or race and class (Boyd-Franklin & Karger, 2012). These locational differences may result in different degrees of assumed privilege and influence or lack of influence and voice in the relationship—for instance, when a cisgender lesbian exerts power over her FTM (female-to-male) trans partner by threatening to out the partner if they don't do something the lesbian partner demands; or when a white heterosexual man holds the stance that "race doesn't matter" in trying to assure his partner of color that he does not view himself as entitled to more influence.

For instance, in an early session with a white French American man and an African American woman, I asked how they had thought and talked about their differences in race and ethnicity. The man said, to the woman's astonishment, "I don't see you as Black, just as a person," thereby denying a core aspect of her identity, her experiences of race-based power differences in the relationship, as well as her experiences of racism in the world at large. His unacknowledged, unearned white privilege and his emotionally forceful stances on parenting and other issues had led her to feel less inclined to receive his sexual overtures. Intersectional social locations are also often linked to cultural beliefs about relationships, childrearing, sex and other forms of intimacy, religion and spirituality, and other topics, and these differences can become polarized and enter into the withdrawer-pursuer pattern, and so must be explored as part of understanding each partner's stance in a polarization.

Neurobiological differences between partners (Fishbane, 2013), including differences in temperament and arousability (Kagan, 2010; Kagan & Snidman, 2009), must also be addressed. One partner may be easily aroused to fear or anger in general (sympathetic nervous system arousal), and the other remains calm in the face of stress. Although these different temperamental and arousability tendencies are often initially sources of attraction, they become polarized in high-conflict couples. Arguments about such seemingly unrelated topics as how to spend leisure time and each partner's preferred allocation of time alone, time as a couple, and time with friends, may be underpinned by differences in temperament. Differences in cognitive style and capacities—for instance, as in the case below of Sheila and Sam—wherein one partner may have attentional, learning, or receptive language issues—may lead to different styles of coping that enter into polarizations.

Family-of-origin experiences, as well as other experiences during childhood and teen years including trauma, contribute to people's coping styles, ways of orienting and inhabiting time (Fraenkel, 2011), and differences in desires for intimacy and styles of communication and problem solving, as well as how and to what degree they experience and express emotions. Partners may seek to replicate what they experienced in their families, or may seek to avoid problematic models they witnessed (Gerson et al., 1993).

As described in Chapter 3, typical emotional differences include one partner being more emotionally expressive and the other more reserved and logical; one holding a more positive perspective and the other a more negative perspective on life in general and the relationship in particular; one being tough, decisive, and confrontational (not only with the partner, but generally) and the other more gentle, sensitive, tentative, and forgiving; and one preferring excitement-oriented emotions and leisure activities, the other preferring calmer emotions and activities.

As is also described in Chapter 3, typical temporal differences include one being more fast paced, the other slower paced; one being future focused, the other more present or past focused; one being rigorous about punctuality, the other looser about timeliness; differences in daily biological rhythms, with one having more energy in the morning, the other more energy at night; one preferring spending time with friends and family, the other preferring more intimate time with the partner; one being guided by clock and calendar, the other seeking a release from chronological time. Other polarities center on parenting (one more strict, the other more lenient); domestic chores, with one emphasizing high standards of tidiness, the other less concerned if things are a bit messy and disorganized, or one wanting to execute these chores daily before bed, the other less rigorous about getting them done; and degree of ambition in their careers (or, ambition aside, the employer-determined demands of the partner's job), leading to differences in preferences or need for time spent working versus personal time.

These differences, especially those centered on emotional styles, are often an initial source of attraction: The emotionally tough, assertive partner is drawn to the other's sensitivity, and the sensitive partner admires the other's seeming implacability and self-assurance. The more negatively focused partner likes that the more positively focused partner helps them gain perspective, and the more positively focused partner likes that the more negatively focused partner has a critical mind and can see the downside of events and situations. As described in Chapter 3, differences in how partners inhabit time are often linked to these differences in emotional styles: The fast-paced, high-energy partner finds the slow-paced partner soothing, and the slow-paced, calmer partner feels energized and enlivened by the fast-paced partner. The present-focused partner admires and feels more secure due to the future-focused partner's capacity for careful planning, and the future-focused partner welcomes the present-focused partner's emphasis on enjoying life in the moment.

In all couples who seek therapy, these differences usually have become somewhat polarized and underlie many of their disagreements and dissatisfactions. But in high-conflict last chance couples, the polarization is usually quite extreme, and partners have completely lost patience with each other's emotional style, perspective and beliefs, and way of being. They have developed well-honed theories about each other's personality deficits related to these differences. Although this high degree of polarization might at first suggest that the partners are simply too incompatible to continue in a life together, the advantage for the therapist working with last chance couples is that the differences are readily apparent and can therefore be addressed without in-depth assessment to reveal them.

Some of these polarizations—around parenting styles and how to accomplish household chores—are quite overt and can mostly be addressed through a combination of exploring family- and culture-of-origin-based beliefs, cognitive needs, and personality-based preferences, and by helping couples combine the strengths of each of their preferences and compromise where necessary. Todd, an accountant with an active practice, had been raised in a family in which parents commanded respect, whereas Jeffrey, a former photographer who now managed Todd's office, had been raised in a family in which his parents were more indulgent of his and his sibling's angry feelings towards them. Todd got into frequent altercations with Tina, their somewhat obstreperous 15-year-old daughter, leaving Jeffrey exhausted by his role as calming mediator between them. Todd also had a more anxious temperament and was a light sleeper, and preferred a firm evening time structure and clear bedtime for the teens, so that he could count on having undisturbed sleep. Their son Nathaniel was a budding musician who liked to spend much time by himself composing on his electronic keyboard, and would sometimes wander down to the kitchen for a snack late at night, disturbing Todd's sleep.

Todd also wanted to have two hours each evening of family time watching movies with the kids, in contrast to his own upbringing in which he and his parents rarely spent enjoyable time together. Jeffrey also enjoyed this family time, but was more attuned to the kids' need as teens to have private time to text with their friends. Sessions with the whole family and with the teens together and separately revealed that the teens were frustrated with the parents' (especially Todd's) insistence on the nightly together time. They were fine with a few evenings spent with their fathers but needed more time to complete homework and connect with their friends. Tina also wanted to spend time connecting with her boyfriend, and Nathaniel wanted time chatting with his girlfriend. Their social needs were accentuated because the family was seen during the COVID-19 pandemic: The kids attended school largely online and had little in-person time with their friends and respective boyfriend and girlfriend. Like many parents, especially during the COVID pandemic, both parents were concerned with the increased amount of time the kids were spending online and on their phones compared to before COVID.

We devised a revised approach to parenting that drew on teen development research and combined the positive aspects of their respective approaches. I agreed with Todd's wish for a clear daily schedule with periods for doing homework, time for the teens to text with friends and their boyfriend and girlfriend, and time for Nathaniel to play music (Tina didn't have a parallel artistic passion). I also supported the plan for a firm bedtime (with phones and computers out of the room, because the kids would often stay up texting for hours otherwise), in light of the research on teens' greater need for sleep and Todd's need for bedtime quiet. I encouraged Todd to take a different, more soothing approach to Tina's upset, taking some of the onus off Jeffrey, but also to set limits gently on how long he would engage with Tina when it seemed she was set on provoking him despite his attempts to be kindly soothing. The parents also agreed to reduce weekday family movie time to twice a week, which greatly relieved their kids. Not surprisingly, once they stopped insisting rigidly on nightly family time, the kids often chose to join their dads to watch a movie.

In another couple, conflict about how to handle their daughter's forgetful behavior led them to the edge of divorce. Family of origin and class-based culture played a large role in their differences about parenting. Attention to these issues, as well as a few family sessions and individual sessions with the daughter, helped them resolve the conflict.

Catherine, 42, had been raised in a white middle-class family in Portland, Oregon, and Roderick, 43, was raised in a white upper-class family in New York City. The couple founded and ran a successful home design and interior decorating business, and worked well together.

Catherine's upbringing was informal and warm. It was acceptable to have elbows and napkins on the table, and the focus of dinner was on interesting and humorous conversation. The parents took an interest in her and her sister's social lives and were available to talk with them about various moments of heartache as they started dating in high school.

In contrast, Roderick described his upbringing as "quite formal," noting that he and his brother were expected from an early age to sit up straight at the dinner table, handle their eating utensils properly, and place their napkins on their laps. Chores were assigned to each child, and they were expected to complete them without reminder, lest they be firmly chastised. Their rooms were to be kept tidy, with clothes in the closet, and books and toys on their designated shelves. Expression of distressed emotions was discouraged; this led Roderick to keep his experiences of being bullied on the way to and from private school to himself. He was eventually sent to boarding school at age 14 and had few conversations with his parents, who were on various organizations' boards and spent much time at glamorous fundraisers. When he and Catherine had their daughter, Charlotte, he vowed to be a much less formal and much more involved parent than his parents had been with him. He was in part attracted to Catherine because of her "looser" style and imagined they would be good coparents.

However, despite his conscious aspirations to be less formal, once their daughter reached middle childhood, Roderick found that he wished to transmit some of his acquired standards of table manners, tidiness, and responsibility for completing chores to their daughter (her chores were to feed the dog and load dishes into the dishwasher). When she failed to follow Roderick's instructions about these behaviors, he became angry at her, leading Charlotte to burst into tears, which led Roderick to feel remorseful, yet the pattern would repeat over and over. Catherine felt alarmed and frustrated, and asked Roderick to lighten up with Charlotte. He would apologize and vow not to react this way again, but also felt frustrated that Charlotte didn't remember to follow his instructions. Catherine increasingly wondered if their marriage was viable, as she felt the need to protect Charlotte and angry that Roderick continued this behavior despite vows to stop. She felt helpless.

In our sessions, Roderick expressed feeling torn: On the one hand, he recognized that his behavior toward his daughter was creating a rift between them and threatening the marriage. On the other, he felt an almost compulsive need to have her follow what he saw as "perfectly reasonable and simple rules." Catherine was beside herself about his behavior. She agreed that Charlotte should learn to do these things, but felt they should give her more time to put them into practice. I suggested that Roderick had clearly communicated his desires to Charlotte, and that some children simply take longer to develop these sorts of behaviors.

In line with Catherine's perspective, I recommended that Roderick give Charlotte a little time to do so, positively reinforce her on occasions when she followed these requests, and use some mindful breathing when he felt the urge to correct her. I reasoned that the conflict between them was likely interfering with Charlotte developing these skills; as long as he played the role of reminding her, she could not find the energy and motivation to do them herself. I suggested that he carry a small stone in his pocket and hold it at these moments while breathing to help him tolerate the impulse to correct her. He thought this would be helpful, and tried it for a couple of weeks, but was only inconsistently successful.

I suggested that we have a family session with Charlotte. Charlotte was a bright, somewhat dreamy 10-year-old who enjoyed creating art, did well in school, and had many friends. It was clear that she and her father had a loving, connected relationship, and that she was not purposely going against her father's requests. With tears in her eyes, she said, plaintively, "I don't know why I don't do these things!" She agreed to try a bit harder to follow his requests. Yet in a next session with the couple, Catherine looked distraught, and Roderick was remorseful, as he had once again reverted to correcting Charlotte.

Further exploration of his painful family-of-origin experiences led him to realize that his compulsive attempts to shape Charlotte's behavior was a way in which he was trying to "rescue" some positive aspects of his upbringing from the otherwise overridingly unpleasant narrative of his childhood: Despite his many class-based privileges, he had felt neglected and lonely. I suggested that in moments when he felt compelled to correct Charlotte, he envision his parents on his shoulders urging him to do so, politely thank them for their guidance, and ask them nevertheless to allow him to parent as he wished.

To make it a bit easier for Roderick, and hopefully resolve the conflict, I suggested that I meet with Charlotte alone to explore further her challenges in remembering to do the few things her father requested and to see if I could help her keep those behaviors in mind. She was highly engaged in our conversation and at one point declared, with tears, "I love my father sooo much! I wish we didn't fight about these silly little things!" I noted that in our session with her parents, when I asked her a question, she turned her head away slightly with a thoughtful expression. She smiled when I said this, and I commented that I imagined her to be one of those people, like myself, who spend a lot of time in their minds, thinking about things. She said that was exactly true about her—she was often making up stories and dreaming up new art projects. I wondered if that tendency sometimes led her just to forget to do her chores and the other stuff her father requested, and that she didn't object to it in principle. She thought that might be true. I suggested that if she wanted to remember, she could take a deep breath in and out, and say to herself, "Now it's time to . . . " and then complete the sentence with whatever thing she was trying to remember to do. I also suggested that she put an index card with a picture of a dishwasher on the dining table to remind her to clean and load the dishes. She liked this idea and decided to draw a dishwasher on a card.

I asked Charlotte about her impressions of her grandmother (Roderick's mother). She called her "Nana" and said she was nice, although "kind of stiff and formal." I said that was my impression from talking with her dad. I joked with her that I often imagined her father had grown up not in Manhattan, but in a very upper-class home in London. I then launched into a high-class British accent and said that I imagined that when her father was a child, Nana had spoken to him in this sort of accent, telling him, "Roderick, my dear! *Please* sit up straight at the dining table, and use your fork and knife appropriately!" Charlotte thought this was hysterical. I said that it was my impression that when her dad, despite himself, corrected her about her table manners, or about stuff not being put away in her room, or about hanging a wet towel over another towel, that it was like the ghost of Nana (even though she was still alive) was sitting on his shoulder urging him on. She thought this was funny. I suggested that this evening, when she sat down to dinner, she sit upright, hold her fork and knife correctly, and say to her parents in a British accent, "Mummy! Daddy! I would like you to notice my fine table manners!" We rehearsed this a few times, and Charlotte replicated a wonderful British accent (she had seen all the Harry Potter movies, so she had a good sense of the accent).

In the next family session, the family reported that Charlotte was doing her chores, hanging wet towels correctly on a separate hanger, had tidied her room each day, and that Roderick had not corrected her even once. In a couple session two weeks later, Catherine looked much relieved, and Roderick seemed relaxed. Even though Charlotte still occasionally forgot to tidy her room and sit up straight, she was much improved, and Roderick had finally let go of the compulsion to correct her.

Described earlier in relation to their polarization around punctuality, Sam and Sheila, a Jewish American couple in their mid-60s, were married for 35 years and had two adult children, yet were on the brink of divorce because of constant bickering that often led to screaming matches filled with hurtful character assassinations. They were enthusiastic about the communication and problems-solving skills I introduced as a start, but irritation and anger about their differences often overwhelmed their attempts to use the techniques. Many of their fights centered on standards for tidiness, especially in the kitchen, with Sheila insisting on a higher standard than Sam felt important, as well as their previously described conflicts around punctuality: Sam became furious when Sheila was not ready to leave the house on time, despite having agreed in the morning or the day before on the necessary departure time.

Exploration of Sheila's need for rigorous tidiness revealed that she had an undiagnosed attentional problem that had affected her academic achievement but had not been identified by teachers (the now commonly diagnosed condition of attention-deficit hyperactivity disorder was not in the *DSM* when she was a school-aged child). As an adult, she often lost track of what she was doing, leading to frustration and negative feelings about her own cognitive competence. She had been treated aggressively for breast cancer a few years earlier, and the treatment had worsened her focus and memory, compounding her existing attentional issues. To compensate, she liked to have an extremely organized home, especially a tidy kitchen, and if Sam forgot to put something away—a dish, a carton of milk—she would fly into a rage, which Sam found absurd and patronizing: "She talks to me like I'm some incompetent little kid!"

My empathic exploration of the lifelong effects of her attentional issues and the impact of cancer treatment on her memory provided for Sam an "honorable explanation" for Sheila's need for order in the home. In addition, Sheila was a talented visual artist and had exhibited her work in several galleries—something Sam spoke of with great pride and admiration. I suggested that perhaps her artistic talents added even more impetus to her wish to maintain a visually calming personal space. Based on these explanations, Sam agreed to compromise with Sheila and go with her wishes about putting things away in the kitchen.

We also explored each partner's families of origin and childhood experiences with peers to understand how each felt the impetus to relentlessly assert their needs and points of view. Sheila's father was extremely dominant, and she was scared to voice her feelings. When she finally began to do so as a teen, she found herself in intense conflict with her father but was determined to hold her ground. She saw standing up for herself as critical to her identity as a strong woman. Sam, who was short in stature, grew up being picked on by peers because of his small size, and found he had to be "verbally strong" to fend them off.

As often happens in an intimate pairing, I suggested that each seemed to have selected the other in part to continue to master these old experiences of being dominated and silenced. Both Sam and Sheila had dated less assertive people with whom they could easily have been the dominant partner. But as I've witnessed hundreds of times with couples, they found these people "boring," seemingly because these people did not provide an opportunity to work through childhood struggles. Instead, they found each other's strong views and ability to speak up for themselves initially appealing, but over time, unable to become the dominant voice in the relationship, their shared strengths became a source of irritation. Understanding how the attraction to one another was in part an attempt to master old issues around strength and voice helped them revalue and respect each other's ability to stand up for themselves, and to see this as a strength of their marriage.

In contrast to these sorts of practical polarizations, those centered around different emotional styles represent the core of the couple's psycho-relational bond, are felt but not clearly articulated in consciousness, and require more in-depth psychological work than just creative problem solving (although the above examples of working with practical polarizations demonstrate that partners' psychological and family-historical issues also must be addressed even with seemingly simple, practical differences). As described in Chapter 3, partners often unconsciously recruit one another to regulate, or "modulate" (Jurist, 2018) and express their own emotions (Fraenkel, 2011, 2020). As I noted in Chapter 3, an early article by Don Jackson (1965) titled "Family Rules: Marital Quid Pro Quo" described how couples early on form an implicit, usually unspoken contract to distribute tasks and roles. Although he never explicated what he meant by "the nature of the relationship,"

Jackson seemed to be pointing to how partners form an implicit contract to handle each other's emotional needs and look to one another to perform emotion tasks or roles for which they have less skill.

For instance, the logical, emotionally reserved partner relies on the emotionally expressive partner to draw out her emotions, and to express emotions for both of them, and the emotionally expressive partner relies on the logical partner to help her (and them together) think through situations that are emotionally confusing. The tough, assertive partner models strength for the sensitive, gentler partner, and the sensitive, gentler partner helps the tough partner learn to be more compassionate. Although these two patterns are often gendered in heterosexual couples due to larger cultural beliefs that men should be strong, logical, and unemotional and women should be sensitive and emotionally expressive, as I wrote these two general scenarios I had in mind two lesbian couples with whom I'd worked.

Likewise, the more positively oriented partner relies on the more negatively oriented partner to represent a more critical perspective on events and express the negative emotions he finds challenging or even unacceptable, and the more negatively oriented partner relies on the more positive partner to help her sustain hope, to not see situations as so dire, and to express a more positive view that she finds paradoxically scary to hold lest she once again be disappointed by life. The partner who generally seeks excitement implicitly relies on the other to reign in her thrill seeking, whereas the more placid partner relies on the other to draw him into exciting adventures.

In high-conflict last chance couples, this initial emotional contract has come to be experienced as an emotional prison sentence. Once I helped them recognize how they had distributed responsibility between them for negative versus positive emotions, Talia, the negatively oriented partner, insisted that Moishe, the more positively oriented partner, was out of touch with reality, and Talia resented having to give voice to "the negative for both of us." Moishe felt dragged down by Talia's negativity and that her view was equally distorted. He said, "Your view of our life is based on selective memory, and it's like a drawing with only charcoal, with no color." In one lesbian couple, Erika, the more expressive partner, complained that Sandra's relentlessly calm, logical style enraged her, because she felt sure Sandra had stronger feelings than she acknowledged. Sandra blamed Erika for their conflicts, complaining that Erika was too emotionally volatile, and even suggested to Erika (just as they got into bed one night) that she fit the diagnosis of borderline personality disorder. Sleeping didn't go well that night!

The psychodynamic concept of projective identification (Crisp, 1987; Nielsen, 2016a; Siegel, 2015) is useful in understanding some forms of emotional polarization. Projective identification occurs when a partner is uncomfortable with an emotion—for instance, anger or anxiety—and unconsciously engages the other partner to experience and express that emotion. Often, the process of projective identification begins with simple projection.

For instance, the partner who has difficulty accepting his own anger sees the other partner as angry, and denies his own anger. The projected-upon partner denies having the feeling, but the projecting partner insists his perception is accurate. Over time and repetition, the projected-upon partner comes to resent being told she is angry, and gets angry about it, which then confirms the projecting partner's perception. Or, as in the case of Erika and Sandra, Erika sensed that Sandra was angry about issues with her parents and yet did not express or act on that feeling. Feeling the need to protect Sandra, Erika expressed the anger she felt Sandra was entitled to feel about the parents' demands, which led Sandra to tell Erika that she was overreacting and didn't understand her relationship with her parents. Sandra attributed Erika's anger to Erika's difficulty feeling comfortable with Sandra spending time with other people. This led Erika to become livid, saying that her anger was all about her concern for Sandra, to which Sandra responded in a calm but somewhat dismissive fashion. The issue escalated to the point that Sandra became angry, and the couple engaged in physical violence, with Erika punching Sandra and throwing plates against the wall. Eventually, the couple broke up, which they'd done many times over their five-year relationship around the same emotion-based polarization, albeit around different topics. (My work with them on the violence in their relationship is described in Chapter 7.)

ADDRESSING POLARIZATIONS: REVEAL, REVALUE, REVISE, REHEARSE

As described in Chapter 3 about time-based polarizations, the steps in working to reduce emotion-based and the often-related temporal polarizations are fourfold: *reveal, revalue, revise,* and *rehearse.* Revealing means discerning and pointing out to the couple their emotional contract. Revaluing means going back to what the couple said about what attracted each partner to the other—just as Jackson (1965) suggested, the beginnings of the emotional contract always lie in those initial impressions of the partner. Noting that emotional differences are inevitable and even positive in relationships, the project of transformation then becomes how to help each partner re-respect and benefit from their partner's style, but without relying on the other to regulate or modulate their own emotions. Each can learn from and adopt part of what the other brings in terms of ways of handling emotions, so that both partners can become more emotionally complete and skilled within themselves. With Moishe and Talia, their relationship changed markedly when Moishe started taking the lead in acknowledging the negative aspects of their history and of events going forward, which freed up Talia to take a chance on holding more positive feelings. Each came to feel that they no longer needed to be the flag bearer for positive or negative emotions.

It is also useful to explore the roots of each partner's emotional style in personal temperament and family and culture of origin. As noted earlier, Geetika came from a warm, highly involved family where talking was constant, and open and frequent expression of emotions was expected, whereas Aadesh grew up in a family in which shared activities (intellectual discussions, sports, watching movies together) formed the means of connection, and emotional expression was essentially forbidden. Depolarizing this couple around their different expectations about intimacy was enhanced by each partner understanding the other's family backgrounds within the same overall culture, and forging a combined, compromise pattern in which they had regular times each day to share feelings, as well as time together without talking, as well as time alone.

Partners may come from similar family and cultural backgrounds, but may differ about whether they wish to replicate or be different from those backgrounds. Mia and Wilson, an African American couple, were both raised in lower-middle-class, urban, Christian families. However, Mia, who was a meditation and yoga teacher, had come to distance herself from what she saw as a restrictive, socially and sexually conservative background, especially as it related to women's roles and identity, and wished to explore pantheistic spirituality and a wider range of sexual activities than were endorsed by her upbringing. Wilson, a mid-level government employee who had a secure managerial job, was focused mostly on being a responsible Black father and husband, different from what he had experienced with his father, who left the family when he was a child, and to distinguish himself from racist stereotypes about Black men. Although not a regular churchgoer, he still found his religious background served as a guide. He was fine with Mia's explorations of spirituality, and noted that he practiced Qigong as a kind of movement meditation. However, he was initially not enthusiastic about Mia's desires for greater sexual experimentation, and not keen to have an open marriage. With greater empathy for how they each related to their similar upbringing, the couple was able to slowly explore and play with less traditional sexual practices, especially once I observed that Wilson approached sex as another responsibility, rather than as an opportunity to create a play space, an observation he found extremely helpful.

ADDRESSING PARTNERS' EMOTIONAL ISSUES AND COMMUNICATION STYLES

Although research has not found that certain personality styles aside from neuroticism (a generally negative view of the world) are reliably associated with relationship distress, partners certainly bring their respective long-standing styles of communicating, handling emotion, and issues with anxiety, depression, trauma, and other individual psychological issues to the relationship. This section discusses how to address these challenges with a mixture of insight-oriented and action-oriented techniques.

Partners' Problematic Communication Styles

The Speaker-Listener Technique is highly useful for equalizing the length of each partner's speaking turns and therefore, their communicative power. But couples cannot talk with each other constantly in this structured format. When one or both partners bring a lifelong dominating style of talking to the relationship, we must work with them to see the impact and help them change. Two frequent styles are particularly problematic: What I call "firehosing" and "catastrophizing." Sad to say to my cisgender heterosexual male counterparts, I find these styles most often exhibited by this category of men.

Firehosing. This is a style in which the partner speaks in rapid, relentless sentences, seemingly without breathing, at a fairly high volume and in an even, sometimes unwittingly abrasive tone. The term was suggested to me by a female partner, Rachel, who, after yet another instance of her husband Josh speaking this way, turned to me helplessly with tears in her eyes and declared, "I feel like I'm being firehosed with words." This couple was described in Chapter 1 in reference to challenges in maintaining the therapeutic alliance when the therapist needs to point out problematic nonverbal behavior. As I described there, after exploring how he had refined this style of speech as a high school debating champion, and then through musical analogies of fast-paced and slower-paced, more spacious jazz trumpet playing, use of a metronome to help him practice speaking slower, and through discussion of the speech rhythms of great orators like President Barack Obama, I was able to help Josh recognize and alter his pace, spacing, and amount of speech. Rachel was much relieved.

Firehosing can also have a basis in culture. Heschel, an Orthodox Jewish husband with a somewhat slower but equally relentless verbal style that silenced even his quite talkative, expressive wife, Judy, explained that he had learned this style in the yeshiva (Orthodox religious school) as a student of the Talmud, where it was expected that one would keep talking as long as possible and interrupt others when they spoke. As an attending physician responsible for supervising residents, he spent his days correcting and providing on-the-spot minilectures to ensure good patient care. These lectures often included repeating points to make sure that the residents grasped them. As a result, he was quite comfortable with and valued his success with this style, but came to see that it led to frustration with Judy. I encouraged him to experiment with a style of inviting Judy to speak first, reflecting back what he heard (even when not explicitly practicing the Speaker-Listener Technique), and then to try making his point once, rather than with his average four to five repetitions.

Catastrophizing. Catastrophizing is when the partner moves from a smaller topic or circumstance about which they are anxious or otherwise upset to stating the most dramatic, worst outcome or implication of the event. Sometimes the partner's tone is irritated or mildly angry, but the desperate tenseness and agitation in their voice, pressured speech, and worried facial expressions suggest that the predominant feeling is anxiety. Especially with people who have difficulty accepting their own anxiety and then repeatedly seek soothing, their thoughts become disconnected from the feelings. With their thoughts now untethered from their reaction to a specific incident, the person's capacity for fearful fantasies takes over, leading to a catastrophic endpoint that in some way provides imagined relief from the circumstance that evoked their anxiety in the first place. After all, if this incident indicates that the marriage must be dissolved, the fantasy of that dissolution (and therefore no further upsetting incidents) can be calming in part.

Underlying this tendency to catastrophize is usually at least one traumatic event, often from childhood. It can also be amplified by a cognitive-intellectual style in which the person's capacity to imagine possibilities—including positive ones—interfaces with negative emotions and trauma that the person has not processed.

Richard was a highly successful 52-year-old litigator married to Janice, a 40-year-old interior decorator. They had two young sons. When the couple came to me, they were on the brink of divorce due to conflict over complex legal issues between Janice and her family. Richard had taken over her case believing he could resolve it quickly, but it had dragged on and became an enormous wedge between them when Richard's attempt to protect her from lawsuits pitted him against her father, to whom she continued to be loyal despite the father's problematic financial decisions that put her at risk. Janice had become angry and rejecting of Richard emotionally and physically, and he felt betrayed by her, given that he had taken on this time-consuming and expensive burden to protect her. Yet he persisted in trying to obtain the best outcome for Janice, even though a less perfect resolution was available. He acknowledged that his insistence was in part due to outrage at how her family was treating her, and him as well.

For her part, Janice believed that if Richard would give up trying to resolve the case perfectly, their previously strong attraction and enjoyment of each other would reemerge. However, she noted that it might take some time for her to get over the intense daily anxiety generated by the case, which was amplified by Richard's catastrophic ways of talking about it. She spoke of his tendency to repeat himself in a rapid, agitated manner (essentially, firehosing), and to describe each development in the case as "the end of the world"—a style that I witnessed many times in sessions. She knew from talking about the case with his legal partners that there could be a simpler resolution.

Richard's intellectual capacity for thinking 10 steps ahead in legal cases contributed to his success as a lawyer, but when fueled by emotional upset that he found difficult to admit and then to soothe, this cognitive capacity led him to imagine the worst outcomes. He thought of himself as someone who could stay calm even when faced with great challenges: Although he was highly effective under stress, his investment in being implacable led him to minimize upset feelings. In initially doing the Speaker-Listener Technique with Janice, the strongest feeling he could acknowledge was being "a bit nervous," although his demeanor and manner of speaking belied a great deal of anxiety and also hurt feelings. When I asked if he might be feeling something stronger than nervous, he said, "No, just a bit nervous."

I suggested that until these legal issues were resolved, it would be difficult to work on other issues in the marriage and determine if they wanted to remain together. Two weeks of multiple individual sessions with Richard helped him recognize the link between the traumatic cutoff his parents instigated with him ("they disowned me") in his early 20s when he chose law school over a career in medicine, and his outrage over Janice's father's behavior, which fueled his futile attempt to "teach her father a lesson." I was able to help him recognize how painful this cutoff from his parents had been, how hurt and alone he had felt, and how Janice's upset and pulling away from him when he thought he was doing the honorable thing for her brought similar feelings of being hurt, betrayed, and abandoned. He allowed me to provide him a first experience of empathy and care about those feelings, and to feel soothed.

I also suggested that his high-pressured style of speech and catastrophic conclusions might result from an unfortunate pairing of his intellectual capacity to imagine future outcomes, his general loquaciousness (which he said characterized him as soon as he learned to speak), his self-described tendency to think out loud, the previously unacknowledged depth of his pain over the traumatic cutoff from his parents, and his tendency to minimize upset feelings. I offered a metaphor he found useful—it was like he was flying a bunch of kites (catastrophic thoughts), holding the strings, and then letting them fly off and bump up against each other, no longer moored by his grip (the emotions he denied).

Richard came to see that this continued struggle was damaging his relationship to Janice, and that he had a choice to make: continue to pursue Janice's father (and other family members involved) or possibly save his marriage. He grudgingly came to a satisfactory although not perfect settlement of the legal issues. Janice expressed gratitude.

Although changes in interactional behavior and attitudes go a long way toward improving couple relationships, partners often bring psychological challenges and behavioral styles that affect the quality of communication and couple satisfaction. In some instances—for example, a partner suffering from serious depression, anxiety, or trauma—a referral for individual therapy or medication may be warranted. But even these issues can sometimes be ameliorated within the context of couple therapy. Other behavioral and communication styles that predate the relationship—such as a tendency toward explosive anger, difficulty naming and expressing emotions—can often readily be effectively addressed in couple therapy.

Working With Partners' Psychological Issues

Chronic anxiety. Anxiety is the most prevalent psychological disorder worldwide (ADAA, 2021). Although teaching couples how to provide mutual soothing can help reduce a partner's anxiety, the partner attempting to provide soothing may feel frustrated because they are unable to fully meet the needs of a chronically anxious partner, resulting in couple conflict. Couple therapy provides a useful context within which to explore the history of the anxiety in family-of-origin and other childhood, teen, or adult experiences, the current factors that trigger it (work demands, social situations, being alone, particular stimuli that elicit phobic reactions, and so on), and the strategies the anxious partner has attempted. Exploring this history in the presence of the other partner can provide more empathy for the anxious partner's struggles. Along with coming to a better understanding of the sources of anxiety, challenging the problematic beliefs that contribute to it, and encouraging experiments in facing the feared situation (along the lines of cognitive–behavioral exposure therapy), the anxious partner will need to engage in self-soothing practices such as mindful breathing to take the "soothing load" off the other partner.

For instance, Cindy was a 51-year-old physician who had been in psychoanalytic psychotherapy for decades, with no appreciable effect on her level of anxiety. Asked what the focus of her therapy had been, she reported that the therapist had explored with her childhood experiences of feeling abandoned by her emotionally reserved lawyer mother and her physician father who was, she said, "nice to me, but rarely home because he was always at the hospital treating patients. His patients loved him because he was so kind, different from many 'colder' doctors—but I rarely saw him." Like her father, her husband Charles, a 52-year-old highly successful plastic surgeon, was warm and compassionate but often preoccupied with his medical practice. Also like her father, Charles had a reputation for being an emotionally soothing physician. From the beginning of their relationship, they established a pattern in which Cindy would become distraught and Charles would soothe her, which would temporarily calm and reassure her, but the effects of his calming were not long lasting.

Charles had grown up in Oklahoma on a farm, and his family was proud of their roots in the pioneer phase of American history where, despite initial poverty, they managed to raise horses and eventually became financially established, expanding into growing crops. Charles took pains to note that his family had always been friendly and not exploitative of the Native American community and had even established partnerships with them that were mutually profitable. As for many families who farmed, there were many tasks to accomplish and much hard labor and, he explained, little attention given to "complaints" or any other "negative feelings." Yet, growing up as a more sensitive young man, he longed for a relationship in which he could express his feelings. As a result, he was initially attracted to Cindy's "emotionality" and liked that she could express her feelings and that he could calm her. He also liked that she was from a northeastern city, which he always imagined as a teenager was a more intellectually sophisticated region than the Southwest. Charles was the first member of his family to go to college. Not surprisingly, he chose one in a northeastern city and then went to medical school in that city, where he and Cindy met.

I noted that their emotional contract from the beginning had centered on Cindy modeling for Charles the ability to express vulnerable emotions, and on Charles providing her soothing in a more consistent manner than she had received from her parents. At one point, I noted with a touch of humor that it seemed he valued being a kind of American "knight in shining armor" for Cindy, "riding in on his horse to rescue the damsel in distress." But I noted that over time, when Charles felt his efforts to soothe Cindy were ultimately ineffective, he began to withdraw from her and spent even more time on his career, leading Cindy to feel abandoned, as she had felt with her parents. In addition, Charles typically withheld his own vulnerable feelings from Cindy, feeling that there was "little room" for him to express himself and receive soothing from Cindy, because he had to attend to her frequent bouts of upset. Cindy wanted to provide soothing for Charles and did not like having the role of the "anxious basket case" in the relationship, which did not fit with the image of being a strong, self-reliant woman to which she aspired, and which her mother had embodied. Yet the frequency and intensity of her anxiety tended to overwhelm their conversations.

The couple found these insights helpful, but Cindy's anxieties persisted. Along the lines of the Creative Relational Movement principles of change described earlier, I suggested that insight alone rarely leads to substantial changes in action—including the internal action of self-soothing—and that it would be important for Cindy to take greater charge of her own anxious temperament. I mentioned the extensive research on the stability of temperament styles from childbirth through adulthood (Kagan, 2010; Kagan & Snidman, 2009), and Cindy confirmed that this was true for her: She reported that her parents had told her that she was "anxious from birth."

With their assent, I taught both partners the research-based approach to mindful breathing described earlier and led them through some Qigong exercises. So as to change the narrative that only Cindy needed soothing (Charles reported experiencing plenty of emotional distress across his demanding workday), I encouraged them to practice these calming activities together in the morning and evening, but also to practice them when apart. Over a period of only a few weeks, both partners, especially Cindy, reported notable changes in their levels of anxiety. With Cindy now better able to soothe herself, nightly conversations were no longer dominated by her anxieties of the day. Cindy felt good about her increased emotional self-reliance, and Charles now felt there was more space to bring his distress to her and receive soothing from her.

Trauma. Similarly, a partner's trauma history can be usefully explored in couple therapy (Monson & Fredman, 2015), and often helps the other partner understand the traumatized partner's strong fear or anger responses to certain seemingly innocuous situations. A series of individual sessions with the traumatized partner can also be useful, with the partner and therapist bringing back to the couple therapy insights gained and implications for further changes in the relationship. Not infrequently, when one partner reveals a history of trauma, it leads the other partner to reveal their own traumatic history, one that may never have been discussed together.

In Chapter 1, I described work with Tanya, an African American woman with a severe history of childhood sexual trauma, and Ramon, a Dominican American man with a history of physical and emotional abuse by his father. That therapy included a combination of individual sessions with each partner and conjoint sessions to improve communication skills and emotion regulation, and to develop mutual appreciation of the impact of each of their traumatic family-of-origin histories, which helped them prevent those histories from exploding into high conflict and possible divorce.

With another couple, one partner's traumatic upbringing contributed to the emotional polarization between them. Ava, 34, was a second-generation Syrian American upper-middle-class woman and Doug, 34, was a fourth-generation Irish American man who had grown up working class and was the first in his family to go to college, never mind graduate school. Married for four years, the couple was on the brink of divorce because of several unremitting challenges. Ava found Doug often "messy and dirty"—for instance, she reported that whenever he used a sauce like ketchup or hot sauce, the area around his plate on the table would be covered in splotches, which he seemed not to notice and did not clean up after meals. She was also bothered by his practice of looking at his phone and texting during movies they watched together.

Doug liked to spend time with friends, often in noisy, exciting activities (for instance, he loved big parties and rock concerts), whereas Ava wished for more quiet, contemplative time together. Doug felt hurt that Ava did not want to join him in these activities. Ava found Doug impatient with her when she talked about upsetting events during the day, feeling as a result that they had little emotional intimacy. Ava also said that during lovemaking, Doug held her too forcefully—she noted, "He's a big guy, and strong, and I'm small and not so physical."

In our third session, Doug reported that after the previous session, they both felt quite despairing about the relationship. I was somewhat surprised, because although it had been centered on their differences around preferred leisure activities, and on my introduction of the concept of hidden issues or broader relationship struggles described in Chapter 4 (power and control, closeness and caring, and so on), I sensed that they had come to some useful understandings and compromises. However, Ava left the session feeling that they had problems around all of the hidden issues, and her upset led Doug, who initially felt the session was productive, to feel, he said, "sadder and more hopeless than I've ever felt in this relationship."

Interestingly, Ava said that although she didn't want Doug to be so sad, "in a way, I felt better, because we were feeling the same thing, instead of Doug being so positive all the time." I suggested that perhaps Ava felt less alone in that moment, with Doug sharing her sadness, and she agreed. Based on my observations of them from the beginning of our work together, I wondered aloud whether there was an underlying emotion-based pattern between them, in which Ava specialized in naming negative feelings for them and Doug's role was to counter with positive, hopeful feelings. Both partners heartily agreed with this idea and laughed, because it seemed to capture something essential to their relationship that they hadn't consciously recognized.

I asked each to tell me about the roles they played in their families growing up. Ava related that her father was periodically verbally and physically abusive to her mother, and that this frightened her. She said that even as a young girl, she wished her parents would get divorced so that there would be no more scary conflict. Preoccupied with one another, the parents paid little attention to her during these moments and in general, and Ava's older sister, Ava said, "basically raised me, and would tell our parents to stop because they were scaring me." The parents would then stop, only for the father at a later time to engage in abusive behavior again.

Ava related that her parents were in some ways quite traditionally Syrian in their gender roles and expectations about marriage, and in the entitlement that many men in that culture feel to be aggressive toward their wives, with wives staying with the husbands to avoid the shame of exposing their conflicts to the extended family and community, who would generally encourage women to stay in the marriage and "work it out." Ava cried as she related this history of trauma, and Doug put his arm around her. I noted how traumatic her experience sounded, and suggested that this may have led her to develop a more negative outlook on relationship problems, and a hopelessness about changing them. She said this made much sense to her, as did Doug. I also noted that she may have learned through her experiences that expressing vulnerable feelings leads violence or other conflict to stop, as happened when her sister would tell the parents that Ava was scared. I wondered if she was now transferring this learning from her family of origin into their relationship, leading her to at times overemphasize her upset feelings to lead Doug to change his behavior. Furthermore, whereas in her family her sister had to give voice to Ava's feelings before the parents would stop fighting, with Doug, Ava hoped she could be effective in stopping Doug's upsetting behavior by communicating her feelings herself. This idea also made sense to them.

Doug related that in his large working-class family, priority was placed on "staying positive" and avoiding complaints, as they struggled to meet their financial challenges. He had little experience experiencing and expressing fear, hurt, or other vulnerable feelings, or in receiving soothing. He related that when he met Ava and sensed her capacity for sorrow and vulnerability, he was "intrigued."

I noted that when Ava decided to be with Doug, she chose a man who, like her father, had "forceful energy" but who was kind and would never hurt her. I suggested that perhaps Doug could go a little lighter in his physicality toward Ava, especially as his "strength of touch" unwittingly reminded her of her father's forcefulness. Both partners smiled at this suggestion and seemed greatly relieved. I suggested that if Doug were able to voice both his positive but also negative feelings more frequently, that might free Ava up to voice positive feelings and lead her not to feel the need to overemphasize the negative.

I also reminded them of the Speaker-Listener Technique, which I had introduced to them in the first session, and how regular use of the technique might lead them both to feel heard. I emphasized the importance of the kind of soothing Doug was doing of Ava spontaneously in the session and suggested that if he became more comfortable sharing upset feelings, Ava might provide him with the new experience of being soothed and comforted.

This session was the turning point for the couple. In subsequent sessions, we systematically addressed issues around doing domestic chores, Doug's occasional "over-partying" with alcohol and drugs despite his assurance that he wouldn't, and others, and the couple fairly quickly decided that they did not have as many hidden issues as they initially thought.

Depression. A large body of research and clinical literature has documented the connection between relationship distress and depression (see Whisman & Beach, 2015, for an excellent review). Depression can be precipitated and sustained by ongoing relationship conflicts, and also contributes to those conflicts. Medication and individual therapy may be advised for people with more than moderate levels of depression. However, couple therapy has been shown effective in ameliorating depression without supplementary treatment (Whisman & Beach, 2015).

For instance, Rob, a 36-year-old white professional guitarist, and Jill, a 32-year-old white assistant director of an art gallery, came to therapy because of high conflict that led Jill to question the future of the relationship. Married six years, they had met in a rehab center, as both had struggled with alcohol and drug addictions. Conflicts centered around Rob being frequently out of work as a musician, and his refusal to get a day job, leaving Jill to support them on her medium-level salary. They frequently argued about many topics, and Rob tended to become sarcastic and at times intimidating, which silenced Jill.

Both partners described histories of childhood trauma: Jill's mother had verbally abused her, and Rob's father had been physically abusive—on one occasion that led Rob to leave home at 16, the father broke his guitar because Rob had not taken out the garbage. Jill described experiencing depression from her teenage years onward, was taking an antidepressant, and had been in extensive individual therapy, without much positive effect.

After an initial intake session, the next two sessions focused on teaching them the Speaker-Listener and Problem-Solving Techniques. In a fourth session, Jill reported that Rob had expressed a desire to end the therapy, feeling that they could now communicate well. However, Jill said she wanted to continue and remarked that for the first time in years, she did not feel depressed. She attributed this change to feeling that therapy, and the techniques I had taught them, had provided them a structure for more egalitarian, less coercive, and emotionally safer communication. She also said she felt that having someone to observe, comment on, and work with their interaction styles made her feel safer.

My hypothesis was that Rob's desire to end was due to the therapy equalizing their voices. Rob had expressed his alignment with Men's Movement ideas about the biologically determined "power" that men had and that women needed to accept. Rather than confronting him directly about these ideas, which I sensed would lead to a power struggle between us and to Rob feeling put down by me, I explored with him the feelings of shame that he said underlay his tendency to get angry and domineering.

Based on my sense of both partners as imaginative, creative types, and by a comment Rob had made that when they spend time apart, "demons appear, and cause us to take each other's negative inventory," I suggested that we might work to externalize his sense of shame by giving that shame a name. Rob became intrigued with this suggestion, and named his shame "V the Dark Knight," and even imagined a figure on a horse in tattered gray leather clothes with a coat of arms. I suggested that when he "sensed the presence of the Dark Knight" he could take steps to keep the Knight from recruiting him into condescending, coercive styles of arguing with Jill, and that Jill could help him when she noticed the beginning signs that he was entering into these styles by saying, "I feel the presence of the Dark Knight."

Jill went on to describe spontaneously an externalization or personification of her tendency to withdraw and feel "squashed," which she named "Rotunda," whom she described as an enormous female creature, "like the Michelin Tire Man, only female, with a pink bow on her head." She related that her abusive mother had been extremely obese, like this imaginary figure. I suggested that Rob could help Jill not get crushed by Rotunda by noticing when she seemed to become silent during their conversations, and by changing how he was speaking with her. Over a few more sessions, the couple stabilized in their new patterns of communicating, and Jill reported that she was no longer depressed. She gradually stopped taking the antidepressant under the guidance of her psychiatrist,

Explosive anger. Partners sometimes come to the relationship with a habitual tendency to become dysregulated and defensively angry and critical. As noted earlier, helping them identify situations that trigger anger and the primary feeling of being attacked, hurt, or scared, which then leads to the "fight" side of sympathetic nervous system fight-or-flight arousal, can help them modulate their anger and talk about the primary, vulnerable feeling with their partner.

As I did with Bahir (see Chapter 4), exploring and honoring their positive, empowering relationship to their anger and the rewarding effects it has in certain circumstances, but helping them decide to "reserve their firepower" for moments outside the relationship when it could be useful, can be quite helpful. It is relieving to the anger-prone partner when a therapist takes this stance toward their anger, as they usually expect a "therapist type" to tell them that their anger is a problem and simply to stop being angry entirely. Indeed, some popular psychology books, often influenced by the mindfulness movement and Buddhist principles, name anger as one of the "destructive" emotions that should be eliminated (Dalai Lama & Goleman, 2003). On the other hand, it should be noted that even the venerable Vietnamese monk, Buddhist leader, and antiwar activist Thich Nhat Hanh, when asked in a wonderful interview with Oprah Winfrey (2016) if he ever gets angry, quickly and strongly declared, "Of course!" and spoke about his anger around social and political injustice.

Finding an analogy that works for the person about the need to choose how much energy to put into a situation or activity is also useful. For instance, ask marathon runners if they adjust how fast they run at different moments in the race, or ask musicians how they vary the volume of their playing from soft to loud depending on the music.

Exploring the role anger has played in a partner's family-of-origin relationships, as well as their identity based on their social location and culture, is also useful. For instance, Carissa, a 34-year-old lawyer, and Gabriella, a 34-year-old corporate consultant, engaged in high-conflict fights in which Carissa would become explosively angry and occasionally throw dishes against the wall. Gabriella would initially stay calm but often quietly made critical and contemptuous comments that agitated Carissa. Carissa would especially become outraged when Gabriella insisted on a certain plan for their leisure time, or that Carissa help more with housework. Carissa felt frustrated that because of her angry outbursts, she was being labeled "the crazy one" in the relationship; Gabriella shrugged her shoulders and said, "What do you expect?"

Carissa described coming from a family in which, as the one female child of three, her culturally traditional Greek American parents expected her to be more compliant with their requests than her two older brothers. Carissa said her father was prone to anger and often dominated her mother. Carissa identified more with her father's power and, as a teen recognizing that she was lesbian and therefore "different," was determined not to be a "weak pushover" like her mother, and as she believed the dominant culture encouraged women to be. As a successful lawyer, Carissa used her capacity for anger and outrage to energize her work, but knew that outbursts in court would cast her as unprofessional.

I validated Carissa's identification as a strong woman and the role that anger played in her identity, and noted that Gabriella had said in a first session how drawn she was to Carissa's strength. However, I wondered if she might consider reserving her firepower for contexts outside the relationship. I empathized with her frustration about being labeled "the crazy one" but noted that her aggressive behavior undermined her power with Gabriella, who would dismiss her point of view due to the way she expressed it. This reframe of her explosivity as weakening rather than strengthening her influence with Gabriella had a remarkable effect on reducing her reactivity, along with a commitment to practicing mindfulness techniques to reduce her baseline level of negative arousal.

With all my clients who struggle with overwhelming anger, I teach mindful breathing and some Qigong, and recommend two books, both based on Buddhist practices: Vietnamese Buddhist leader Thich Nhat Hanh's (2001) *Anger: Wisdom for Cooling the Flames*, and Leonard Scheff's book *The Cow in the Parking Lot: A Zen Approach to Overcoming Anger* (Scheff & Edmiston, 2010). Scheff was a high-powered, aggressive Type-A lawyer whose friends and family worried that his relentless rages would result in a heart attack. They bought him a ticket to see the Dalai Lama in Los Angeles, an event that launched him on the practice of Zen Buddhism.

If a partner's anger tends to escalate to the point of verbal or physical violence, I engage the ideas and practices for working with interpersonal violence described in Chapter 7. However, the ideas and practices named in this section are always useful in working with interpersonal violence, and sometimes are sufficient to help a partner modulate their anger.

Difficulty experiencing and expressing emotions. Some people have difficulty allowing themselves to experience vulnerable emotions, or to differentiate and name specific emotional states. Instead, they experience a general sense of physiological arousal. The term *alexithymia* was coined by Sifneos (1991) to capture this difficulty distinguishing and naming emotions; naming them can help to distinguish one state from another, and practice in differentiating those states can help refine a person's emotional vocabulary. Difficulty discriminating different emotions in oneself results in difficulty empathizing with others. The other partner may experience the alexithymic partner as cold, uninterested in their feelings, robotic, and overly rational, as they typically assume that the alexithymic partner has feelings but simply refuses to express them.

Although some researchers have hypothesized that alexithymia is primarily the result of a disconnection between the limbic emotion center and the verbal prefrontal cortex of the brain (Sifneos, 1991), it can also be due to family- and culture-of-origin socialization.

Reginald, a 36-year-old second-generation Korean American man who worked in finance, and Mariana, a 35-year-old Mexican American woman who managed a law firm, were on the brink of ending their six-year relationship, largely because Mariana found Reginald to be persistently unemotional, especially when she wished to engage him in talking about problems. Reginald was somewhat expressive when it came to positive feelings, but claimed not to have any negative feelings. Mariana found this impossible to imagine, having been raised in the generally highly expressive Latinx culture. She assumed that "he just doesn't care about me and my feelings."

Hypothesizing that, like many cisgender heterosexual men, Reginald simply felt anxious and overwhelmed when faced with listening to Mariana's emotion-laden complaints, I taught the couple the Speaker-Listener Technique. Both partners found this helpful, but Reginald often had little to share about his feelings on topics—even those around which it was likely he would have strong feelings. When Mariana would express a feeling even in a mild fashion, he typically would say that he needed some time to "process" what she had said, but that often meant a day or two of thinking about the situation, which Mariana found frustrating. In one session, he said, with a facial expression of genuine bafflement, that he just didn't know what he felt. He truly seemed at a loss.

Exploration of Reginald's family- and culture-of-origin revealed that, like many traditional Korean families (as he asserted, and as I've learned from my Korean colleagues and students), there was virtually no verbal expression of either positive or negative emotion. However, his family life constituted a more extreme version of this cultural norm. He related that his parents immigrated from Korea penniless, and spent years working long shifts in Korean dry-cleaning establishments. Reginald described a family life that was solely centered around financial security and hard work, with no time given even to small moments of pleasure. His parents never asked him how he felt, and never expressed their own feelings. As a young adult, he adopted his parents' single-mindedness about making money, and had been quite successful. Although Reginald was attracted to Mariana in part because she was warm and lively, and she—having experienced a great deal of chaos and instability growing up—found his sense of responsibility and implacability attractive, Reginald had not been able to come forward to meet her in emotional intimacy.

I said that because of his family experience combined with cultural beliefs about the lack of value in expressing emotions, it seemed he had not had much practice in discerning and naming what he felt. With an expression of anxious eagerness, he asked if I had any "methods or tools" to help him develop this capacity. I suggested that he set an alarm on his phone for five times a day, and when it rang, to jot down what was happening in the moment and how he might be feeling. Reginald applied his hard-working diligent attitude to this task of self-discovery. Over a period of a few weeks, Reginald became better able to name his feelings, and by two months later, appeared much more relaxed and emotionally open, which delighted Mariana. I also suggested Daniel Goleman's book, *Emotional Intelligence: Why It Can Matter More than IQ* (Goleman, 1995), and another book on career success that, although not directly focused on emotional intelligence, included tips that centered around managing relationships in a more sensitive manner (Goldsmith, 2007).

In a last session with the couple, Mariana and Reginald both shared that what had helped them most in the therapy was our work on getting to know better each other's minds and emotional states—an outcome that supports the importance of fostering mentalization (Asen & Fonagy, 2012, 2021) and intersubjectivity (Benjamin, 1995, 2017). Both noted that the communication skills I taught them facilitated this outcome. Reginald added—to both Mariana's and my surprise and delight—that once the issue of his difficulty identifying and naming his own emotions had been identified, he had worked earnestly during sessions (without telling us that he was doing so) to imagine what Mariana felt like when she named specific emotions. He noted, "Yeah, for instance, when Mariana said she felt sad, or hurt, I thought of times when I felt sad or hurt, so that I could feel what she was feeling. I always had understood the emotion words she was saying, and her perspective, but it was totally different to feel something like she was feeling in the moment."

One of the other issues the couple had discussed during sessions was Mariana's anxiety about Reginald staying out late at times with friends, drinking. He had curtailed this activity, which led her to feel more secure and that they were partners on the "same page about how we spend our time." The couple spent the remaining session time discussing, with much laughter, the complexities of organizing their wedding, including how to have a ceremony and reception that would blend their respective cultures and families.

SUMMARY

This chapter demonstrates how to utilize the full Therapeutic Palette of insight- and action-oriented techniques to reveal and transform the many sorts of polarizations that high-conflict last chance couples present. It also addresses various problematic communication and interaction styles that partners learned and developed before beginning the relationship and that contribute to conflict, as well as the psychological problems of anxiety, depression, trauma, explosive anger, and inability to recognize and name feelings, all of which can underlie polarizations. In the next two chapters, I address some of the most challenging problems experienced by last chance couples: value- and safety-violating behaviors, including affairs, interpersonal violence, and overuse of alcohol or substances. In addressing these problems, all of the ideas and techniques described thus far are brought to bear, along with some additional specialized techniques.

CHAPTER 6

VIOLATIONS OF VALUES AND SAFETY

Affairs

THIS CHAPTER AND THE NEXT one provide guidance to work with couples on the brink of relationship dissolution due to one or both partners engaging in behavior that violates partners' values, expectations, and assumptions about relationships. Violating relational expectations results inevitably in damage to the sense of trust, which is crucial to well-functioning, satisfying relationships (Gottman, 2011), and thereby challenges partners' level of emotional attunement, security, and commitment. In some cases, these violations also involve behaviors that threaten the safety—emotional, sexual, physical—of one or both partners.

Oftentimes, these behaviors have resulted in trauma reactions—intrusions of unbidden thoughts, feelings, and memories (flashbacks), which can also be triggered by stimuli of various types (media accounts, films, even colors and particular clothing associated with the behavior, times of the year, and more), hypervigilance, and on the other end of the arousal spectrum, numbing (Herman, 1992; Gordon et al., 2015; Janoff-Bulman, 1992; Resick et al., 2007; Spring, 2020; Tedeschi & Calhoun, 2004; van der Kolk, 2014). Anxiety, depression, and other psychological symptoms (for instance, psychosomatic symptoms) can be precipitated or, when these symptoms already exist in a partner, amplified by these behaviors and the couple's struggles around them. These symptoms can be experienced by the nonoffending partner as well as by the partner who engaged in these behaviors. Thus, last chance couples that come to therapy due to value and safety violations require an integrative approach that addresses the relational issues as well as partners' often-significant psychological distress.

This chapter addresses one common form of value and safety violations: affairs, or infidelity. The following chapter addresses interpersonal aggression and violence (formerly called domestic violence) and a partner's use of alcohol or other substances. There are large literatures on each of these issues, which have been discussed not only in articles and chapters but in entire books. My approach to working with these issues draws heavily upon the work of my esteemed colleagues, and I am not presenting completely new, innovative approaches. Rather, my intent is to present a brief, practical guide that summarizes the best of what already exists in the field, with some innovative techniques that I have found usefully supplement the extant treatment literature. The approach I've described in previous chapters to forming a useful, collaborative treatment alliance with last chance couples forms the basis of this work and is also useful for working with couples even when they are not considering divorce or its unmarried equivalent. However, the vignettes in this chapter are all of couples in which value and safety violations resulted in one or both partners considering separation or permanent ending of the relationship.

A MORAL PERSPECTIVE

Work with couples in which values and safety have been violated requires us to engage issues of morality. Although these issues are important in work with any couple, the crises presented by couples in which values and/or safety have been violated require therapists to engage a moral stance about problematic behavior. As Goldner (2004) writes,

> Although this specific set of concerns is particular to abuse cases, the approach raises larger questions about the place of the moral work of psychotherapy in our therapy-saturated society. The introduction of the concept of morality into the clinical situation seems odd to many practitioners, but the formulaic splitting of moral and clinical discourses in our professional culture is theoretically meaningless and psychologically inauthentic. Moral issues are psychologically real to everyone. Each party to a relationship is always aware (or defensively unaware) of

the balance of fairness. Are we being recognized for who we are and appreciated for what we do and give, or are we being neglected and misused? Are we being unfair to our partner, or are we mistreating our partner? Clearly, morality is a relational category. (p. 348)

The therapist needs to bring such moral considerations to bear and also to engage couples to reflect on their sociocultural beliefs about gender, sexual orientation and gender identity, race, ethnicity, and other dimensions of social locations that afford relative privilege or oppression and disempowerment in relationships (Knudson-Martin, 2013, 2015; Knudson-Martin & Huenergardt, 2010; Williams & Knudson-Martin, 2013). The therapist must view the couple's interactions and each partner's beliefs about the other and about relationships more generally through the lens of fairness and social justice.

For instance, the familiar concepts of circular interaction and equal responsibility for problems cannot be applied in these situations to both explain and excuse the behavior of a partner who perpetrates violence, conducts an extradyadic relationship, or engages in substance-abusing behavior despite alarm expressed by the other partner (and often by children or other family members). As Goldner et al. (1990) argued in their classic work on couples engaged in interpersonal violence, the application of theories must be reconciled and guided by explicit moral principles about equity, fairness, and compassion. To do otherwise engages in blaming the victim for their own victimization, and diminishes the other partner's willingness to accept responsibility for their behavior, colluding with their explanation that the victim "gave me no choice."

Instead, violence, affairs, or substance abuse must be viewed as a linear, "power-over" act that shuts out the objections of the other partner and leads them to feel powerless. As I will describe, both a circular and linear view of influence between partners can be engaged without contradiction, if we accept the notion that the appropriateness of theoretical constructs must be evaluated through a moral lens.

I draw heavily upon the following authors in my work with extradyadic affairs: Spring (2020), Gordon et al. (2015), Perel (2017), and Scheinkman (2005). I strongly encourage readers to expand their knowledge of this complex work by reading these publications and others.

PREVALENCE AND EFFECTS OF INFIDELITY

Controlled community studies indicate that 20–40% of cisgender heterosexual men and 20–25% of cisgender heterosexual women will engage in extramarital affairs (Greeley [1994] and Laumann et al. [1994], as reviewed by Whisman & Snyder, [2007]). Given that these statistics are almost 30 years old, it is likely that the rates are even higher now, given changes in women's gender norms around sexuality and increased economic and social power (Lammers et al., 2011), the rise of polyamory as an acceptable alternative to monogamous relationships (Perel, 2017), and the increased access to available partners through technologies and apps on mobile phones and computers and the phenomenon of cybersex (Schneider, 2002). Interestingly, a more recent study did not reveal higher rates of infidelity: It found that 23.2% of men and 19.2% of women reported engaging in extradyadic sex (Mark et al., 2011).

However, it is important to note that the definition of *infidelity* may determine reporting rates and also reactions of the affaired-on partner—also termed the "nonparticipating spouse" (Gordon et al., 2015) or "noninvolved spouse" (Atkins et al., 2005): Especially for women, affairs may be more centered on emotional connection, and therefore rates would be higher (especially because an emotional affair can be conducted without the complexities of arranging for physical contact), whereas for men, sexual contact is more frequently involved (Gordon et al., 2015). Glass (2002) provided the broadest definition of infidelity: "a secret, sexual, romantic or emotional involvement that violates the commitment to an exclusive relationship" (p. 489). Reported rates of infidelity also depend on the methodology used to assess it: Whisman and Snyder (2007) found higher rates of reporting through computer-assisted self-interviews than through in-person interviews.

Across several decades, infidelity has been ranked the highest reason for divorce (Allen & Atkins, 2012; Amato & Rogers, 1997). Infidelity is associated with mental health issues, including anxiety and depression (Cano & Leary, 2000). As noted, the partner who has been affaired on often experiences full-blown symptoms of trauma, and the affairing partner (also termed the *participating spouse*; note that the term *cheating spouse* is not used in the professional literature because of its obvious moralistic connotation) may also experience these symptoms, once they emerge from the secret bubble of the extradyadic relationship and fully face the way in which their behavior violated their own religious, relational, and ethical values, and how it has precipitated a crisis in their primary relationship.

Vignette: Tamara and Terry

Tamara had a two-year affair with Jim, an electrician who had done work on the house she owned with her husband, Terry, and lived in with their three young children. A devout Christian, she said, "I knew what I was doing was wrong, but I was so intoxicated by the attention Jim gave me I kinda ignored my gut. Now that it's been revealed, I feel like I've woken up from a dream, and it's now a nightmare. I never meant to hurt Terry, and I really believe in faithfulness and monogamy. I can barely sleep or eat, and eating is important to me, and I go over and over in my mind, how could I have done this?" Meanwhile, Terry, who shared Tamara's religious faith and who had never experienced mental health issues, found himself with intrusions, nightmares, and such high levels of anxiety that he could barely sleep and focus on his demanding work as a litigator. In the first session, he said that although he wanted to try to keep the marriage and family together, he didn't know if he could get over this, and couldn't get out of his mind that when they first met, he and Tamara both spoke strongly about the one thing that might lead them to divorce: an affair.

If you've found couples in which there's been an affair difficult to work with, you are not alone: a survey by Whisman et al. (1997) (as reviewed by Gordon et al., 2015) found that therapists rank affairs "as the third most difficult problem to treat" (Gordon et al., 2015, p. 412). As was noted, affairs are one of the major reasons couples divorce (see review in Gordon et al., 2015), although some couples respond to an affair as a wake-up bell that inspires them to address long-standing problems (Atkins et al., 2005; Perel, 2017). Moreover, the sense of betrayal of relationship expectations for intimacy may be experienced not only by the partner who has been affaired on: The partner who had the affair may have done so due to a sense that the other has become emotionally and sexually unavailable for some time despite requests to rectify the problem (Perel, 2017). Scheinkman (2005) and Welter-Enderlin (1993) note that affairs may be motivated by a need to "individuate," to reclaim a sense of self that has been overshadowed by the affairing partner's role in the marriage or as a parent, and as "a way of counteracting disappointment, emptiness, or constraint. Affairs can also be about fantasy and illusions, or even related to feelings of anger and revenge" (Scheinkman, 2005, p. 230).

If therapy for affairs is to be successful, it is necessary to fully understand not only the negative effects on the affaired-on partner but the motivations and longings of the affairing partner. Compassionately hosting a conversation about the unmet needs of the affairing partner can be challenging in the face of the trauma experienced by the affaired-on partner but is necessary to identify areas where the relationship needs to improve if the couple is to recover from an affair and thrive. As Scheinkman (2005) notes, "Deceiving and hurting the partner are indeed serious consequences, and the very high price an individual pays for the choice of having an affair, but deception and betrayal are rarely primary motivations" (p. 230). Given that 30% of couples who come to therapy do so because of an affair (Whisman et al., 1997), couple therapists will inevitably need the skills and knowledge to work with them.

FACTORS AFFECTING THE IMPACT OF AN AFFAIR

A number of factors affect the degree of disruption caused by an affair and the degree to which couples engage successfully in therapy (Gordon et al., 2015).

Preexisting Relationship Satisfaction and Length of Relationship

On the high end of upset are couples in which an affair results in initiation of separation or divorce; shorter length of relationship and less commitment, and lower satisfaction predict less engagement in attempts at salvaging the relationship and greater likelihood of dissolution. On the other hand, affairing partners who view the marriage more positively are more likely to experience greater remorse, which in turn can result in more engagement in therapy. As might be obvious, the higher the couple's satisfaction with and commitment to the relationship (affected also by whether or not they have children), the greater the chance that they will engage enthusiastically in treatment.

Vignette: Tamara and Terry

This latter state of the marriage was the case for Tamara and Terry. Although Tamara noted that Terry could often be "tough on" her, holding her to high standards of caring for the kids, maintaining the home, and often being critical of her lateness (he was highly punctual), she was overall fairly satisfied with the marriage, as was Terry, despite his criticisms of her. Like many couples with young children in the transition to parenthood, they seemed to have put to the side time for intimacy due to his long work hours and commute and her frequent feeling of overwhelm managing the children's lives. Painful as it was, her affair became the stimulus to make more time for the relationship, and for them to develop new communication and problem-solving skills to address differences in standards about child-rearing, home care, and punctuality.

Degree of Openness of Affairing Partner About Details of Affair

Another predictor of outcomes of therapy is whether the couple can discuss the specifics of the affair openly and in as much detail as the affaired-on partner requests (Gordon et al., 2015). When the affairing partner refuses to disclose details of what happened, where encounters occurred, how they genuinely felt about the extradyadic partner, why they initiated and maintained the affair, and even details about the sex or other aspects of intimacy requested by the affaired-on partner, this bodes poorly for the relationship.

Since the affair is often revealed by the affaired-on partner discovering emails, texts, photos, messages exchanged on Instagram or other social media platforms, or credit card charges, the affaired-on partner often requests free access to the affairing partner's phone, computer, and financial records. The affairing partner is often perplexed that the affaired-on partner would want to view and hear more information about the affair, believing this will only exacerbate the affaired-on partner's upset. Yet clinical experience suggests that partners almost always want more information, as they want to know the full truth about the partner's deceptive behavior so as to make a clearer decision about whether or not to stay in the marriage—and often because their fantasies about what the partner did are so acutely vivid and painful that grounding themselves in the actual facts feels less distressing (Perel, 2017).

This seemingly obsessive "detective work" may also be a way in which the brain attempts to calm itself after a traumatic experience. Just as families who've lost a home in a hurricane or tornado want to go back to see the damage and see what's left to salvage, when the relational "home" has been violated, partners feel compelled to examine the wreckage and see what's left. Sometimes the search leads to a particularly painful discovery. For instance, Terry found an email from

Tamara to Jim on his 33rd birthday, in which Tamara listed 33 things she loved about him, including "You're the most handsome man I've ever met," "I love how your lips feel when you kiss me," "I love how you touch me," and, finally, "I love you." Of all the communications Terry had seen from the two-year relationship, he experienced these as the most painful.

Like Perel (2017), I normalize this intense need of the affaired-on partner to gather these data, as painful and further disruptive to the chances of rebuilding the marriage as they might be, but I also suggest that hopefully, over the course of therapy as the couple comes to terms with the facts of the affair and engages in relationship-strengthening activities, this need for more facts will diminish. I emphasize that this need to gather more information is a normal albeit counterintuitive way that the brain copes with trauma, but that as we work in other ways to diminish the trauma (mindfulness practices, journaling, and others to be discussed later), hopefully the affaired-on partner will be able to desist from further data gathering.

Gender of the Affairing Partner and Gender Role Beliefs

In cisgender heterosexual couples, the gender of the partner who had the affair can also influence the emotions of each partner and relationship outcomes. Research shows that when women have an affair, they experience more guilt than do men when they have the affair (Carpenter, 2012; Miller & Maner, 2008), and affairs by women are more likely to lead to divorce than affairs by men (Allen & Atkins, 2012). This is likely due to cross-culturally shared notions that men (and sometimes women) believe that men are more entitled to engage in such affairs than women, and that women are not entitled to have extradyadic relationships, an aspect of the enduring power differences between men and women, which have been found largely unattended to in the literature on infidelity (Williams & Knudson-Martin, 2013).

As noted earlier, women's affairs have been found generally to involve more emotional connection and fulfilling unmet relational needs (Lewandowski & Ackerman, 2006; Scheinkman, 2005), or to emphasize emotional connection over sexual activity when sex also occurs. As Scheinkman (2005) writes, "As for the women having affairs, their motivation may be more often related to romantic ideals or to disappointments with their bargain in the marriage, or rebelliousness related to a sense of constriction associated with the burdens of domesticity" (p. 238). The male affaired-on partner who has little sense of his partner's dissatisfaction may respond with shock and a litany of reasons why she should be satisfied with her role. The "male code" (Garfield, 2016) that forbids experiencing and expressing vulnerability may limit his willingness or ability to empathize with the female partner's unhappiness in the marriage. Likewise, the socioculturally based expectation that women put their needs aside to serve those of others can result in a woman not expressing her desires and unhappiness in the marriage for fear that it will upset and challenge her male partner to give her something he feels unable to give (Williams, 2011), but her yearning for connection and soothing about her unhappiness may lead her to seek solace and connection with a more sympathetic man.

For women, an affair may be based on a desire to escape the humdrum nature of child-rearing and domestic labor, and the sense of being subservient to their male partners, and unappreciated for what they do for the relationship and family (Williams & Knudson-Martin, 2013). In contrast, men's affairs are often largely limited to sex (Allen & Rhoades, 2008; Scheinkman, 2005). They may view their marriage as satisfactory and treat it as a secure base from which to venture out and experience the excitement of a new sex partner.

Vignette: Gladys and Nathan

For instance, Nathan, 54, married to Gladys, 49, had an affair with Tina, a coworker who was 20 years his junior. Both he and Gladys reported that their marriage was fairly satisfying, although for both, sex had become boring and infrequent. Nathan said that when Tina showed interest in him, he "went for it," and "It felt good to have someone be attracted to me—I felt young again." Indeed, Glass and Wright (1985, 1992) found that more than half of men who had extradyadic sex did so not because their marriages were unhappy, but because they sought excitement and novelty, not for emotional intimacy. This appears to be true for both heterosexual and gay men, whereas for both heterosexual and lesbian women, seeking emotional intimacy is the primary reason for extradyadic affairs (Leigh, 1989).

However, these are broad generalizations which may not apply to a particular affairing partner. Steven was a 48-year-old businessman who felt "trapped" in his 23-year marriage to Ella, with whom they had two college-aged children. Steven described feeling extremely lonely, because Ella spent much of her time exercising and meditating, and showed little interest in his feelings and business. Steven felt that he was Ella's emotional caretaker, and that he received little emotional caretaking from her. He had a 3-year affair with a younger woman, Sasha, with whom he worked. Although he was drawn to Sasha physically and enjoyed sex with her, he primarily valued their relationship because of their shared experiences in the business, and relied on her greatly for daily emotional soothing, including around his unhappy marriage. Likewise, Leisha, discussed in more detail below, had an affair with David, who worked for her at her company, that was largely centered on sex. She did not talk much about her feelings with David, finding him "somewhat shallow emotionally." For her, the affair was all about fun, affirmation of her physical attractiveness, and a release from the pressures of work and raising the children, as well as from the emotional constraints of her marriage to Bruce, who was chronically anxious.

Vignette: Tamara and Terry

Although Terry initially didn't believe her, Tamara insisted that her primary reason for engaging in an affair with Jim was that he made her feel "seen again," "attractive," "respected," and "cherished and adored"—"he made me feel special"—and that their sexual contact was limited to "heavy making out." From Terry's typically male perspective, it made no sense to engage in a long-term affair without having intercourse, but he acknowledged that he rarely complimented Tamara or made her feel cherished anymore. Women may thus be more emotionally attached to the affair partner and struggle with the idea of trying to replace what they experienced with the affair partner with their husband, especially if the absence of these qualities was a major reason they engaged in the affair in the first place. They may have a harder time ending the relationship because they deeply care about the affair partner and don't want to hurt him if he desires to continue. In Tamara's case, despite his wife just having had a child, Jim promised he would leave her for Tamara if she wanted to be with him. This emotional attachment between the affairing partner and the person with whom they're having the affair can pose a challenge to rebuilding the marriage.

Gender and Power

The dynamics of power between men and women are often complex. Therapists who ascribe to feminist values—as I do—may hear women describe how they have gained power in traditionally gendered ways that arouse feelings of dismay in the therapist. Working within a multicultural frame, therapists may hear women genuinely ascribe to a one-down position compared to men because of religious or other cultural beliefs. As will be described, Tamara viewed her ability to arouse men as a source of power; as a devout Christian, she also largely accepted her role as subordinate to Terry. Yet we must understand how women, denied as much power as men in most domains of life, may seek power through avenues that the sociocultural context allows and may also accommodate to cultural prescriptions and proscriptions regarding women's power relative to men. Therapists may want to challenge these normative gender roles, as I did with Tamara, but must do so without suggesting that women are failing to "liberate themselves" by acceding to or even endorsing differential power between them and their husbands.

Due to sociocultural beliefs, men, who generally earn more than women even for the same job, tend to assert that their role as the main provider entitles them to the freedom to use their leisure time as they wish—which may include having an affair. In contrast, without the same earning power and career status that would accord them power, some women may mostly experience themselves as powerful through what they provide relationally and sexually.

Vignette: Tamara and Terry

Tamara spoke of how, beginning at 14 when she developed secondary sex characteristics, she became aware of and enjoyed her power to attract men. Now at 41, and still feeling good about her beauty, she acknowledged that she enjoyed men flirting with her when she passed them at construction sites or in other public spaces, and felt reaffirmed in this aspect of herself. She stated this in a confident manner that suggested that all women would enjoy such attentions. When I suggested that some women might react with revulsion and anger when strange men commented on their bodies, Tamara noted, with a shrug, "I guess I'm not much of a feminist that way, that my looks and male attention are so important to me."

Early in their marriage, Tamara and Terry had agreed that she would give up her career as an office manager and be a full-time parent. She saw this as in keeping with her family-of-origin traditions and her devout Christianity. But the isolation she experienced in this role left her lonely and, with Terry failing to notice her attractiveness, Jim's attention revived this long-standing sense of self and relational power.

Tamara's admission greatly upset Terry. He cried, "Why is it so important for you to be attractive to other men?" I noted that her desire for attention had not been fulfilled for many years by him, and that their ability to move forward would need to include more attention from him. In addition, his frequent criticisms of how she was doing her job as a mother and housewife managing the home reduced her self-esteem; because she was not working outside the home and therefore did not have an opportunity to experience positive regard from others in a work setting, her role as mother and homemaker was her sole opportunity to get compliments and appreciation for her efforts. Terry needed to stop criticizing her, and instead, they were instructed to use the Speaker-Listener and Problem-Solving Techniques to discuss their expectations around all things domestic and come to compromises that worked well for each of them. In addition, I suggested that they engage in daily statements of appreciation, admiration, and fondness. These practices were quite helpful for the couple in eliminating this source of tension and in beginning to rebuild a positive feeling between them.

Affairs in Same-Sex Couples

In working with gay male couples, it is essential to ascertain whether they have a consensual open relationship or expect monogamy. LaSala (2005) found that gay male couples who agreed on extradyadic sex were no different in relationship satisfaction than gay male couples committed to monogamy. However, in couples in which partners agreed to be monogamous but one or both partners had extradyadic sex ("broken agreement" couples), the relationship had lower dyadic adjustment, affectional expression, and satisfaction. Greenan and Tunnel (2002) suggest that the conditions for extradyadic relationships are generally that these will be sex-focused and that the primary partner remains the one for love and emotional intimacy. Lesbian couples tend to ascribe to monogamy, given that sex is generally viewed by them as linked to emotional intimacy. When a lesbian partner seeks greater emotional intimacy with a friend—even without sexual contact—it may arouse jealousy and upset with the relationship partner.

For instance, Clara and Linda were a committed lesbian couple, and Linda had a wide network of close friends, with some of whom she shared intimate details of her life. Clara was hurt and would fly into a rage when Linda chose to spend time with these friends, and threatened to end the relationship if she continued.

This was difficult for Linda, who had coped with coming out as a lesbian in high school without disclosing her sexual orientation to her traditional Maltese American parents—whom she feared would reject her—by seeking other lesbian friends. For her part, Clara had coped with coming out by isolating herself and immersing in her work as a high-school art teacher.

Power issues may also emerge in same-sex couples that contribute to a partner having an affair. Marisol, a 38-year-old Filipina American, was married to Teresa, a 52-year-old white Anglo-American woman, for six years. Teresa had the higher income and paid for most of the couple's expenses, and bought their house and paid the mortgage. According to Marisol, Teresa made many demands for emotional intimacy, especially when she went through a period of intensive medical treatment. Marisol felt Teresa controlled her, and engaged in an affair with a woman closer to her age and economic status, in part to be with someone equal in relational power. Teresa felt betrayed and insisted that Marisol end the affair, which she did, but ultimately, she decided to leave Teresa because she felt Teresa could not share power with her.

Psychological Well-Being and Relational Beliefs of the Affaired-on Partner

The level of psychological health of the affaired-on partner also affects their reaction to an affair. Partners' level of self-esteem; presence of preexisting psychological issues such as anxiety, depression, and history of trauma; and degree of confidence in their physical attractiveness, body image, and sexual abilities, all can affect the impact of an affair. Their attitudes and values about monogamy and the consequences of infidelity, which are often related to cultural backgrounds, as well as attitudes and beliefs about being emotionally intimate with someone other than the partner, even in the absence of sexual behavior and sexually tinged communication; their relationship histories prior to the current relationship and especially whether they experienced infidelity or rejection from previous partners; their family-of-origin experiences around relationship stability and monogamy (i.e., did a sibling, parent, grandparent, or other adult family member engage in an affair?); and other personal and historical factors can influence how traumatic the affair will be.

These factors may also influence the decision of the affairing partner to engage in an affair. For instance, an affair might be experienced as an antidote to anxiety or depression, as a means to gain reassurance about one's physical attractiveness and desirability, as a rejection of family-of-origin religious and moral constraints around sexuality, and even as an attempt to gain mastery over painful memories and scripts about a parent's affair or a previous partner's rejection or affair.

Vignette: Tamara and Terry

For instance, Terry recounted, and Tamara agreed, that they had discussed the importance of fidelity and monogamy when they were dating, and that both had emphasized how important these values and practices were to them. Terry also related in the first phone call that he came from a "broken home," and despite his thoughts about ending the marriage, did not want to have his children experience what he'd experienced. As noted, Tamara related that she had relied on her physical attractiveness as a source of self-esteem, and after giving birth to two children, felt her body was not as "sexy" as in her youth. The relentless adulation from Jim led her to feel "good about [herself] again this way," and she began dressing up in a way that she hadn't in years as a stay-at-home mom, where she spent much of her days dressed in sweatpants and T-shirts. For his part, Terry had always struggled with his weight, and felt his attractiveness was more about his personality and career success; as noted earlier, he was deeply upset and winced when he read the portion of Tamara's birthday email to Jim where she called him "the most handsome man I've ever met." The therapist must ascertain the push and pull of factors that lead partners to want to preserve commitment to the marriage and those that threaten to tear it apart.

Furthermore, as we explored what led Tamara to engage in and maintain the affair, it became clear that this was also a way in which she acted against her strict religious and moral upbringing. She (and Terry) came to recognize that she had chafed against these restrictions, and that the affair allowed her to do something pleasurable and secret, to be, as she said, a "bad girl for a change," which had a tantalizing, exciting aura for her, because forbidden. This quality was accentuated by the settings in which she and Jim would meet— "mostly in his car, or in out-of-the-way little bars" outside of town.

Impact of Online Affairs and Sexting

In line with the expanded definition of affairs (Glass, 2002), some extradyadic relationships may involve no actual in-person contact and no physical sex, and may be limited to interactions online and in text messages (Hertlein & Piercy, 2005, 2006). Some of these relationships may be limited to emotional intimacy, whereas others involve engaging in mutual sexual fantasies and sometimes, mutual masturbation ("sexting"). Nevertheless, such relationships are typically viewed as a form of infidelity (Henline et al., 2007) and have negative effects on the partner and their desire for sex with the affairing partner (Schneider, 2002). In addition, a large percentage (65%) of relationships that begin online end up with actual physical contact (Rietmeijer et al., 2001). Others may involve a partner connecting with someone (through "direct messaging") who posts erotic photos and sexually explicit, inviting messages on erotic websites, and where a paid subscription is usually required. The other partner may react with upset and disgust that their partner is not only engaging in an extradyadic relationship, but is involved in cybersex (Schneider, 2002). Especially when it is a man engaging in such behavior who overtly ascribes to feminist values, a woman partner may find his behavior reveals a lack of true commitment to respectful treatment of women. Other partners may view this behavior as a safe way for the partner to engage in fantasy and may not see the behavior as violating expectations of monogamy or other values.

TREATMENT OF AFFAIRS

My approach to working with affairs has been refined over 30 years, beginning in 1989 when, as a postdoctoral intern at NYU's Family Studies Unit, I saw my first couple, Sidney and Marcia, in which there had been an affair. At that time, little had been written about this complex work. Interestingly, with some important differences in how couple therapists have conceptualized the causes, impact, and path forward for these couples, there is a great deal of what researchers call "convergent validity"—similarities developed independently—across published perspectives (as noted earlier, see especially Spring, 2020; Gordon et al., 2015; Perel, 2017; Scheinkman, 2005).

Vignette: Sidney and Marcia

Sidney and Marcia were a Jewish American middle-class cisgender heterosexual couple in their early 30s when they came to therapy. On the couple's honeymoon, feeling terribly guilty, Marcia told Sidney that the day before their wedding, she had sex with her boss, Roger.

She said that Roger, a tall, handsome, accomplished man, had pursued her intensely, and she finally gave in, thinking this would be her last chance to have sex with someone other than Sidney. Sidney was completely devastated, and the honeymoon was miserable for them both. Having met her boss, he experienced almost constant intrusions, was alternately angry and tearful; Marcia was wracked with guilt, and said she now felt it was "crazy" for her to engage in this one-time sexual encounter. She considered not telling Sidney, but felt that it would be dishonest and that she couldn't live with the secret.

Sidney, who was short, balding, and wiry in build, felt that this proved Marcia was not really attracted to him. Marcia insisted this was not true. He asked her many questions about Roger, culminating in a question that almost led him to end the marriage: "How big was his penis?" Marcia's answer was, "Too big to fit in my mouth." This incident well illustrates that, although the general guideline in working with couples and affairs is that the affairing partner should answer the affaired-on partner honestly, the results of this honesty can at least temporarily devastate the affaired-on partner. Marcia hoped that by answering Sidney's questions, they could quickly move on from this incident and continue to build their life together. But Sidney was traumatized and could not stop thinking about the affair and asking questions.

Perel (2017) describes three phases of working with couples and affairs: "crisis, meaning making, and visioning" (p. 58), with "visioning" referring to helping the couple chart a course toward a future together, if they've decided to sustain the relationship. Likewise, Gordon et al. (2015) describes three stages, following an initial session focused on building the therapeutic alliance, assessment of the couple and of outside stressors and resources, and treatment planning and goal setting: The three stages are dealing with the impact of the affair, finding meaning, and moving on. Gordon et al. additionally specify in Step 1 the substeps of forming an approach to problem solving and damage control, encouraging time-outs and teaching venting techniques, discussing the impact of the affair, imparting strategies of self-care, including ways to cope with flashbacks, dealing with partners who are dysregulated or volatile and defensive as well as those who do not express feelings. In Step 2, substeps include exploring factors that contributed to the affair, problem-solving, and cognitive restructuring of relationship issues; and in Step 3, summarizing what has been learned in previous sessions and formulating a coherent explanation about why the affair occurred, exploring the possibility of forgiveness, and evaluating the viability of the relationship.

Although I agree that these different phases and the components of each of the steps are essential aspects of the work, I find that elements of all three of these phases often occur even in the first session. In the spirit of the Therapeutic Palette integrative approach discussed in Chapter 2, the therapist needs to address whatever is offered as a need and opening presented by the couple rather than sticking to a step-wise sequence. For instance, to reduce the affaired-on partner's upset, the therapist may need to explore with the affairing partner in the first session at least a preliminary understanding of why the affairing partner engaged in the affair. Without such a beginning explanation, affaired-on partners may be too distraught to commit to further sessions and to staying in the relationship.

Likewise, whereas Gordon et al. (2015) state that the topic of forgiveness "is not introduced to the couple until near the end of treatment . . . when the anger has died down and the person's understanding of the betrayal has increased" (p. 431), in reality, affaired-on partners often state in a first session that they feel it may be impossible to forgive the affairing partner and therefore, the only logical path forward is divorce. Or affairing partners may despair because they can't imagine the other partner could ever forgive them—or, now out of the secret bubble and trance state of the affair and considering their own ethical or religious values, may feel shame and guilt that leads them to feel they can never forgive themselves. I concur with Gordon and colleagues that couples cannot engage in possible forgiveness before addressing the impact of the affair, understanding the reasons for it, exploring the problems in the relationship that may have prompted it, gaining greater mutual empathy, and decreasing upset and conflict.

However, when the issue of forgiveness is raised in a first session, to encourage couples to engage in the process of recovery and stick with the therapy, I suggest that the affaired-on partner may indeed never be able to fully forgive the affairing partner—but that I've seen couples able to stay together and move on to a better future if they can fully accept that it happened, that it's irrevocably changed the story of their relationship, and if they can view these events as the stimulus that led them to address issues so as to improve the relationship. Full acceptance of the fact of the affair (and its details) is often challenging in itself, especially when the affaired-on partner had strong faith in the vows of fidelity that both partners affirmed when dating and deciding to marry.

If the challenge of forgiving is raised in a first session, is important to explore with partners, at least preliminarily, the meaning of forgiveness. Oftentimes, one or both partners describe forgiveness as a spiritual act, often linked to religious beliefs, and one or both partners may feel that adultery cannot be forgiven on this deep, spiritual basis. Religions and cultures vary markedly on views about what can and cannot be forgiven. As Perel (2017) notes, adultery is the only sin that is mentioned twice in the Ten Commandments: "one for doing it, and one just for thinking about it" (p. 3). In contrast, "acceptance" connotes more the psychological and relational act of fully acknowledging that a traumatic even has occurred, and that it is now a part of the couple's history. Like the act of forgiveness, acceptance of the affair as a reality must include letting go of the anger and bitterness that, if maintained and acted upon in punishing comments or acts, can impede partners from recovering (Seybold et al., 2001).

With last chance couples who by definition always raise the question of whether the relationship can continue in light of the affair, I note that somewhere along the way of a life together, many if not most couples experience "a test of trust and commitment," and that they can either grow from it or disband. I often use a metaphor of their lives together as a "broad highway" and the affair as potentially a "side road and cul de sac"—a road that ends with no additional roads leading back to the main highway—and that if we can figure out how to move on, over time, the affair, although never forgotten, can recede into the past and become less prominent in their memories and their lives. I've found these interventions effectively allow the partners to put the issue of forgiveness and how they will be able to move on to the side, and to engage in the therapy.

Thus, the therapist needs to be ready to address any element of partners' responses to an affair at any moment. What follows is my typical approach to working with affairs, which mirrors much of what has been discussed in the literature.

The First Session

Setting the therapeutic frame. As with all last chance couples, the first session must focus on creating a frame for the therapy that acknowledges the possibility that they will end the relationship; that we will be engaging in experiments in possibility; that they should not feel compelled to remain in the relationship even if it improves; and that although the therapist's bias is to help couples work things out, the therapist will be mindful of this bias and invites the couple to tell the therapist if they feel pressured by the therapist to stay together (or to separate). What differentiates a first session with an affair couple (or with any couple in which one partner has violated the values and/or safety of the other partner) from those in which the contributions to the present problems are more equally distributed is that the affaired-on partner's pain is privileged a bit more than that of the affairing partner.

Discussing the story of how the affair was revealed. The couple (usually, with the affaired-on partner taking the lead) will want to describe how the affair was discovered, and how each partner feels about it. This revealing of the affair is a central aspect of the sense of crisis that couples are experiencing—the crisis of violated values, agreements, and expectations about fidelity. Usually, in our contemporary world of smart phones, social media, and the internet, it is revealed by texts (phone or social media) or emails seen by the affaired-on partner (or someone else who reports it to the partner), or by unexplained or unexpected expenditures, often on business or other trips. Occasionally, the partner of the person with whom the affairing partner had the affair contacts the affaired-on partner. But other sources of discovery exist. In some cases, the affaired-on partner has noticed emotional distance and lack of enthusiasm for sexual contact with the affairing partner, and confrontation leads the affairing partner to acknowledge the affair, often after a period of vehement denial. In still other cases, especially when the affairing partner is quite unhappy with the marriage, they may disclose the affair as part of revealing the wish to separate. But there are other, albeit more unusual ways in which an affair may be discovered.

Vignette: Leisha and Bruce

Leisha, a 34-year-old Lebanese American woman with a high position in a finance company, and Bruce, a 34-year-old white Anglo-American man who was a software engineer, were married for six years and together for eight years, and had two young children. They lived in an apartment in Manhattan, with the children sharing a room with Zuzanna, a Polish au pair who cared for the kids during the day. Leisha had engaged in an affair for about eight months with David, one of her "reports" in the company. Most of their encounters occurred during her frequent business trips. These trips often involved entertaining clients, with many late nights in restaurants and bars where Leisha drank considerably.

One night, David came to her neighborhood somewhat drunk, and texted her asking to come up. Leisha had also been drinking, and invited him up. She asked the au pair to stay with the children in their room. Leisha and David shared some more beers, and they ended up having sex in Leisha and Bruce's bed. Bruce was away on business, and when he returned the next day, he noticed the large number of beer bottles in the garbage the day after these were usually brought down to the recycling bin. Curious about whether someone had been over, he asked Zuzanna if Leisha had had a friend over. Zuzanna looked extremely uncomfortable and said yes, a man had come in. Bruce then asked the building super to allow him to see the video of the front door from the night before and saw that it was a man he didn't recognize. He confronted Leisha, and she acknowledged the affair.

Explaining why the affaired-on partner wants more details: Introducing the trauma frame. No matter how much the affairing partner has already revealed, the affaired-on partner almost always will press the other to disclose more details of the affair. Oftentimes, the affairing partner is reluctant to share these details, due to a combination of guilt or shame, and a belief that more information will only upset the other partner even more and decrease their wish to repair their relationship. The affairing partner may wonder why the affaired-on partner is so insistent on learning the "gory details."

I use this moment to introduce the explanation that the affaired-on partner is likely experiencing trauma symptoms, and the affaired-on partner always concurs. I explain that trauma occurs when our expectations about the world are violated in a marked, emotionally disturbing way. I use the analogy of a family that has lost their home due to a natural disaster: They know their home has been destroyed, but they want to return to the home to assess the degree of damage and see what's left to be salvaged. Often, the scenarios that the affaired-on partner imagines occurred during the affair—including explicit images of their partner having sex with the affair partner— are worse than what actually occurred, and hearing the details may be somewhat reassuring. Of course, in some instances, as with Leisha and Bruce, and Sidney and Marcia, the details of the contact between the affairing partner and the affair partner are even more upsetting than the affaired-on partner has imagined. Sometimes, the affairing partner will reveal that the relationship discovered is not the first time they have had extradyadic relationships.

Vignette: Lev and Alina

Lev and Alina were Russian Jewish American actuaries in their late 40s, who had met in school in the United States. Lev ran a division of an actuarial consulting firm, while Alina worked in-house at an insurance company. Alina had discovered purchases for jewelry that she hadn't received on Lev's credit card, as well as charges for dinners at high-end restaurants in cities where Lev had gone to present at actuarial conferences. Alina knew that Lev had brought one of his actuarial assistants, a Chinese American woman named Shi Jing, to these conferences, but until then had accepted his explanation that he needed her to assist him in putting together his presentations. For months prior to the discovery of the jewelry purchase, Lev denied having an affair with Shi Jing, but when confronted with this expenditure, acknowledged that he had an affair with her for the past six months. Alina was devasted and extremely traumatized: The couple had two teenaged children, and Alina did not want to separate from Lev and have to explain why to the children and to their extended family, but she also felt a complete loss of trust in him and wondered if it was best for her mental health to leave.

After four months of treatment, having viewed the affair as a wake-up call to improve their connection, the couple was doing quite well, although Alina periodically was plagued with intrusive memories of the affair. One day, she visited Lev's office and spoke with a senior actuarial associate in Lev's division, another Chinese American woman named Iris, and noticed that Iris didn't make eye contact with her. She suspected that Lev may have been having an affair with Iris, and confronted him. Lev reluctantly shared that before the affair with Shi Jing he had conducted an eight-year affair with Iris, which she had ended because she felt guilty about being unfaithful to her husband. Of course, this was a major setback for Alina and for the couple. I also noted that I was disappointed with Lev that, in our individual sessions, he had not previously disclosed this earlier affair and allowed me to help him disclose it.

Alina felt torn: On the one hand, she felt she would never get over the trauma of these affairs, and wondered if it would be best for her to end the marriage. On the other, as she had felt upon revelation of the affair with Shi Jing, she did not want to reveal it to their sons, and to initiate a breakup of the family. In the end, she decided to stay with Lev. However, the work we had done to improve their marriage, and Lev's (seemingly) honest assertion that there were no further affairs to be discovered allowed the couple to bounce back fairly quickly.

As with this couple, I always further explain that trauma sets off a process in the brain in which it must reorganize how the person sees their partner, their memories, and their feelings. I also frequently describe the research of the Gestalt cognitive–perceptual psychologists from the 1940s and 1950s, in which they demonstrated how the brain automatically looks for connections among disparate but possibly related stimuli. For instance, in this research (noted earlier), subjects were exposed subliminally to images of dots in a row or three dots arranged to represent the points in a triangle, and when asked what they saw, they would report seeing a line or a triangle. This explanation of how the brain functions normally and in responding to trauma helps couples understand the affaired-on partner's often relentless need to know all the facts, even though they realize the information may cause further trauma, and their tendency to be triggered by stimuli associated with the affair partner's behavior. For instance, Alina felt revulsed seeing the sports jacket that Lev usually wore when traveling to conferences; he decided to throw the jacket out.

Putting brain functioning and adjustment aside, I also remind the affairing partner that the affaired-on partner in a last chance couple is trying to determine whether to stay or leave the relationship. To be fair to that partner, it is incumbent on the affairing partner to let their partner know the details of what happened. The affaired-on partner also wants to be reassured through direct examination of cell phones, tablets, and computers that there is no ongoing contact with the affair partner or other potential affair partners. This is the basis for my recommendation that the affairing partner allow the affaired-on partner to have access to electronic devices and financial records.

However, there is a point in recovery from an affair, by which time the affairing partner has disclosed everything they can remember (or says so, anyway), when it makes sense to suggest that the affaired-on partner start to decrease the frequency of examining these sources of information and eventually end the monitoring and detective work as part of trying to rebuild trust and move on from the affair. Even if it reveals nothing new, monitoring information brings a level of anxiety and sustains the state of hypervigilance associated with trauma, so it is in the best interest of the affaired-on partner to eventually stop so as to recover more fully from the trauma.

Although clinical experience indicates that many affaired-on partners experience trauma, Scheinkman (2005) has pointed out from a multicultural perspective that the occurrence and intensity of traumatic reactions is to a large extent a result of larger societal beliefs about the sanctity of monogamy and ethical beliefs about marriage or other committed relationships. Coming from Latin America, she reflects on how different cultures may view affairs differently in terms of the degree of acceptability, and points to the manner in which treatment of affairs in the United States tends to invoke a moralistic script of "perpetrator" and "traumatized victim" (for instance, Glass, 2003; Madden, 2014; Pittman, 1989). As Scheinkman (2005) writes,

> when we consider that love and the vagaries of desire are fueled by an infinite number of emotional forces, it becomes our job to understand and grasp the meaning of these undercurrents rather than to infuse particular moral ideas into the love experience. By overfocusing on the impact of affairs, we get away from this fuller understanding about the motives, contextual forces, and cultural ideas that may propel individuals into affairs in the first place. (p. 228)

As a result of a dominant focus on the effects of the affair, therapy may not invite couples to reflect on the powerful force of desire and the challenges of maintaining desire in long-term relationships. Perel (2007, 2017) has offered similar critiques of the literature on affairs, and emphasizes the importance of addressing these challenges. Scheinkman and Perel balance the field's dominant focus on the traumatic effects of betrayal with equal attention to the longings and "yearning" (Scheinkman, 2005, p. 230) of the affairing partner. Scheinkman writes, "The yearning can be for a particular kind of emotional connection, assurance, self-discovery, novelty, or freedom; it may also involve a wish to recapture lost parts of the self, or an attempt to bring back vitality in the face of loss or tragedy" (p. 230).

I concur with these authors and adopt a "both-and" approach, addressing the traumatic effects of the affair while also making space for a nonjudgmental exploration of how for both the affairing and affaired-on partner, desires may have been suppressed by cultural, societal, and family-of-origin-based beliefs about the place of desire in marriage, as well as by the often-overwhelming responsibilities couples face in raising children, maintaining income and pursuing careers, and supporting a family.

Helping the affairing partner take 100% responsibility: Distinction between explanation and excuse. In starting to answer the questions of the affaired-on partner about why the affairing partner had the affair, the affairing partner will often point to issues in the relationship that led them to feel criticized, dominated, unappreciated, unloved, rejected, and disconnected from the affaired-on partner. I note that we will want to use the affair to examine the problems in the relationship that prompted engaging in the affair, and I make it clear that this will help us explain at least in part why the affairing partner went outside the relationship for what they needed. But I also draw a distinction between developing an explanation and seeing that explanation as an excuse for having the affair. This is a critical step, because the affaired-on partner will likely otherwise feel blamed for what the affairing partner did. I make it clear that the affairing partner had other options: raising the issues, seeking couple counseling, and, if those choices did not lead to changes, suggesting that the relationship end. The affairing partner needs to take 100% responsibility for their choice to engage in an extradyadic relationship before the following apology ritual can be genuine and effective. This step sometimes takes a few sessions to be achieved, and may also involve individual sessions with the affairing partner.

Sharing the emotional distress of the affaired-on partner: The daily apology ritual. Typically, once the affair is revealed, the affairing partner wants to move on, and often feels relieved that the secret is now disclosed, but because it has traumatized the affaired-on partner, the latter cannot move on so quickly. The affaired-on partner is hurt and angry, and feels the request of the affairing partner to simply move on minimizes the traumatic effects of the affair. Therefore, as part of helping couples navigate the crisis of disclosure, in a first session, I suggest they eventually engage in a daily apology ritual in which the affairing partner demonstrates that they are mindful that the affaired-on partner will likely suffer from intrusions during the day and confirms on a daily basis that they are sorry for having had the affair and for the effects it's now having on their partner (Fraenkel, 2011).

I suggest that the couple do this apology ritual in the morning and, if requested by the affaired-on partner, in the evening as well. The apology can go something like this: "[Name of partner], I want again to say how sorry I am for having had the affair, and I know that at some point today you may be having thoughts and feelings about what I did, and I am sorry for the effect that my actions have on you." I've found that the affaired-on partner deeply appreciates this ritual, as it helps them feel less alone in their trauma symptoms, and shows them that the affairing partner continues to keep them in mind and take responsibility. I suggest that the ritual continue until such time as the affaired-on partner feels it is no longer necessary.

Managing trauma symptoms. Psychoeducation about trauma and the brain is useful for both partners, both for the affaired-on partner experiencing the intrusions, hypervigilance, triggering, reactivity, and numbing, as well as for the affairing partner who doesn't understand why their partner sometimes seems okay but can suddenly be overcome with anger, hurt, questions, sleeplessness, and other trauma reactions, and who also may now be experiencing trauma themselves. I suggest two practical tools for reducing trauma. First, I teach both couples mindful breathing and also introduce them to Qigong, a Chinese movement meditation particularly well-suited for people who are agitated and may have difficulty engaging in sitting meditation. As discussed in Chapter 4, I recommend doing three repetitions of mindful breathing and three repetitions of a Qigong move five times a day to help train the nervous system to be less arousable and to sustain a feeling of relative calm and serenity across the day.

Second, I suggest that the affaired-on partner do a journaling activity twice a day as follows (and I provide a written guide): Purchase a blank journal or diary that is aesthetically appealing, and use a specific pen or pencil for this activity, also one that is aesthetically appealing, with the idea that having tools that bring aesthetic pleasure makes doing difficult work a bit more enjoyable. Spend five minutes in the morning writing all the intrusive feelings, thoughts, and memories associated with the affair. Then put the journal away and out of sight, so that the sight of it doesn't inadvertently trigger them. During the day, when the intrusions inevitably appear (as they will at first), the person should address them in an internal dialogue, and say that they know those thoughts and feelings are still there and that they are important, but "I don't have time to do you justice right now—I'll see you later at our evening writing time." To enhance the separation between the person and the trauma symptoms, I suggest a therapeutic practice from narrative therapy—externalizing (White, 1988)—wherein they give the thoughts and feelings a name that captures their effects, almost as if the collective thoughts and feelings are a creature or being that visits them. Affaired-on partners have used such names as the Soul Crusher, the Whirlwind, and the Tornado.

I also sometimes refer to a concept and practice from internal family systems therapy (Schwartz & Sweezy, 2020)—the notion that symptoms can be understood as a part of one's internal world whose function is to protect the core self. Trauma symptoms—especially hypervigilance—can be understood as a way that the protective part seeks to avoid another shock to the self. The person can thank the externalized thoughts and feelings for the attempt to help them not receive another shock, but, at least for today until the evening, give that part permission to pull back and let the person go on with their day, knowing that there will be another five-minute writing time in the evening (a few hours before bed, so that the exercise and the negative arousal it incurs do not disrupt sleep). Importantly, even if the person wakes up in the morning or arrives at the evening writing time without the presence of these disruptive intrusions, they should nevertheless conjure them up and write them down.

This technique integrates several therapeutic theories. It involves the long-supported behavior therapy technique of exposure; paradoxical intervention—inviting symptoms deliberately as a way of changing the power relationship between the self and the intrusions, a technique invented by Victor Frankl (2019) and developed by master hypnotherapist Milton Erickson (Haley, 1993); externalizing; internal family systems therapy; and the well-documented positive effects of journaling in ameliorating both psychological and physical health symptoms that are worsened by stress (Esterling et al., 1999; Pennebaker, 1997, 2004; Smyth et al., 2008). It is also supported by similar therapeutic suggestions described by Grayson (2014) in working with clients with obsessive–compulsive disorders that involve high degrees of anxious rumination.

Addressing high conflict and violence. The discovery of an affair can provoke high degrees of conflict (Gordon et al., 2015). Some couples may already have been engaging in the types of destructive interactions detailed in Chapter 4; for other, more emotionally disengaged couples, the affair may result in new or renewed patterns of conflict that led them to disengage (see Chapter 9). Suggesting in a first session that you will teach the couple communication and problem-solving skills usually provides a sense of hope and can in itself reduce conflict. If the couple is willing to have a two-hour session, you can launch into teaching the skills.

Gordon et al. (2015) also note the importance of assessing whether or not violence or any behavior on the continuum of excessive force and control are occurring or a risk. In more than 30 years of working with couples and affairs, I've never encountered such a couple in which violence or aggression were present or a risk, but of course, the therapist should be attuned to that possibility in hearing about the nature of the couple's interactions. Chapter 7 addresses how to work with couples where there has been violence or less extreme forms of intimation and aggression.

Limiting times to talk about the affair between sessions. Because of the traumatic effect of the affair, the affaired-on partner may find themselves wanting at all hours (including the middle of the night) to engage the affairing partner to talk about it. This can create more emotional dysregulation and loss of sleep for both partners. I recommend that the couple specify times during the day to talk about it and encourage the affaired-on partner to add the use of the journaling exercise to discharge feelings and thoughts about the affair. This suggestion is met with relief from both partners. The couple should be urged to use the therapy sessions, which initially may need to occur more than once a week, to process the affair, with the idea that their conversations without therapeutic guidance may not go so well.

Deciding with whom to discuss the affair. As Gordon et al. (2015) suggest, it is important to discuss with the couple to whom in their network of family and friends they want to disclose the affair. Others' knowledge about the affair (for instance, family members of the affaired-on partner, friends of the couple) can have long-lasting negative repercussions in terms of how these others view the affairing partner, the affaired-on partner who decides to stay in the marriage, and the viability of the marriage. This can interfere with the couple's recovery. Yet the affaired-on partner often feels isolated with this information and their feelings, so it is useful to discuss with whom they can share what happened and gain support confidentially. By the time of their first session, the affaired-on partner may already have shared information with family and friends, and then the plan for recovery will need to include how to talk with those people once the couple is making progress and decides to stay together, if indeed that is the direction the therapy goes.

Discussing a plan to end contact with the affair partner. One of the main concerns of the affaired-on partner will be that the affairing partner might have continued contact with the affair partner. If the affair relationship is with someone outside of work, the affairing partner needs to end contact entirely with the affair partner and demonstrate that there is no further contact, through making phone and computer available to the affaired-on partner, or even by installing a tracking app on the affairing partner's phone to show where they are during the day. if that partner so desires. Sometimes the affairing partner has difficulty ending the relationship, or is ambivalent about doing so, because they care about that person or worry that the affair partner will retaliate in some manner. These are complicated situations and must be addressed on a case-by-case basis.

Vignette: Tamara and Terry

For instance, Tamara's affair partner Jim had an office in the town where Tamara and Terry lived. On a few occasions, Jim saw Tamara in her car in a parking lot and pulled up next to her to start a conversation. Tamara viewed herself as a "nice person" and didn't want to be rude to Jim, so initially she engaged in brief conversations, which she then reported to Terry, who was furious and hurt. I honored her intentions to be a nice person but noted that Jim was putting her in a difficult situation, which suggested he didn't care as much for her feelings as she imagined, especially since she'd already been clear with him that she wanted to end their relationship. She sighed, and agreed. With my support, Tamara eventually texted Jim to tell him that she was working on repairing her marriage and that she did not want any further contact with him. On a later occasion when he parked outside her home and tried to give her a letter, she shook her head and drove away. That was the last time Jim attempted contact with her. Fortunately, he did not continue to engage in behavior that could be considered stalking, because the couple was reluctant to contact the police, as Jim was friendly with a number of officers.

If the affair was with someone at work, the affairing partner must do whatever possible to end the work relationship with that person. Sometimes this is quite complicated, because efforts to dismiss or move a junior colleague or employee could result in a lawsuit or disclosure of the inappropriate relationship. When the affair partner is someone at equal level in the company hierarchy, or higher, such a move may jeopardize the affairing partner's career.

Vignette: Leisha and Bruce

For instance, Leisha stopped having David accompany her on business trips. Having told David that their affair had been discovered, she asked him to stop contacting her, and he readily agreed, saying he did not want to disrupt her marriage and family life. Eventually, she had David reassigned to another group at work and had his desk moved (previously, their desks had been side by side), and he was agreeable. She also shortened the time she spent at client dinners, which during the period of the affair had kept her out at times until after midnight. Leisha also recognized that her drinking at these events lowered her inhibitions and made her vulnerable to engaging in flirtatious and sexual behavior (like dancing on a bar), and she cut back dramatically.

Although Bruce welcomed these changes, he felt it was not enough. He wanted to confront David himself and "beat him up" (not a great plan, as Bruce had no experience with physical fighting and David was a much larger man who had been a boxer in college) and also wanted to call Leisha's boss to report the affair (especially since it was with a colleague whom Leisha supervised, a clearly unethical practice). I said that I understood his desire for revenge, but drew his attention to the serious negative consequences these moves would likely have for Leisha's career, and their financial well-being as a couple, and that these actions and effects might set them back in their attempts at recovery. He decided not to pursue these paths, but over the course of therapy, when his trauma symptoms increased, would sometimes again threaten to take these steps, requiring me to again empathize with his anger but remind him of the likely negative consequences.

Vignette: Lev and Alina

In contrast, Lev refused to fire Iris or Shi Jing, claiming they had special skill sets that he required to successfully run his division. He also accurately worried that they might sue the company and reveal their intimate affairs with him to HR. No degree of urging him to reconsider this decision from me was successful, and Alina had to decide whether she could accept this arrangement. However, Lev did not have Shi Jing continue to accompany him on trips, and Alina continued to check his phone and computer for some time. In addition, as we explored the reasons for Lev's affairs (see below), Alina came to believe that he was changing and could be trusted again.

Handling disclosures of unrevealed and ongoing affairs. If in a first phone call or a confidential individual session, a partner reveals that they are having an affair, I do not require that partner to reveal it. So that I do not end up in a position of holding this secret with the affairing partner, I emphasize to both partners that phone calls and individual sessions with each partner individually are completely confidential. As Scheinkman's 2005 review of the literature on affairs indicates, some therapists hold the position that the affair must be revealed or else the therapy will end.

Along with Scheinkman (2005) and Perel (2017), I find this approach problematic, because it means that the couple will not be able to work to improve the relationship so as to make the affair unnecessary for the affairing partner, especially when the motivations for the affair center on the partner's need to recover a sense of self or is a response to other problems in the relationship that have led to feelings of resentment, distance, powerlessness, and loneliness. As Spring (2020) writes in her book for couples, "Even if you're committed to rebuilding the relationship, there is no one clear way to proceed. For some couples the truth can have adverse, even destructive, consequences. For others it's essential for restoring a damaged relationship . . . in grappling for the best strategy, therefore, it may help to ask, 'Best for whom?'" (p. 301).

When one partner believes strongly that the other is having an affair and even has clear evidence, yet the other denies it, I will meet with the "suspected" partner for a confidential session, ask if this is true, and, if they acknowledge it, I explore their reasons for not disclosing it. Usually, the affairing partner believes that disclosure will only make things worse with their spouse and states that they wish to continue the marriage. However, I strongly suggest that in most cases, it is the ongoing loss of trust based on the partner's denial of clear evidence that is most damaging to a marriage, and that I have a good success rate in assisting couples to recover from an affair.

Vignette: Gladys and Nathan

This occurred in the case of Gladys and Nathan. Gladys contacted me first, reporting that she had found multiple texts and sexting between Nathan and another woman. She confronted Nathan about these, and he denied the affair. Gladys noted that she had no intention of dissolving the marriage if Nathan would admit to the affair; if he didn't, she was considering asking for a separation. I asked her to invite him to contact me by phone. I told him that our call was confidential and asked him if he was having an affair. He said yes, but did not see the point of acknowledging it to Gladys, as it was now over and the disclosure would only lead to divorce. I told him that my impression in speaking with Gladys was that she was quite committed to their marriage but that her continuing doubt about his truthfulness could create an irreparable rift between them. He understood my point, and in our first couple session, he acknowledged the affair and also said he was committed to working on their marriage. Gladys responded as I expected she would: "Well, at least now I know I'm not crazy!" She affirmed her desire to work on the marriage and even noted that her overuse of alcohol over the past two years, which she had stopped in the prior month, might have driven Nathan away, which he confirmed. The couple was able fairly quickly to work through the affair and restore their sexual relationship.

However, if the affair is ongoing and the affairing partner is reluctant to end it, I do ask that partner to at least "take a vacation" from the affair so that they can more fully immerse in the marital relationship and the therapy. (It is noteworthy that this is not the only approach: For instance, Perel [2017] does not make this request as a condition for therapy.) I remind the affairing partner that my approach is to engage couples in "experiments in possibility," and that these experiments may be half-hearted attempts if the affair is ongoing and the partner is getting some of their needs met with the affair partner. In order to fully examine whether changes in the marriage can correct whatever patterns prompted the affair (emotional isolation and loneliness, power differences, sexual dissatisfactions, and others), the affairing partner needs to be emotionally and energetically present in the therapy. To date, all partners to whom I've suggested this approach have told me (ostensibly honestly) that they ended or took a break from the affair. I should also note that in my experience, this situation is extremely rare: In most cases, the affair has been disclosed and ended.

Summary of first-session goals. The couple should leave the first session with a sense of a map for how therapy will proceed and how it may assist them to cope with the crisis of the affair and heal from it. Having a sense of the path forward reassures the couple that the treatment you will provide is credible (as noted in Chapter 1, essential to build the therapeutic alliance) and potentially useful, and can help the partners calm down. The session must create a liminal space for experimenting with possibilities; provide an opportunity to discuss how the affair was revealed and to begin exploring the reasons for it; introduce the distinction between formulating an explanation versus validating excuses for the affair, and encourage the affairing partner to take 100% responsibility for choosing to respond to relationship issues by having an affair; and should introduce the frame that an affair is experienced by the affaired-on partner as a trauma, which explains their emotional reactions.

The session should introduce the apology ritual and have the couple try it (only if the affairing partner has taken 100% responsibility), and teach the couple the journaling exercise to help especially the affaired-on partner manage trauma symptoms, along with instructing both partners in mindfulness activities to decrease negative physiological and emotional arousal. The first session should also validate the affaired-on partner's resulting need for more information and to continue to have access to the affairing partner's phone and other electronic devices; empathize with their desires for revenge but help them think through the ramifications of acting on these desires; discuss with whom they will reveal the affair; encourage the couple to set specific times during the day to discuss the affair; discuss a plan with the affairing partner to end contact with the affair partner; address increased conflict by teaching structured communication skills; and assess and decrease the risk of violence or other forms of interpersonal aggression.

Further Sessions

Like the approach described by Gordon et al. (2005, 2015), my approach integrates the action-oriented techniques described with exploration of each partner's relational and family-of-origin pasts to develop greater insight into the reasons for the affair. The second and subsequent sessions include checking in to see the progress partners have made with the various aspects of the recovery plan (for instance, has the affairing partner ended contact with the affair partner? Has the couple used the apology ritual, and if not, why not?) and how each partner is doing emotionally and as a couple in their interactions.

These sessions center on further exploration of the reasons for the affair—both as a response to perceived deficits in the primary relationship, and in terms of psychological issues the affairing partner struggles with—as well as the meaning of the affair for the affaired-on partner and the nature of their specific reactions to it. This work involves exploring family-of-origin experiences, partners' relationships with their sociocultural backgrounds, including articulated or unarticulated assumptions about gender, power, and the value of equality (Williams & Knudson-Martin, 2013), the previous adult relationships of each partner, and issues of adult development, sense of self, and how each partner is adjusting to their current place in the life cycle. Couples are encouraged to engage in a variety of experiments in possibility to strengthen the relationship and address experienced deficits and longings, and these experiments in turn often evoke narratives, beliefs, and emotions about values, family-of-origin experiences, and cultural context, such that new action results in new insights, and new insights provide the platform to try new action to experiment with transforming partners' relationships to their histories and accumulated meaning systems.

Family- and culture-of-origin themes in affairs and relational power. For instance, Leisha came from a family in which her mother, who was a physician, represented being a responsible, hard-working, ambitious woman who, as a first-generation immigrant from Lebanon, broke out of what she viewed as the culture's expectations of the subservient role Lebanese women were forced to adopt in their families. Leisha modeled her drive for academic and career achievement after her mother. But she also admired her father's adventuresomeness and enjoyment of sensual pleasures. Leisha reported that as a teenager and young adult growing up in a large city in California, she relied on her physical beauty and willingness to engage boys and men in sex as a way to bolster her self-esteem and sense of belonging in a largely white peer culture, in which she often felt marginalized or treated as "exotic."

Although she loved Bruce and was attracted to him, as the years went by and they had two children, she often found him "uptight and nervous"—qualities that I also sensed about Bruce and that he confirmed. David had offered her a more carefree sexual relationship, and allowed her to sustain her sense of adventure and fed her need to be seen as "sexy," which she no longer experienced with Bruce, who was often preoccupied with his work and who often had nightmares and night sweats.

As therapy progressed, Bruce vacillated about regaining trust in Leisha, but at times was plagued by his intrusive feelings and thoughts about whether she had possibly had other affairs. He eventually confronted her about other close work relationships she'd had with men, and she acknowledged having sex with two other men before David.

Interestingly, Leisha's decision to conduct an affair came from a sense of both power—she had long experienced the power of her attractiveness to engage men, and her affair partner was one of her staff whom she supervised—and powerlessness—her feeling growing up of being marginalized in her peer group as a woman of color and child of immigrant parents. Leisha's case suggests that it is having power, rather than gender itself, that may facilitate partners engaging in affairs, but that at least in some cases, that power is used to rectify a sense of powerlessness. As noted earlier, as women gain greater economic and other sources of power, it may contribute to a greater sense of freedom to have affairs. This may help explain why Mark et al. (2011) found no statistically significant difference in the self-reported rate of affairs between men and women.

Vignette: Lev and Alina

For Lev, there was a similar mix of insecurity/relational powerlessness, and an exploitation of his power as a man and boss. Lev was a rather plain-looking man who had difficulty attracting women as a teenager, and who saw himself as a "nerd." Alina was a quite stunning woman, and his ability to attract her surprised and initially delighted him. Over the years of their marriage, he often felt criticized by Alina, mostly around his failing to do household chores that he agreed should be his responsibility. These criticisms and power over him led him to feel "emasculated" and reduced his sexual desire for her.

Additionally, the partners came from quite different places in Russia: Lev was raised in Moscow, and said that being a Muscovite often required lying to get ahead or even to procure basic needs like food, and he had to put up a "tough front" to deal with bullying by non-Jewish Russian boys. We agreed that his long-time "practice" in being deceptive prepared him to lie to Alina effectively about his affairs. His self-described cynical attitude ("everybody lies to get what they want") and his sense of entitlement as a man to seek sexual contacts when he could get them enabled him to have the affairs. In addition, he held a stereotype of East Asian women often held by white men—that they were oriented towards pleasing men, and passive, and not likely to criticize him in the ways that Alina did. Of course, the fact that both Iris and Shi Jing were his subordinates gave him power over them which, as I pointed out, would make it hard for them to resist his advances. Examining the mix of his insecurities and his sexist and racist attitudes were ultimately transformative for him, and he began to accept Alina's valid criticisms of him, and to accept her as an equal partner yet still be attracted to her.

In contrast, Alina described being raised in a small Jewish village, where she felt quite protected from the self-seeking and corrupt attitudes and behaviors that both said were dominant in larger Russian cities. She maintained a kind of innocence and faith in the sanctity of marriage that Lev did not hold, and along with her feeling betrayed by Lev, couldn't understand how someone could even feel attracted to someone else besides their marital partner, never mind have an affair. As a result, her trauma was amplified by her cultural context because it forced her to recognize that her innocent, trusting beliefs about complete devotion and singularity of attraction in married persons was not held by many persons. This was a painful realization for Alina, but as Lev became truly faithful, she was able to move beyond her newfound cynicism and enjoy their relationship again. Interestingly, the couple started taking ballroom dance lessons, which allowed Lev to "lead" but in a pleasurable and consensual manner. They came to specialize in the tango, which of all the ballroom styles of dance, involves more of a back-and-forth between partners in who is "leading" or directing the flow of the dance. Their interest in dance and tango in particular provided an opening for me to use partner dancing as a metaphor for how they could reconfigure their relationship as one that was engaged and more equal in power.

Vignette: Tamara and Terry

Tamara's psychological reasons for her affair with Jim also reflected this dialectic between powerlessness and power, and low versus high self-esteem. As noted earlier, she was raised in a devout Christian family that forbid her to have sex before marriage. In high school, many boys sought to date her, but the family's religious beliefs led her to turn them down. In her relationship with Terry, she was finally able to act on a man's attraction to her, and she felt powerful through his desire for her. But over time, as the couple had children and Terry's attention turned increasingly toward his career while she tended to the children and home (she had decided to be a full-time mom), she lost her sense of herself as attractive and the power she gained in having men pursue her.

When Jim approached her for sex, she felt a wave of restored self-esteem, amplified by her sense that Terry was often critical of her work as a mother and manager of the home. Therapy addressed Terry's critical attitude and led him to assume more of the home-based chores and parenting. In line with the Gottmans' research-based suggestions on strengthening the "fondness and admiration system" (Gottman & Gottman, 2018, pp. 147–148), I also encouraged the partners to make at least one statement of appreciation and admiration a day. These interventions led the partners to feel more equal and appreciated by one another, and restarted their mutual sexual attraction.

The affaired-on partner may also struggle to move beyond the affair due to beliefs and expectations derived from family-of-origin, culture-of-origin, and broader sociocultural beliefs and experiences.

For instance, with some cisgender heterosexual men whose women partners have had an extradyadic relationship, the affair may reveal previously unspoken beliefs and feelings about assumed control over women and their sexuality.

In an early session, Terry spoke with great outrage and pain that Tamara was "sharing her sexuality with the world—I don't want her to, and she wants to!" because she had acknowledged enjoying getting attention from men about her looks. "She feels put down by the fact that I think she dresses promiscuously, and I feel hurt by her dressing the ways she does to get that attention from people who are not Terry Johnston." Tamara said, "I don't think it's as bad as he thinks it is." The couple then discussed how Tamara had struggled with bulimia since she was 16; Terry said, "So she doesn't feel good about herself and her body." Terry noted that after Tamara had their second child, he paid for breast enhancement and a "tummy tuck" at Tamara's request: "And the irony is that she went somewhere else with that love." Tamara interjected, "I don't think I dress so over the top." Speaking to me— as if by speaking "man to man," I might come to agree with him—he countered, "Since she has bulimia, she clearly has body dysmorphic issues, and she doesn't see the way she actually looks; so as a result, she doesn't realize how sexy she looks when she dresses up."

Tamara was puzzled by this line of reasoning, and I felt increasing concern about what appeared to be Terry's assumption that only he should be able to gaze appreciatively at his wife. Indeed, a bit later, he cried out, "Every piece of the word 'sex' that is my wife should be mine! And if I want to share that with the world, I can, but I don't want to! I don't want to share any of her sexiness with the world! I didn't think I had to, and I thought once I got married, it would be mine alone, and I love the shit out of it. I don't want other people to share it—that's the problem." Tamara interjected, "He only loves it in the bedroom, though," and went on to say that she frequently tried to get Terry come out with her to social events where she hoped he would treat her "as a trophy wife" and let other people know that he was proud to be with her. Terry countered that he didn't like doing social events, and was too busy with work. He noted, "Here's the equation, Peter. I'm a 250-pound 5-feet 9-inch guy. I'm not an Adonis, but I'm a good man and a good person." Terry went on to tell how he and Tamara often joked about how she's "much better looking than me"—even noting that at a store cashier's checkout line, "the cashier placed a bar between us, because obviously she couldn't imagine we were together."

In fact, although somewhat overweight, Terry was a very good-looking man, but clearly believed that Tamara found the affair partner more attractive. Despite Tamara's birthday email to Jim when she said "You're the most handsome man I've ever met," which confirmed Terry's belief that Tamara thought Jim better looking than him, Terry had clearly not understood that Tamara's attraction to Jim was mainly due to the incessant attention and adulation he gave her. Tamara explained that calling Jim "the most handsome man" was due to "how he looked at me, not his physical looks." I extended Tamara's explanation, saying, "As I understand it, your looks might have been the initial reason Jim noticed you, but his interest in you as a person is what you found most attractive. Unfortunately, in our society, this is the way it goes for many women—their looks are their initial 'currency' or 'portal' in getting a man's attention, and then you hope he'll be a nice guy who's interested in your mind and other aspects of being a person! And Terry, that emotional connection has been missing between you and Tamara, I think." Although he acknowledged once again that his appreciative gaze and emotional connection had been missing from their relationship, Terry went on to compare his sexual prowess—especially his skill at giving oral sex—with Tamara's sexy appearance "when she wears low-cut blouses and a short skirt." He said vehemently, "If I told my female coworker Judy that I love going down on my wife, I love eating pussy, that would be like you dressing sexy, sharing my sex with the world." Tamara rightly objected to this comparison.

As a male feminist couple therapist who believes that it is crucial to address men's sexist and controlling attitudes toward women (Knudson-Martin, 2015), I found myself troubled by Terry's traditional male perspective that his wife's beauty could be shared with him and him alone. I felt there was a need to distinguish between her having an affair—acting on a man's desire for her—and the attentions she frequently received for her looks. For me, Terry's beliefs fed into his sense of entitlement that he could control Tamara as his wife and, moreover, seemed unrealistic—Tamara was a beautiful woman, and both men and women, in different ways, often noticed her and commented on her beauty—which bolstered Tamara's self-esteem.

Although as noted earlier, I felt sad that Tamara had absorbed the larger culture's overvaluation of women's appearance as central to their self-esteem—especially her stated desire to be viewed by Terry and their friends as a "trophy wife"—I felt the most important focus should be on Terry's male possessiveness. Sensing that this was a moment when what I felt was necessary to say might anger Terry and rupture our alliance, I started by naming this concern, with a little laugh to lighten the message: "Terry, I'm trying to think of a way to say this that won't piss you off, but there's something a little bit scary about the degree to which you want to have Tamara's sexiness as 'mine'—that feels a little proprietary." Terry sat back and took a deep breath, and said he agreed with me, but that I had to understand that when she dressed up to go out with her group of female friends, "Tamara always dresses much more sexy than they do. I realize I might be biased, but that's how it looks to me. You should see the photos!" Sensing that it might be a useful opportunity to model a different way of looking at women—acknowledging their beauty without a sexualized gaze—I countered, "If you want to send me photos, I'll take a look!" Tamara said she would appreciate my comments on the photos. Terry agreed, and Tamara sent them to me.

There were several photos of Tamara and her 10 friends, all very attractive women lined up in a row on a pier wall by the ocean, clearly having fun together being all dressed up, and all wearing short dresses showing their legs and fancy high heels. I said, "Well, Tamara, you and your friends all look lovely, and I guess I'm wondering whom did you all dress up for—the men who might see you in the restaurant, or each other?" Tamara laughed and said, "We dress up for each other—Terry doesn't understand that when women go out on the town, it's like a fashion show for each other, and we comment on each other's dresses and shoes, talk about hair, stuff like that. It's a mutual appreciation society!" I said, "Yes, that's what I've come to understand as well."

Terry looked pensive and said this was a new realization for him. I went on to say that even if Tamara dressed more conservatively, she likely would still get attention because of her face, and I noted, "You can't expect her to wear a bag over her head when she goes out so that no one but you sees how pretty she is." This seemed to reach Terry, and he agreed it would be preposterous for him to ask Tamara to wear a bag over her head. I went on to say that, given Tamara's struggles with bulimia, I imagined that looking good was an important part of how she felt about herself. Tamara agreed.

In that session, I also inquired more about Tamara's long-standing bulimia and her high focus on her physical attractiveness as a source of self-confidence. She noted that, like her mother, she felt the need to be highly "in control all day"—of the kids and of the home—and that at night, she said, "all the wheels go off and I binge, and then purge. . . . I love food, love to eat, but I want to control my weight." She related that her bulimia was not a result of critical comments from her parents, or inappropriate sexualized comments from her father— "it was just that me and my cousins [all women, and with whom she was quite close] were always super concerned with our figures, and now it's just a habit, and actually, it feels good. I just hope I don't die from it!" She'd had therapy around the behavior, but it had no impact.

I suggested that if she and Terry could engage regularly in conversations about topics that might help her develop other sources of self-esteem (she was bright, and had a masters' degree in occupational therapy), and if she received forms of admiration from Terry other than appreciation of her looks and her competence as a mother, and if she tried mindful or slow eating to enjoy food but let her body recognize when it was sated, she might be able to break her bulimia habit. In a short time, Tamara was able to end her decades-long bulimia.

A day after this session, Terry sent me an email with the subject line, "Hey man!" In it, he reflected on what he'd learned in the session and asked if I thought it was a good idea for him to take Tamara on a surprise trip to Paris, or whether it was "too soon" in our work together. I said that was a great idea—and suggested that on the trip, they go together to a nice Parisian boutique, so that he could enjoy Tamara's enjoyment of trying on and purchasing some French clothes—and that he could respond if she asked what he liked, but not impose his desires for more conservative dressing on her.

Life-cycle challenges and affairs. Challenges in accepting one's stage in the life cycle may also contribute to having an affair. With two young children whom she adored, Leisha nevertheless acknowledged having difficulty accepting the greater constraints on time and freedom that accompany the transition to parenthood. Up until the affair was discovered, she had led two lives—one centered on her responsibilities at work and with her children, and one still free to "party" (as she said) at night (rationalized as being part of her work) and to act on her sexual desires for other men and experience their attraction to her. We worked on improving her and Bruce's sexual relationship, and Bruce worked hard (and, in his studious way, read several books on meditation and managing anxiety) to become more the free-spirited sexual partner Leisha desired, and which he had been early in their relationship.

In one session, I worked with the couple's sexual relationship by playing some funky music and having them dance. Leisha danced in a relaxed, sensual manner, whereas Bruce danced in a tight way; with playful humor, I commented on their different styles of dancing and demonstrated to Bruce a looser way of moving. The couple found this to be one of our most helpful sessions (Fraenkel, 2020), and their sex life became more "loose," playful, and adventurous.

SUMMARY: VISIONING AND EVALUATING THE VIABILITY OF THE RELATIONSHIP

As noted earlier, Perel (2017) and Gordon et al. (2015) specify the third step in treatment of an affair as engaging the couple to reflect on the therapy process and changes made in the relationship in response to the crisis of infidelity to determine whether the relationship can or cannot be continued. I find that the couple's conclusion about the viability of their relationship occurs spontaneously through their ongoing evaluation of the outcomes of the experiments in possibility, and that there is no need for a separate step to determine their sense of whether they desire to stay in the relationship. But certainly, there is a point at which the couple reflects on the value of the therapy and decides whether they have received enough assistance to decide whether to stay together or disband. I have had good success with the integrative approach described above: to date, none of the many couples I've worked with where there had been an affair decided to end the relationship.

CHAPTER 7

VIOLATIONS OF VALUES AND SAFETY

Interpersonal Violence and Addictions

IN THIS CHAPTER, I PROVIDE guidance on how to work with couples in which there has been interpersonal violence, aggression, or intimidation, and in which one partner engages in overuse of a substance, particularly alcohol. If you have skipped to this chapter and have not yet read Chapter 6, please go back to that chapter's first few pages, as I address there two important overarching considerations for working with any sort of value and safety violation: the importance of engaging a moral perspective in our work and the importance of exploring the ways in which power between partners often becomes unequal based in part on gender, gender identity, race, ethnicity, social class, citizenship status, and other social locations that afford unearned privilege and power to some people and oppression and less power to others.

VIOLENCE AND INTIMIDATION

As with affairs, there is a large literature on working with couples in which there has been violence and intimidation (see review by Fraenkel et al., 2022; Goldner, 1998, 2004; Goldner et al., 1990; Holtzworth-Munroe et al., 2003; Stith et al., 2004, 2011). These approaches all have at their base the feminist family therapy agenda of equalizing power, influence, and voice between partners (Hare-Mustin, 1978; Goldner, 1985). Although historically the work on what was formerly called "domestic violence" and is now termed "interpersonal violence" centered on cisgender heterosexual partners and focused on the sociocultural gender beliefs that privilege men over women (Knudson-Martin, 2013, 2015), the feminist emphasis on power equality is now also the base in work with GLBTQ couples. Work with couples in which at least one partner inhabits minoritized social locations based on sexual orientation and gender identity, race, ethnicity, immigration history or citizenship status, and other locations that result in marginalization and oppression also addresses the power inequities and internalized oppressive beliefs between the larger, dominant white heterosexual majority and individuals and couples inhabiting these less powerful locations that can result in risk factors for intimidation and violence in couples (Almeida & Durkin, 1999; Carvalho et al., 2011).

Work with couples in which one or both partners engage in acts of aggression, intimidation, and physical or emotional violence requires an integrative approach that assists couples to develop nonviolent approaches to communication and problem solving (Holtzworth-Munroe et al., 2003; Stith et al., 2011). The therapy must promote more effective dyadic coping with daily hassles and larger issues of work, finances, medical issues, and others (Falconier et al., 2015); encourage couples to envision in detail what their relationship could be like without aggression and set goals and take steps toward that vision, à la solution-focused therapy (Stith et al., 2011); encourage couples to decrease substance use that disinhibits aggression (see next section); and must explore each partner's family and cultures of origin to identify beliefs about intimate relationships, power and its intersection with gender and other social locations, and the models partners have experienced around use of violence and intimidation in relationships and the complex identifications with parent figures that are often outside of awareness (Goldner et al., 1990).

Because in Chapter 4 I described in detail action-oriented, nonaggressive approaches to improving communication, problem solving, and dyadic coping that are central to working with these couples, I do not repeat this material here, and instead turn to the approach pioneered by Goldner et al. (1990) to explore gender-power dynamics as well as family-of-origin and related psychodynamic themes of attachment and identification that set the stage for violence and intimidation.

An Integrative Approach to Discerning and Altering Family- and Culture-Based Roots of Violence

The work of Goldner (2004) and Goldner and colleagues (1990) remains the most nuanced, detailed theory of how gender beliefs and identifications with family-of-origin figures represent risk factors for some men to engage in violence against women. Although their work focused on cisgender heterosexual partners, much of their thinking can be transposed to Queer couples, where power discrepancies exist due to a number of factors—for instance, where one partner is a cisgender lesbian and the other is a trans man, as trans persons experience less acceptance in society than lesbians and gay men, or where one partner is out and the other closeted, and the out partner uses the closeted partner's fear of having their sexual orientation and gender identity revealed to family, friends, and the workplace as an instrument of relational power.

In this theory, men at risk for violence or other behaviors on the continuum of aggressiveness and intimidation often grew up in families in which the father also behaved in a violent or intimidating fashion. Sometimes that behavior was solely directed at the wife/mother, and sometimes also at the children. Boys are torn between upset and fear that their mothers (and themselves) are targets of violence, and their desire to identify with their powerful fathers. As part of this identification, the frequent pattern of boys separating from their mothers and choosing to emulate their fathers—a cornerstone of the psychodynamic theory of gender identity—becomes amplified and even more polarized, such that the parts of themselves that are viewed as feminine—vulnerable feelings of fear, anxiety, loneliness, and worries associated with insecure attachment and about commitment, loyalty, and stability of the relationship—become disowned.

When a woman partner expresses dissatisfaction with aspects of the relationship, or even threatens to leave, feelings of vulnerability are experienced by the man partner, and because he views these as feminine and not male, he responds with aggressive, controlling, and dominating behavior to assert his maleness and to keep the woman in the relationship. His behavior is validated, consciously or unconsciously, by the broader sociocultural beliefs that men should be in control and are entitled to behave aggressively, even with their intimate partners and children. In the denouement of this pattern, he will apologize profusely, sometimes with tears, gifts, and promises to do better, pleading that she not leave him and that she forgive him.

For her part, the woman partner also often experienced violence and other control strategies exerted by her father. This can lead to two coexisting scripts: first, a wish to be able in the current relationship to master the script of a man who dominates a woman; second, even more importantly, she understands and empathizes with the "hurt part" of the male partner and feels compelled to reaffirm the relationship. The bond between the man and woman is therefore predicated on both of them being survivors of abuse and trauma, and their sense of having a special connection that others cannot understand. In addition, the woman may have experienced emotional neglect in her family of origin, including by her mother, who was preoccupied with monitoring and attempting to diminish her husband's aggressiveness.

As a result, the male partner's anxious and angry preoccupation with her—often exhibited by high levels of jealousy, and monitoring and controlling her comings and goings—may be experienced by the woman as attention that corrects for her family-of-origin-based sense that no one cares for her—even if it is exhibited in aggressive, threat-based control and constraint. Interestingly, a doctoral student of mine, Jody Brandt, conducted an in-depth qualitative study to explore the reasons women survivors of domestic violence leave the relationship, in contrast to the majority of studies that explore the reasons women stay. The study was conducted in a New York City shelter for low- to no-income women and their children, mostly women of color, who were homeless as a result of escaping domestic violence, and the level of abuse experienced was extreme. The two main reasons women gave for what made them decide to leave were threats to take away the children, and a partner who had had an affair with a friend or family member. In other words, women would often put up with severe abuse if that was part of the couple's bond but would not tolerate betrayal or unfaithfulness (Brandt, 2005).

As with all approaches to working with interpersonal violence (see, for instance, Stith et al., 2011), Goldner et al.'s (1990) model for therapy begins with assessing whether there is ongoing abuse or risk of abuse and making safety plans for the woman (and to prevent opportunities for the man to be violent), including temporary separation and agreement by the perpetrating partner that he will not seek to determine her whereabouts (if she prefers an undisclosed location, including possibly a shelter) or, if he does know where she's going, will not try to make contact with her or stalk her. Therapy then elicits the history and specific details of the abuse and other controlling behaviors and the story of what brought the couple together, and the role of their respective abuse histories in that bonding. It then moves to helping the male who has perpetrated violence to recognize how he acted upon both sociocultural beliefs about male entitlement to be violent and dominant as well as his particular family-of-origin experiences and identification with the father as central to establishing his male identity.

The therapist explores the patterns of conflict between the partners to which the male partner responds with control strategies. This exploration is designed to guide him to more fully recognize the negative impact on the woman, her safety and personal integrity (as well as the effects on children), and to take 100% responsibility for his choice to respond to upset in the relationship with threats and violence, versus other nonviolent approaches. As with affairs, the therapist makes the distinction between formulating psychological or relational explanations for the abuse versus establishing excuses for it. Individual sessions with both partners are often central at this stage, until the man authentically takes responsibility. Sessions with the woman center on the impact of the abuse, which often includes trauma symptoms, and the nature of her intense bond with the man and her level of self-esteem and self-efficacy, as well as other factors that may have discouraged her from leaving the relationship, such as financial dependency or more extreme threats to her life, and encouragement from family and community (including her religious community) to stay and work things out.

The therapist works with the couple to develop a nonaggressive, equitable, compassionate approach to communication, including techniques for modulating negative emotions and arousal. It is at this point that I introduce the Speaker-Listener and Problem-Solving Techniques, as well as material from PREP on exploring expectations and hidden issues, as discussed in Chapter 4, and as used in CBT-based approaches to interpersonal violence (Epstein et al., 2015; Holtzworth-Munroe et al., 2003). Once it is clear (assessed over a period of weeks to months) that the man is no longer apt to engage in violent or other forms of controlling behavior, and the woman feels safe, the couple is encouraged to experiment with regaining sources of intimacy and pleasure. However, as with all last chance couples, the therapist makes clear that improvement in the relationship does not guarantee that the partners will decide to remain together, especially if the woman, now more empowered, decides to leave.

Vignette: Matt and Julie

Matt and Julie, both 41, requested couple therapy due to arguments in which Matt would become verbally abusive and threatening toward

Julie. Although he had never struck her, Matt engaged in character assassinations when angry, calling Julie "stupid," a "bitch," and a "liar," and would shout and stomp around the house while Julie tried to engage him in a soft-spoken manner, to no avail. At 6 feet 5 inches and with a heavy beard, and an intense scowl when angry, Matt was extremely intimidating, and Julie, who was much shorter, became silenced and frightened. The couple had two young children who cried when witnessing these fights and became inconsolable when Matt became abusive, leading him to feel ashamed of his behavior, and to vow never to act this way again, only to be followed a week or so later with more abusive behavior. When I met them, Julie had left Matt, had taken the kids, and was living in their New York City apartment, while Matt was in their new home in the town where he grew up outside of New Haven, Connecticut. Matt was contrite and desperate to try to make a fresh start and have Julie and the kids return.

Aside from their differences in physical size and gender, there were other social-locational sources of significant power discrepancies between them. Matt was a white man raised as an only child by his mother (he never knew his father) in a wealthy suburb of New Haven. He had inherited enough money to never have to work. He was not working when I began working with them, but had previously produced graphic designs in his art studio. Julie was an African American woman raised in Brooklyn in a lower-middle-class family. She had worked as an event coordinator but was now by choice a full-time mother. However, she had plans to become a social worker or a lawyer, so that she could serve the African American community. They met at Matt's graphic design studio, and were attracted by each other's political views and interests in art, literature, and spirituality. Julie was also drawn to Matt's "powerful energy, his ability to hold a room's attention" and his adventuresome nature. Matt was enamored by Julie's "beauty and intelligence," and said, "I felt like I knew her immediately."

In the first session, which occurred online and with each of them in their different homes, Matt readily acknowledged his abusive behavior, although he said that he was frequently annoyed at Julie when she disagreed with him. I noted that we would be looking at the conflict patterns that occurred between the two of them, but that a major first step was for Matt to recognize that his behavior was a choice to power over Julie, and led her to feel unsafe and silenced. Julie appreciated my statement and said she felt she needed "to get [her] strength and power back" in the relationship. Both Julie and Matt reported that they did not have models from their respective families of origin for productive and equitable conversation about problems. Julie said that her father had been similarly explosive and intimidating toward her mother, despite his religious endorsement of equitable relationships and nonviolence. Although Matt had never met his father, he heard from his mother that she left him before Matt was born because of the father's explosive, threatening temper. I asked Matt if he thought that his explosively angry behavior might in part be a way that he connected with the father he never had; this was a novel idea for Matt, and he reflected that it might be true. I also wondered if he was behaving in ways similar to what he heard about his father and mother's relationship as a way of unconsciously reenacting the parents' dynamic and trying to improve on it. He liked this hypothesis and saw that it gave him an opportunity to do better with his spouse than his father had done with his mother.

Feeling safer with Matt and that the therapy might be helpful, Julie returned with the kids to their home near New Haven. I taught the couple the Speaker-Listener Technique as well as a mindful breathing practice to use when either of them, especially Matt, felt negatively aroused, and then, based on their shared endorsement of Buddhist principles, I introduced them to the Beginning Anew mindfulness-based approach to couple communication, described in Chapter 4. The couple liked both these techniques, and for two weeks they had no conflict and no eruptions by Matt.

In the third session, I asked how they thought about being an interracial and interethnic couple. As often happens in my experience, they said they had never explicitly discussed the effects of differences in race and ethnicity in their relationship and how it might be related to power differences between them. Like most interracial and interethnic couples I've worked with, these issues are often left unspoken, and the emphasis is on interests and attitudes that they share. Julie said that although her family had a strong base in the African American religious and cultural community, she had been raised in a mostly white neighborhood and attended a school with mostly white peers, and she often felt more comfortable among white than Black people, as she sometimes felt the attitude of Black people about whites as the oppressor put her in an uncomfortable position with her white classmates and friends.

Like many white people I've encountered, Matt did not focus much on his whiteness as a social location, nor had he reflected on the unearned privilege being white provided him. Matt also added that being raised in a socially and politically liberal Jewish home, he considered himself "enlightened" about respecting persons of color and of different ethnicities. The couple reemphasized that their bond came from their shared interests. However, I wondered aloud about how Matt's moments of being verbally abusive and aggressive were possibly supported by his unexamined white privilege and larger sociocultural narratives about race and assumed superiority of white people, as well as by his class privilege. Julie gave me an appreciative glance and said she was glad I raised these issues; Matt was more circumspect, but said he was willing to consider them.

In a subsequent session, the couple reported they had experienced no conflicts in the past week. One of the topics the couple then discussed using the Speaker-Listener Technique centered on a major difference they had about how they wanted to live their lives: Julie wanted to settle down, go back to school, and raise the kids in a supportive community. Matt said that he wanted more "freedom" to travel and live in different countries and considered himself a "citizen of the world" (although he had traveled little and never lived abroad). The session ended on this note, with some tension around this major difference.

In the next session, to which Matt was late, Julie began by saying they had been getting along well. She spoke about adjusting to their new home in the semirural suburb and her wish to meet more people and establish a sense of community, and how she still longed in part to return to her community in Brooklyn, where her mother and friends lived. However, she looked relaxed and happy, and their baby was sitting on her lap.

However, when Matt appeared, he was in a highly agitated state. Wearing a baseball cap backward in hip-hop style, he was in another room online, talking loudly and gesturing like a rap artist singing an angry song, and peppering his outbursts toward Julie with "Yo, dude!" I found his behavior offensive on two levels: that he was acting like a rapper, which he was not, and with the knowledge that most rap music is performed by Black artists—so in this way, he was imitating a tough Black man, which he was not; and, of course, that he was speaking to Julie in an abusive manner. I modulated my own upset and asked what was leading him to be so upset, but he ignored me. It was clear that I had a choice—either to stop the session or allow it to continue and see this spontaneous enactment of his abusive behavior. I chose the latter approach, at least for the time being, knowing that at least Matt was in another room of the house than where Julie and the baby sat.

Matt restated, but now aggressively, his desire to "be free of the routines of school vacations" and travel the world. He accused Julie of "lying" (because, he claimed, she had expressed a similar desire early in their relationship, which she quietly said she had not), and repeatedly called her a "square." Julie attempted to maintain her outward composure and soft-spoken voice but raised important points for Matt to consider, in the hope that he would settle down and move off his diatribe—for instance, that they had to consider the children's school life and that she did not want to homeschool them as some of their friends were doing.

My attempts to get Matt to modulate his affect and speech were ineffective, and he talked over me. Seeing that Julie was getting increasingly upset, I raised my voice and said that his aggressive style of talking was shutting her down and disempowering me as well. His response was, "How am I doing that?" I reiterated that I could not get a word in edgewise, and so could not be helpful to him. When he insisted on continuing in this style, I became firmer and said that, as we'd discussed before (but I'd never witnessed in session), his aggressive, insulting way of speaking to Julie would lead nowhere good. The session ended with me saying that he needed to decide whether he really wanted to work with me and make the necessary changes in the power dynamics between them, that they needed to discuss whether they wanted to continue with therapy, and that I would wait for their call.

Later that day, I sensed that I might have gotten through to Matt, because when he sent the fee for the session through Venmo, he included a heart emoji. A few days later, Julie emailed me, saying, "I apologize that our session got out of hand, but I am grateful that you saw an honest, raw episode. I appreciate all the tools you've offered thus far. I feel heard and safe during the sessions. Thank you for holding that space." I responded that she was welcome, but that she was not at fault for the session getting out of hand, just Matt, and that I was still open to working with them and would wait to hear from them. I mentioned that he had sent me a heart emoji; she knew, and wrote, "I'd like to keep going but I'd like to double check with Matt. We'll reach out."

The couple contacted me early the next week and said they wished to continue. In the session, Matt apologized to Julie and to me (he'd already apologized to her) and was quite remorseful. I accepted his apology, and Julie had as well, with the condition that he work more earnestly on managing his anger and avoiding abusive behavior. I asked whether this cycle of abusive behavior by Matt followed by a remorseful apology had occurred before; both partners reported that this was their pattern. I asked Matt what he could do to stop this cycle;

he said that he needed to make a stronger commitment to modulating his frustration and avoiding such behavior at all costs. I reminded him about our discussion about how his behavior might be fueled by his wish to emulate what he'd heard about his father, and that he had an opportunity now to behave differently than his father had with his mother, and thereby keep Julie from divorcing him.

We also discussed in more depth Matt's strong desire to be free of regular constraints on time and living location due to the kids' need to attend school. He related that he had never been a good student and that he responded to his academic difficulties by creating a persona centered on creativity and "breaking out" of normal expectations of school and career. He was proud of having rejected normal temporal and spatial constraints of life. However, he acknowledged that he had not been very successful in his creative endeavors, and considered going back to school to learn more about graphic design.

I commented that while I appreciated his critical questioning of the often-automatic, unquestioned expectations and routines of life as lived by many people, this stance clearly did not fit with Julie's goals and needs for temporal regularity and belonging to a community. I wondered aloud whether his multiple intersecting privileges—as a tall, white, heterosexual man who was financially independent—led him to ignore Julie's needs as an African American woman who had faced racism at times at a mostly white school, and as a member of the African American community, which has experienced relentless marginalization and disempowerment. These were issues that the couple had never discussed as being related to their respective social locations and their different ideas and desires for their lives.

Julie's goal of becoming a lawyer and serving the African American community, and her desire to ensure a good education for their kids, required "spatial stability" (living in one place), in contrast to his fantasy of an itinerant, "free" life. In addition, the overwhelming intensity of his affect as he spoke about his goals resulted in intimidating and silencing Julie. Julie nodded in appreciation of what I said; Matt looked a bit defensive but then became remorseful. He said to Julie, in quiet tones, "I've always thought of you as my equal, and as strong; so I guess I didn't track how I overpower you when I talk like this." Julie responded, "I am strong, but you get scary, and you're tall." Matt nodded and, for the first time, realized how oppressive and self-centered his behavior had been in these moments.

This was the turning point in our work together. The couple re-embraced the communication and problem-solving skills I had taught them, and decided to meditate together on a daily basis. Matt began to consider how he could build a career in graphic design in which he had opportunities to travel but without demanding that Julie accompany him when she did not want to. Julie enjoyed traveling and adventure, and the couple started to make plans to spend some portion of the summer months after the kids' school ended to live abroad. Julie reflected that she could go to school and eventually pursue her career in part online.

WHEN THE VIOLENCE DOESN'T END

In some cases, the person perpetrating violence does not accept guidance to examine and end their behavior. This suggests that the partners will need to separate at least temporarily, and may need to end the relationship. Two short vignettes illustrate how these decisions are made and how to encourage couples to end the relationship amicably, and without escalating to dangerous violence before finally deciding to do so.

Vignette: Erika and Sandra

Erika, a 33-year-old lesbian, and Sandra, a 32-year-old lesbian, both second-generation Greek Americans, had engaged in high conflict throughout their six tumultuous years together. I was their fourth couple therapist. As I described in Chapter 5, Erika acknowledged her volatile temper, but blamed Sandra for triggering her with her attempts to be calm in the face of Erika's upset, and viewed Sandra's not getting equally aroused as a sign of disconnection. Additionally, Erika felt that Sandra's calmer temperament and insistence on solving problems "logically" was Sandra's way of trying to "act superior" to her. I suggested that something about Sandra's attempts not to join Erika in her upset triggered a sense of abandonment in Erika. We explored her family-of-origin history, and it seemed that when Erika realized she was attracted to women as a teen, she withdrew somewhat from her highly engaged family, because she worried that coming out would lead to rejection. However, when she did tell her parents about her sexual orientation, they were quite accepting. It never became clear what had resulted in Erika's hypersensitivity to possible abandonment.

Sandra disagreed with Erika's beliefs about her attempts to stay calm in the face of emotional upset. She said that even as a child, she had adopted a more emotionally restrained style as a way of coping with her parents' frequent arguments. An only child, she often found herself mediating her parents' conflicts to calm them down. Erika largely rejected Sandra's explanation of herself, insisting that she "*must* be angry" at her parents, and was just too "repressed" to acknowledge these feelings. Erika grew up in an emotionally volatile family, although she reported there had been no violence. She was comfortable with high levels of expressed negative affect, said that this style was "typical of Greeks," and saw such behavior as more "honest" than Sandra's cool demeanor during conflict.

As noted in Chapter 5, Erika insisted that Sandra was usually angrier than she let on, which Sandra acknowledged was true—yet she still believed in modulating her anger and wished that Erika would do so as well. My work with them to identify a pattern of projective identification (described in Chapter 5), in which Sandra disavowed her anger and Erika came to express that anger for her, temporarily led to a period of greater calm between them, as Sandra became better able to express her own anger. But eventually, their pattern of rapid escalation resumed.

Erika begrudgingly and half-heartedly accepted my attempts to help her modulate her anger, as well as my encouragement for the couple to employ the Speaker-Listener Technique when discussing problems. I taught the couple mindful breathing and some Qigong as techniques to modulate their arousal, and although they appreciated these techniques, and the relationship improved markedly for a few weeks, Erika returned to her aggressive, threatening behavior during a vacation, in an argument about which room of the house they had rented each would work in during the day. During this fight, Erika punched Sandra and threw plates. Sandra was alarmed. The couple decided that it was best for them to finally separate and thanked me for my attempts to help them. As I did not have contact with them after this session, I do not know if they actually separated or eventually got back together.

Vignette: Cherisse and Christopher

Cherisse, a mixed-race cisgender heterosexual woman whose father was from the Bahamas, and Christopher, an Anglo-American cisgender heterosexual man, both 31 years old, requested couple therapy because of high levels of conflict. When they met, they were attracted by their shared interest in philosophy, and enjoyed debating ideas. But they described their relationship as volatile from the start. As they recounted examples of their fights, I was immediately concerned by a pattern in which Cherisse would assert something, and Christopher would persistently state that her position made no sense, often drawing inaccurately on philosophical ideas (as I was a philosophy-psychology double major in college, I was aware of the ideas he attempted to recruit and how he often did so inaccurately).

Cherisse, a successful trade negotiator who had attended a top business school, would not back down. When she reasserted her perspective on a topic, Christopher would call her a "liar," even though she was simply stating her opinion. Cherisse would inevitably then step back from the argument temporarily, as if speechless at this accusation, but eventually would reengage with Christopher to assert herself, and their fights escalated. On several occasions, Christopher struck Cherisse, and she would strike back in self-defense.

Compounding their conflict was that, in part because their sex life had ended two years earlier due to conflict, Cherisse had a female lover. Christopher claimed to be open minded about her relationship, but from his dismayed affect it was clear that he felt upset about it. As is often the case, there was a disconnect between his stated positions and values, and his emotions. He eventually acknowledged that he felt "diminished as a man" in Cherisse's eyes due to her affair.

In the first session, I strongly urged them to adopt a no-violence policy, and encouraged Cherisse to leave their home if Christopher seemed to be escalating in his aggressiveness. Despite my efforts in conjoint and individual sessions with him, Christopher refused to take 100% responsibility for his abusive language and physical aggression. I also pointed out his pattern of moving away from his feelings and rationalizing them by recruiting high-level moral philosophical principles, which always involved him taking the higher moral ground compared to Cherisse. I encouraged him to express his feelings directly. He related that this was difficult for him, as he had grown up in a family that discouraged it. I empathized with him, but he remained steadfast in his belief in Stoicism—which he had misunderstood as a stance of not expressing feelings. The actual Stoic philosophy could have been useful to him, as the main principle is to engage in all activities in moderation. When I pointed this out, he argued with me and said that I did not understand the true essence of Stoic philosophy.

Unlike other couples I've worked with where there are racial and ethnic differences between the partners, neither Christopher nor Cherisse engaged in my attempts to highlight the possible power discrepancies between them due to their racial/ethnic locations, because although Cherisse was female and of mixed race, she also had far more economic power than Christopher, who was a claims manager for an insurance company. As I do with all couples, I taught them the Speaker-Listener Technique, mindfulness practices to regulate arousal, and the time-out rule to use if they started to escalate.

However, each partner seemed almost magnetically drawn into their conflicts. In Cherisse's family-of-origin, her father had been abusive to her mother, and while she hated her father's abusiveness, she acknowledged that she identified more with the father's powerfulness than with what she saw as her mother's weakness. Christopher came from a family in which the parents often seemed distant from one another and never engaged in overt conflict.

Although the couple had periods in which they got along better and avoided escalations and violence, these periods of calm continued to be interrupted by periods of high conflict, during which Christopher would revert to calling Cherisse a liar and other insulting names. In an individual session with Cherisse, I wondered aloud what was keeping her in the relationship. She reflected that much as she disliked Christopher's behavior, she felt drawn to defend herself and argue him out of his positions, even though she realized this was futile. She decided to end the relationship.

In a last session, with both partners having agreed to separate, I urged them to do so amicably and without further conflict. They agreed this would be best. Because we had connected around shared interests in music, I also asked them if they had a song that might guide them. Neither could come up with a song, and I suggested an oldie—"It's Too Late," by Carole King, noting that they might not like it (they were both more interested in aggressive hip-hop songs). I played the song in the session, and they liked it, and felt it could provide a frame for an amicable divorce.

Sadly and disturbingly, a few weeks later, I heard from Cherisse's individual therapist, who had referred the couple initially, that Christopher had become violent again, destroying much of the couple's belongings as he prepared to leave, and finally, Cherisse was convinced that she needed to end the relationship with him. These last two vignettes bring home an important point: Some couples may not be able to engage sufficiently in change efforts to maintain the relationship. Especially where threats to safety are involved, this can represent a positive outcome of therapy.

ALCOHOL AND SUBSTANCE USE

When one partner overuses alcohol or other substances, the other partner is often caught in a bind. On the one hand, they want to help the partner address the behavior and the underlying emotional issues driving it, hoping the substance-using partner will gain control of their use or stop altogether if they seem unable to moderate. On the other hand, they wish to protect themselves (and children if there are any) from the negative effects of the partner's usage, which can include aggressiveness and violence (Caetano et al., 2001, 2005; Drapkin et al., 2005) that was often uncharacteristic of the partner before they began overusing substances; underfunctioning in their roles at work and at home; sexual difficulties; and more. There is a circular pattern of trying to help the addicted or otherwise using partner, which may backfire and facilitate or otherwise prompt their substance use, which then leads to more attempts to cajole or force them to stop, which is met with resistance and/or hiding the substance use. In addition, as in the case of Leisha and Bruce, alcohol or other substance use may play a role in a partner having an affair or engaging in intimidation or violence.

Repeated broken promises by the substance-using partner to curtail their usage eventually may lead the other partner to give up on the relationship. In addition, substance use by one partner may be in response to preexisting and ongoing relationship problems. In some cases, both partners are engaged in problematic use. Whatever led a partner (or partners) to engage in substance use, this vicious cycle between relationship problems and usage often results in one or both partners considering ending the relationship.

The initial causes of substance overuse are diverse and vary across those who use. A family history of substance use, psychological or psychiatric problems (Rosenthal, 2013), inadequate stress management and emotion regulation skills, absence of regular pleasurable activities, a work or social context that encourages drinking or other substance use, couple conflict and conflict with other family members, social anxiety—all may contribute to a person turning to substances for pleasure and to cope with challenges. Eventually, a physical addiction may begin, leading to cravings and withdrawal symptoms that drive the person to ingest more of the substance. As McCrady and Epstein (2015) write about people with an alcohol use disorder (AUD),

> the drinking behavior of a person with an AUD is embedded in
> a complex network of factors relating to the individual's physi-

ology and psychology, the family, and other social networks. In each component of the network, there is a reciprocal relation between the drinking and the functioning of the network; the individual's behavior both influences the social network and is influenced by it. (p. 559)

Research has found that behavioral couple therapy results in greater positive change in relationship satisfaction, and decreased frequency of use and negative consequences of use than traditional individual therapy for substance abuse, with most of the research focusing on alcohol use disorders rather than other substances (McCrady & Epstein, 2015; Powers et al., 2008). In this section, I present vignettes of an integrative approach to last chance couples in which a partner is overusing alcohol. This approach incorporates many of the strategies of alcohol behavioral couple therapy (McCrady & Epstein, 2015) but draws upon other perspectives and their associated techniques.

One important way in which this approach differs from that of McCrady and Epstein is that I always recommend that the partner engaged in alcohol overuse join Alcoholics Anonymous, as that program provides a daily support of sobriety that once-a-week therapy cannot offer, and a community of other people committed to the same goal. Even if drinking was originally done in a social context, eventually the problem drinker usually drinks in isolation, especially if they suffer from social anxiety. AA provides an opportunity to make new friends, which can take pressure off the relationship for all the partner's social needs.

Work with last chance couples in which a partner is overusing a substance involves all the elements of the Therapeutic Palette integrative approach: creating a therapeutic frame that acknowledges the possibility that the relationship will end, and encouraging a liminal space in which to engage in experiments in possibility designed to improve the relationship and that provide clearer data upon which to make that decision; addressing present patterns of destructive interaction, including through training in communication and problem-solving skills, and mindfulness activities that reduce negative emotional arousal; examining expectations and hidden issues, as well as the impact of work and other larger systems challenges on the relationship, and developing better individual and joint coping skills; exploration of family- and culture-of-origin factors that contribute to these relational patterns as well as to the partner's substance overuse; and the overusing partner's psychological functioning, including depression, anxiety, or trauma, and difficulties with emotion regulation and social skills that may contribute to their usage, as well as the psychological functioning of the other partner, which is often greatly affected by the partner's overuse. In addition, as with affairs and violence, therapy closely examines the events leading up to the moment in which a partner decides to drink or use drugs, rather than engage in other, healthier means of coping and gaining pleasure, as a means of encouraging the partner to take 100% responsibility for their choices, rather than blaming the other partner.

Vignette: Ana and Michael[3]

Ana, 38, was born and raised in a low-income single mother Catholic household in the Dominican Republic, and Michael, 39, was raised by Irish American upper-middle class parents in Cleveland. Michael was a high-powered attorney, and Ana worked as the head of a nursing department of a major hospital, and both were highly successful in demanding jobs. Together 12 years and married for 10, with 4-year-old twins, both partners were considering divorce, and declared this therapy to be their "last chance." Indeed, they represented three of the types of last chance couples: high conflict, low connection, and one partner engaging in behavior that violated the values and comfort of the other—in this case, Michael's return after seven years of sobriety to active alcohol overuse three months earlier, when he spent three weeks in bed continuously drunk, often angrily denying drinking, and hid his vodka bottles, which Ana would find and confront him about, leading to conflict. In the weeks prior to calling, they had several sessions with another therapist, and quit because, they said, "The therapist just let us argue in the session and talk about how messed up our relationship is, like we do at home. We weren't getting anywhere with that." Neither had been in individual therapy, although Michael's psychiatrist attempted to explore his childhood along with prescribing him antidepressants and antianxiety medication. Michael said he didn't see what his childhood had to do with his feelings of anger and depression, which he attributed solely to his sense that Ana didn't support him around his highly stressful job, or appreciate, he said, "what I go through for this family." When asked about his treatment with the addictions psychiatrist and his issues with alcohol more generally, Michael became defensive, saying he

---

3 This vignette, with slight modifications, was previously published in the following article: Fraenkel, P. (2019). Love in action: An integrative approach to last chance couple therapy. *Family Process, 58,* 569–594. It is replicated with permission from John Wiley & Sons. License number 5277250771904.

was able years ago to stop drinking and that he would be able to stop on his own. He said he had no interest in joining AA, seeing that as a "program for losers."

The couple said they had decided to try therapy one last time because they would prefer not to "break up the family" for their children's sake, but both reported little real motivation, due to their anger and sense of hopelessness. Neither partner believed couple therapy could really help with their issues, which had begun shortly after the birth of their sons, when Michael felt Ana only cared about the children, and Ana felt Michael's resentment led him not to help her with the household chores and childcare. He countered that he tried to participate, especially around disciplining the boys, saying bitterly, "We're not on the same page—when we decide on a strategy, Ana eventually doesn't follow it, and is too indulgent of the kids." Ana frowned and shrugged, saying she was often uncomfortable being punitive in the style Michael preferred, relating that she had been raised with harsh discipline and didn't want to treat her children that way. I noted briefly that research shows many couples lose connection and have difficulty dividing up tasks during the transition to parenthood, and that perhaps we could work on these issues.

I asked about how they met and what attracted each to the other initially. They met through friends, and were strongly attracted physically. Ana said she found Michael's strong work ethic, intellect, organizational abilities (which she said she lacked, despite evidence to the contrary in her work life) and "rationality" appealing; Michael said he was drawn to Ana's liveliness and spontaneity, as well as her intellect and determination. They traveled a lot and enjoyed exploring restaurants and art museums together in the early years. But whereas with less distressed couples, this question about the beginnings of the relationship typically results in a positive shift in affect and connectedness, Ana and Michael remained taciturn and detached, with Ana explaining, "That all seems so long ago, and there's been so much bad water under the bridge, and we're in crisis."

I asked if they had a history of better communication about problems, and they said they did not, even during the early, happier years of their relationship. Nor did either have positive models of problem solving from their families of origin. Ana's mother had ejected her father from the household when Ana was five years old because of his drinking, affairs, and violence. Michael reported that his parents had always seemed distant from one another, rarely affectionate, and he had never seen them talk about issues. I briefly described the action-insight approach to couple therapy and, given what they had described so far, offered to teach them research-based communication and problem-solving skills as a first step toward reducing their level of conflict, noting that even if they did get divorced, these skills would be helpful as they continued on as coparents.

I reflected that indeed, what they seemed to want at that moment, if anything, was a therapy that would demonstrate some possible effectiveness in directly improving their interactions, rather than simply reiterating their painful feelings. They said this seemed like a sensible idea but neither expressed excitement about it. Referring to the Creative Relational Movement principles of change described in Chapter 1, I also noted that it was not necessary that they be highly motivated for now, just that they experiment with some new possibilities—to try to step out of the old patterns. I noted that, given how unsure they were about staying together, even if they experienced improvement, they might still decide to divorce, but that the best way to make that decision was to see if things could get better.

I reviewed briefly the major findings on problematic patterns of communication (noting that I would send some readings to have them review the patterns in more detail if they wished) and, for the first time, they smiled slightly at each other, albeit with a touch of embarrassed chagrin, saying that they engaged in all of these patterns. I taught them the skills, had them try them briefly, and both said these were much preferable to their typical ways of arguing—although they felt rather artificial and awkward. I validated that sense and noted that like all new skills, these would become more fluid with practice. I added that I wouldn't be surprised if the skills not only felt awkward, but when trying to do them at home in a moment of anger, it might almost feel irrational to try, given how upset and mistrusting each was of the other's intentions. They nodded and said they could absolutely imagine feeling this way. I suggested that if those feelings occurred, just to recognize them as a normal part of changing from one set of feelings and beliefs about each other to more positive ones that might follow from repeated success in doing the skills.

With their assent, after determining that neither had reliable practices of self-soothing, I also taught them mindful breathing and two Qigong movements, which I described as movement meditations, to help with reducing negative physiological arousal in general and prior to or during use of the communication skills. I described briefly the manner in which the sympathetic nervous system activates rapidly before and during conflict. Both found the mindfulness techniques calming and the "neuro-education" interesting.

They reminded me that one of their major issues was differences in how to handle their sons—one in particular who was sometimes over-active and oppositional—and asked if I could see them with their sons next time and then offer suggestions. In that second session with the kids, I introduced some playful child-oriented mindfulness practices to help with calming down, suggesting that the whole family could do them together, and offered some ideas about how to reinforce better behavior.

The couple got busy with the end of the year and holidays, but during that time, Michael called one morning because he had again spent a weekend drinking heavily, and overnight had experienced frightening withdrawal symptoms. I urged him to contact his psychiatrist and to go to the Emergency Department, explaining how unpredictable and dangerous withdrawal could be. Michael said he would call the psychiatrist but was reluctant to go to the hospital and said he now recognized he had a more serious problem.

I was on holiday for two weeks, and toward the end of that time Ana contacted me, saying she was "at the end of [her] rope," as Michael had again drunk through a weekend. Saying that she knew how I appreciated music, she sent me the names of two songs capturing her feelings: Puerto Rican salsa-pop singer Marc Anthony's "Vivir Mi Vida," a song expressing a desperate desire to escape adversity and live one's life; and Kesha's "Praying," a song about leaving one's abusive partner. She requested to see me individually, saying Michael was fine with it.

When I returned, we had two sessions where she reported that they had been fighting less and talking more with the aid of the communication skills. But she expressed fears and frustrations about Michael's drinking, and how he blamed her entirely for their problems. She described how her mother had thrown her father's clothes and other possessions out the window after yet another night of carousing with alcohol and other women, and wondered why she didn't have the strength to leave Michael. I commented that she might indeed have that strength, but clearly was trying to see if Michael could stay sober and they could still make a life together. She cried and said, "I still love him. I just hate how he blames me for his problems. He says I'm so cold, so maybe it is my fault."

I affirmed that she was not at fault for Michael's drinking, that he would need to take responsibility for it, and that her emotional withdrawal from him was understandable, given his drinking, depression, and blaming of her for it all. There might be things that she did in the relationship that could change for the better, but these did not excuse drinking—he would have to stop and that would allow us better to determine what role each of them played in their difficulties aside from the alcohol. She seemed relieved and reassured by this empathic explanation.

In the next session with both partners, Michael, who had not had a drink since the previous episode, was nevertheless sullen and resentful, saying, "No one gives me a break, not Ana, not my work colleagues, no one. No one appreciates me." Gentle attempts, through questions, to have him recognize how his behavior led to others' feelings and behavior toward him fell flat. With Ana's permission, I reiterated what I had told Ana in their individual session; that surely there were things each did (and did not do, like positive, affirming, loving statements and actions) that contributed to their difficulties, but said, "I know this might make you angry, Michael, and I'm sorry for that, but your drinking is scary and upsetting to Ana, and confusing for the kids" (who had repeatedly asked Ana, "What's wrong with Daddy? Is he sick?"). I said, "Ana is not to blame for your drinking—there are other ways to deal with your dissatisfaction in the relationship, and with work pressures, and only you can stop the drinking and remove the effects it's having on your family."

Michael listened pensively and, in the next week, decided to enter an intensive outpatient program where he learned dialectical behavior therapy skills including how to identify triggers, and participated in recovery groups. Luckily, after initial reluctance, he found the program useful, and the therapy materials interesting, and had resumed practicing the mindfulness skills I had taught the couple, which fit with some of the practices he was learning in dialectical behavior therapy. On his own initiative, he also started reading books on mindfulness and on coping with career challenges.

In a following session, Michael still angrily complained that Ana didn't appreciate him, including all his current efforts to get help for his drinking. He said he was frustrated that she didn't share her feelings and seemed withdrawn from him, a problem he said had been occurring even before his drinking restarted. Ana was clearly hurt and angry hearing this but acknowledged that in her family and culture more generally, children were taught not to express their negative feelings. She realized she could do better with this, but found it hard to express herself to Michael. I wondered aloud whether Ana's explanation helped Michael understand her reserve, and he said, "Yes, I know about her family history, but it's still difficult when I don't know what she's feeling about me."

I again noted that what I was about to say might anger Michael, but it was my sense that in addition to Ana's upbringing, her reluctance to talk about negative feelings had to do with his intense rage and resentment toward her, which created a wall that I could also feel at times between Michael and myself. Michael, who was very tall and well built, could be rather loud and intimidating when he got angry. I suggested that Michael could "dial it down a bit," using the mindfulness skills he liked, and that perhaps the Speaker-Listener Technique could also help. Michael looked thoughtful and said that this made sense. Ana seemed relieved that I gently pointed this out to Michael.

As the session was about to end, I suggested that because they each felt unappreciated by the other, it might be helpful to try something that research by John Gottman found characterizes happy couples—daily statements of appreciation and admiration. I noted that this might be extremely challenging given their negative feelings, but that if they could try their best to experiment with this practice once a day, it might start to soften things between them. They tried it in the session and said this might be a good thing to do.

The turning point came two weeks later. The couple had gone on holiday to Hawaii, and had not fought, but still felt distant from one another. Once again, Michael launched into his feelings about not being appreciated and being pushed away by Ana. This greatly upset her, because, in an effort to be kind and understanding of his stress, Ana had taken the kids for two days so that he could go scuba diving. She was outraged that he still saw her as inconsiderate, and she felt her efforts were unappreciated. Michael countered that he had thanked her for this break (she did not remember him doing so), but that what upset him was that on a few occasions, he'd tried to help more with the kids—for instance, helping them get dressed—and she had rejected his offer, saying she could do it herself. In those moments he felt unappreciated and excluded.

I noted that they each seemed to be trying to take care of the other, and that the other was not letting them do so. Michael's angry narrative of "you don't appreciate me" still made it difficult for Ana to reach out and listen to his suffering. And noting tentatively that, based in part on what I, as a non-Latino man, had learned from my Latinx colleagues and their writings, I wondered if Ana might be enacting a script learned from her mother, and her culture, of the "strong Latina woman" who, when things are hard, handles them herself, as captured in part by the term *marianismo*. Ana said, "Absolutely! When things are tough in our families, and we don't feel men are helping, we learn to just do everything ourselves." Michael seemed genuinely moved by this, and said, gently, "I really want to help you. I want to help you feel less stressed." Ana looked unsure but said she would welcome that. Michael suggested he could take over breakfast duties and, on the weekend, take the kids for a few hours so that Ana could get back to the gym.

The following week, the couple arrived smiling and relaxed. Michael said, "After that session, we both realized how silly we'd been with each other, and decided to stop being hurtful to each other. We have so much good between us." Ana smiled broadly and agreed. Michael had bought her a gift that she felt was very thoughtful—salamander earrings and a salamander necklace, which she was wearing that day. He explained with a warm smile: "A salamander can regenerate its entire tail. I think our relationship can be like that. We need to grow it back." They spoke of how they were now more ready to use the various practices they'd learned in therapy. There followed a lot of laughter among us on various topics, not all having to do with them specifically.

The following three weeks were similar in emotional tone. We returned to their differences in parenting beliefs and found a workable compromise. We briefly touched on the emotion style differences between them that had attracted them initially (he as more rational and contained, she as more expressive and spontaneous) but that first become polarized and then largely reversed, albeit in a distorted, unpleasant manner, through the impact of Michael's drinking, depression, and rage, leading Ana to become emotionally shut down. They recognized the virtue of each of them being able to be rational and expressive, and they demonstrated this greater flexibility in the sessions. We were also able to return to Michael's feelings of being displaced when the boys were born, which, although not uncommon in the transition to parenthood, were accentuated by attachment issues because he was adopted (it was not an open adoption, and he never learned exactly why his biological mother had given him up). Michael continued to be engaged in his outpatient addictions treatment, now quite enthusiastically, and had remained sober. Ana was now freer to express genuine warmth toward him as well as upset feelings. One year later, the couple contacted me to report they were doing well.

SUMMARY

Therapy with last chance couples in which a partner has violated the values of the other partner (and often, their own values) or has behaved in ways that make the other feel unsafe requires the same approaches to forming the therapeutic alliance, and a contract that honors the ambivalence of at least one partner, that pertain to all such couples. In addition, the partner who has engaged in intimidation, aggression, or violence, or has used substances problematically must take responsibility for their behavior, irrespective of the provocativeness of the other's behavior and their joint dysfunctional communication patterns. These couples require a great deal of adeptness on the part of the therapist, as the therapist moves between addressing the value- and safety-violating behaviors and associated beliefs and psychological issues of one partner while also addressing those patterns in which both partners participate. Yet as the vignettes presented indicate, in many cases, couples can heal from these sorts of serious problems. In others in which one or both partners are unable or unwilling to change, the best outcome is to end the relationship.

CHAPTER 8

COUPLES WITH MISMATCHED PERSONAL LIFE CHRONOLOGIES

THIS CHAPTER ADDRESSES COUPLES ON the brink of relationship dissolution due to partners having different needs and desires about whether or when to achieve certain goals. Partners may disagree about whether to get married or whether to have a child (or another child). They may differ on their goals about what represents career stability and success, or level of financial attainment; whether to move from apartment living to owning a home; or whether to retire. However, many couples agree on these goals (the question of "whether"), but differ on the question of *when* these should be achieved.

I have termed these differences regarding when to reach certain goals as dyssynchronies about "personal life chronologies"—each person's projected timelines (Fraenkel, 1994, 2011; Fraenkel & Wilson, 2000). Couples who get along fairly well and without high conflict, have a satisfactory level of pleasure and passion, and have had no incidents of violation of the values and safety of a partner may nevertheless be on the brink of separation due to mismatched preferences about whether or when to attain certain life goals.

A core concept in family therapy is the notion that families move through a set of developmental stages known as the family life cycle (McGoldrick et al., 2011; McGoldrick & Shibusawa, 2012). The notion of a "normal," homogeneous family life cycle based on middle-class white heterosexual nuclear families has been expanded to recognize different forms of couples and families and differing goals depending on culture and the social locations of the members (for instance, in terms of ethnicity, social class and educational attainment, sexual orientation, and gender identity).

However, it is still the case that most couples make some sort of relationship commitment (formal marriage or otherwise); many have children (either produced biologically or adopted) and launch those children into school, and eventually, when the children reach young adulthood, into some degree of separation and independence from the family of origin. Likewise, partners usually have goals about career and finances, retirement, and other plans. Each of these goals can bring both positive feelings and desired changes in identity, as well as challenges. Partners often differ about what it will mean to reach certain goals, and may differ in their sense of the balance of pros and cons of the changes incurred by attaining these developments.

Frequently, partners may have assumed they were on the same page about these goals when they first entered the relationship, only to discover later that they differ on the question of either whether or when to reach them. In other cases, one partner may have promised to join the other in fulfilling a certain goal, only essentially to renege on that promise, or ask for a delay, frustrating the other partner and leaving them in a sort of identity limbo.

The Therapeutic Palette integrative approach offers a comprehensive perspective and set of interventions with which to address these discrepancies in personal life chronologies. Effective therapy requires examining each partner's respective visions of the near and more distant future, their level of satisfaction with the present and style of handling their conflict about the future, their respective family and cultures of origin, and the degree to which they wish to replicate or avoid what they learned, witnessed, and experienced. The following short vignettes provide illustrations of how to address these discrepancies.

DIFFERENCES ABOUT WHEN TO COMMIT

Vignette: Atafa and Andreas

Atafa, 41, was a Pakistani American woman in public relations, and Andreas, 52, was a Swiss lawyer working for an international law firm. After more than two years together, the couple was on the brink of ending the relationship because Atafa was disappointed and angry at Andreas for continually backtracking on his promise to marry. They

met online, and Atafa noted that it was months into their relationship before she discovered, by seeing a prescription bottle that listed
Andreas' date of birth, that he had lied on his profile about his age (he
had stated that he was 43). Andreas looked anxious and embarrassed
about this fabrication but protested that he believed listing his actual
age would diminish his prospects for attracting women, and that in
any case, he "felt" and looked much younger than his age. Although
this deception led Atafa to become wary about trusting him, she was
willing to overlook this lie because she generally enjoyed being with
Andreas, and envisioned a financially and materially satisfying and
secure life with him.

Atafa came from a working-class family in Lahore that had often
struggled to make ends meet. She was the first in her family to go to
college and graduate school, Within the first two months of the relationship, Andreas showered Atafa with expensive gifts and took her
on expensive vacations. When the topic of marriage arose, Andreas
initially affirmed his desire to marry within the year. But as the
months went on, he seemed increasingly reluctant to set a date, which
led Atafa to express her anger and frustration, and reignited her concerns about his dishonesty. Andreas initially countered that his reluctance had grown due to Atafa's intense expressions of anger; Atafa
responded that her anger was reasonable and due to his seeming to
hedge on his initial promise. The couple was clearly in a vicious cycle
due to divergent plans to commit.

To reduce their level of conflict, I taught them the Speaker-Listener
and Problem-Solving Techniques. Although this led to emotionally
less intense discussions, the fundamental discrepancy in their position on when to marry remained. I explored each of their family and
cultures of origin. Although Atafa had already demonstrated her separation from traditional Pakistani cultural expectations about a woman
needing to marry in her early 20s and to prioritize marriage above
career, she felt tied to her cultural belief about the need to marry one's
intimate partner. In contrast, Andreas noted that many people in his
country and in Europe more generally lived in more informal committed relationships without formal marriage. He also noted that his
parents had been unhappily married and had divorced when he was
young which he experienced as painful.

In a later session, Andreas acknowledged that although he loved
Atafa and was highly responsible in his job, he was having difficulty
taking this next step toward "full adulthood." Atafa's response to this
revelation was initially harsh—she tied it to his lying about his age
on the dating app, and stated she didn't want to be with a man who

refused to "grow up." However, Atafa became more compassionate toward Andreas as I continued to explore his fears that, as happened to his father, he would lose his enthusiasm and ability to have "adventures" (mostly centered on travel). I invited the partners to share their more specific visions of the future and what would change if they were to marry. Both came to realize that little would change, and Andreas heard from Atafa that she too wanted to continue to live an adventuresome life. Reassured that marriage to Atafa would not result in replicating his parents' marriage, Andreas agreed to marry, which the couple did six months later.

DIFFERENCES ON WHEN TO HAVE A FIRST CHILD

Many couples have anxiety about what researchers have called the "transition to parenthood" (Belsky & Rovine, 1990; Cowan & Cowan, 2012; Trillingsgaard et al., 2014), and for good reason. Although usually anticipated as a positive, even joyous experience, research in multiple studies has established that a large percentage of couples experience a decline in relationship and sexual satisfaction after the birth of the first child. Increased financial pressure, the need to relocate to a larger living space, sleep deprivation due to nocturnal feedings and the baby's different sleep rhythms, redirecting loving attention to the baby and away from one another, postpartum depression in a significant number of women, less freedom to venture out for pleasurable couple experiences (Claxton & Perry-Jenkins, 2008), a woman's need to recover physically from childbirth, and other factors contribute to this decline in satisfaction. Messages from one's family of origin about men's and women's respective responsibilities—traditionally, for men to be good providers and for women to sacrifice career ambitions and become full-time mothers, at least when the child is young, can lead to tension between partners who had aspired to balance work and family life and to share equally in childcare and home care tasks, often leading them to retreat to these more traditional roles (Knudson-Martin, 2012).

Vignette: Tom and Susan

Tom and Susan were a white married couple in their mid-30s. Together six years, they had an affectionate, conflict-free relationship until Tom started to express reservations about starting a family. Susan felt frustrated and anxious, saying, "My biological clock is ticking," and that she thought Tom had also wanted to start a family. Tom related that he did want children but worried that they were not financially secure enough to bring a child into the world. Both partners had good salaries in their respective jobs, Susan as a marketing executive for a fashion company, Tom as an information technology consultant to a major bank.

Tom received strong messages from his parents about his need to be a good provider. He did not have a clear sense of exactly what that meant in terms of income and so was left with a vague sense that he was not making enough money, even though he earned a six-figure salary and had opportunities for career advancement. Hearing that Susan wished to spend the first year of their baby's life as a full-time mother raised his anxiety about their future financial well-being and the pressure he would experience to make up for her lack of income.

Tom also sensed that his parents had little emotional intimacy (and although he wasn't sure, imagined they had little sexual intimacy as well). He described his mother as "doting on us kids," and he imagined this partly contributed to his parents' lack of intimate connection. He worried that the same would happen with him and Susan. Susan understood his concerns, and had repeatedly assured him that she would work to keep their relationship strong, to little effect. As a result, she wondered if there was more to his reluctance to have a child soon than what he had revealed. She wondered if he just wasn't prepared to enter this new stage of adulthood and pointed to his love of video games as a sign that he was "still a teenager." As a result, she had become sullen and withdrawn, which only confirmed Tom's worst fears—that even talking about having a kid was resulting in a rift between them. He said he could only imagine what would happen once the baby arrived. As with Atafa and Andreas, this couple had been captured by an unfortunate vicious cycle.

My first step in addressing the couple's issue was to share the research on the transition to parenthood, as a way of validating Tom's concerns (Cowan & Cowan, 2012; Trillingsgaard et al., 2014). This psychoeducational intervention calmed him down, although initially it made Susan anxious that it would overly confirm his fears. However, I quickly noted that knowing ahead of time about the typical challenges, they were in a good place to develop coping skills that would aid them in averting the negative effects of this transition.

Borrowing content of psychoeducational programs designed for couples in this transition (Cowan & Cowan, 2000; Jordan et al., 2001) and other guides to maintaining relationship satisfaction in the face of the demands of parenting (Doherty, 2013), this launched us on a pre-child distress-prevention program. This included learning communication and problem-solving skills, discussing how they would divide up childcare and housework (and initiating some of those changes around household chores), developing better skills around balancing work and relationship time (Fraenkel & Capstick, 2012), establishing clearer "rhythms of relationship"—regular times for intimacy and other pleasurable activities as well as a regular "relationship maintenance meeting" (Fraenkel, 2011), and planning how they would sustain time for couple connection once the baby arrived. I noted that some couples I'd worked with had mistakenly decided that total focus on the child was required in the early years, including never going out as a couple, and noted how important it would be—for both them and their future child(ren)—to nurture their pleasurable, empathic connection to weather the inevitable sleep deprivation and other stresses on them individually and as a unit.

I also noted that, like many cisgender heterosexual couples in which the woman elects to do much of the childcare, Tom's role during Susan's pregnancy and after the birth of the child might often be that of a sous chef, with Susan as master chef, making requests and giving orders as needed. The couple already had a strong "peer marriage" (Schwartz, 1994), with both partners endorsing the notion of sharing household and childcare responsibilities. However, I've sometimes found that men in such marriages insist on equal influence around such daily activities as bathing, feeding, and putting children to bed, even though it is the woman who elected to take the role of primary caretaker and has developed those often-intricate routines (Fraenkel, 1999, 2011). In other words, in the name of perfect equality, men may inadvertently undermine their female partners, or at least argue with them about childcare.

Addressing further Tom's concern about the possible loss of connection between him and Susan, which came from what he witnessed in his parents' marriage, I asked the couple what emotions they might consider "relationship alarm bells"—signals from their bodies that a rift might be growing between them. Susan replied, "Well, certainly irritation, frustration, and anger." I concurred that they needed to pay attention to those emotions and use the communication skills to discuss the source of those feelings. I asked, "What else? What other emotions might be good to notice and act on?" The couple sat silently thinking and turned to me quizzically.

I said, "How about loneliness? Loneliness is an emotion we often don't talk about in regard to marriage, but in fact, at times, being married yet disconnected from one another can be the loneliest place on earth." Susan and Tom glanced knowingly at each other, and at me.

Susan recalled that they'd already experienced periods of loneliness, especially as their conflict grew about when to have a child, amplified by their busy work schedules. Tom said, "Yeah, that's actually what I'm most worried about—ending up in a lonely marriage. Reminds me of that sad song by Carly Simon, where she sings something about her mother sitting alone in the dark and her father reading his magazine in another room or something." We reviewed the importance of setting up regular rhythms of time together and not waiting until one or the other felt ignored and lonely, but if loneliness appeared, to reach out to each other to talk about it and correct course.

Regarding Tom's worries about financial security, I helped him realize that the vague instructions he had received from his parents about being a good provider had left him highly anxious and that forming a concrete plan based on actual numbers would help relieve this anxiety. I then worked with the couple to come up with a plan to save and cut costs to prepare for the year when Susan would take a break from working.

Equipped with an approach to how they would best make the transition to parenthood, Tom's anxieties diminished greatly, to Susan's great relief, and the couple ended therapy with a commitment to getting pregnant.

DIFFERENCES ABOUT WHEN TO LAUNCH AN ADULT CHILD

Vignette: Krysten and Daniel

Krysten, a 72-year-old white woman, and Daniel, a 74-year-old white man, had been in a relationship for six years. Each had been previously married, and each had adult children from those marriages. Although quite happy when spending time as a couple, serious conflicts emerged around Krysten's son Hugo, especially when they all spent time together. Hugo had suffered from major depressive disorder for decades. From Krysten's description of Hugo's behavior, it seemed likely that he also might fit the diagnosis of avoidant personality disorder: He had been socially withdrawn from childhood (despite years of psychotherapy), had no close friendships, had never established an intimate romantic relationship, and for many years had never worked except for a few low-paying music gigs, and spent all of his time in his room, making music (Krysten shared with me some YouTube links of his music, all solo keyboard work, and he was quite talented), or in bed.

Hugo had made several suicide attempts through overdosing on medications (one just weeks before Krysten contacted me for couple therapy), had spent some time in inpatient treatment, and had several mental health professionals working with him sporadically, but without any success in helping him overcome his disorders and establish an independent adult life. I recommended a Boston-based clinic that did high-level comprehensive psychiatric evaluations and that had been extremely helpful to a client of mine whose daughter had experienced a psychotic episode, with the hope that a more thorough evaluation might result in more effective medications and a comprehensive treatment plan, but Krysten reported that Hugo was ambivalent about pursing this course of action.

Daniel felt frustrated with Krysten for not forcing Hugo to move out and get on with his life. Krysten wanted to encourage Hugo to move out, and had tried unsuccessfully to do so, but was frightened that he would react with another suicide attempt, possibly leading to his death. Although he was sympathetic to Krysten's dilemma, Daniel felt that Hugo's presence interfered with his and Krysten's relationship. She initially minimized Daniel's concerns, but with the aid of the Speaker-Listener Technique, the couple became better able to discuss the situation without Daniel becoming rageful and Krysten retreating.

I suggested that we meet together with Hugo, in the hope that I might be able to work with him to get on with his life. Krysten approached Hugo with this idea, and he refused. However, he did agree to meet with me alone for one session. During this session, I found him quiet but engaged. I shared with him that I'd listened to his music videos and found them quite remarkable. He was pleased to hear my appreciative comments, and we talked about the challenges of being a professional musician (as noted earlier, I had originally planned to become a full-time musician and attended a conservatory for my first year of college). I urged him to send some recordings to a record company that promoted the sort of ambient, peaceful music he created, and he liked this idea.

Hugo asked if he could comment on one of Daniel's behaviors that troubled him. I said of course, and he described how Daniel sometimes drove too fast and engaged in road rage behavior. This worried him, especially because it might jeopardize his mother's safety. I asked if I could share his concerns in my next session with his mother and Daniel, and he said yes.

In that next couple session, I remarked that I found Hugo pleasant to talk with; Krysten seemed relieved, and Daniel concurred that at times he also found Hugo pleasant. I noted that Hugo had shared a concern about Daniel and had given me permission to share it. Daniel's initial reaction was dismissive: "Who is he to tell me anything! He doesn't even have a life!" I smiled and said I could understand his reaction, but that the issue Hugo raised might be useful for me to raise nonetheless. Daniel settled down, and I shared Hugo's concerns about Daniel's speeding and angry behavior in the car. Krysten smiled and said this was a concern of hers, and Daniel acknowledged that he did at times behave in these ways, and that he would make a renewed attempt to slow down and avoid angry gestures at other drivers.

Interestingly, this exchange—aided by my emphasizing some of Hugo's strengths despite his disabling psychiatric conditions—seemed to soften Daniel's pathologizing attitude toward Hugo. With Daniel putting less pressure on Krysten to eject Hugo from the home, Krysten seemed to be released from the loyalty bind between Daniel and Hugo, and started more actively brainstorming ways that she could encourage Hugo to move out of the home. She had an additional apartment from her previous marriage that had been uninhabited for years (her husband had died and left it to her), and began working on renovating it so that Hugo could live there. These actions, along with activities to strengthen the couple's pleasurable connection, and the softened, more respectful attitude Daniel adopted in interactions with Hugo, to which Hugo responded in kind, led to a significant improvement in the couple's relationship.

However, there was one further issue that challenged their commitment to the relationship: their different desires around the issue of retirement.

DIFFERENCES ABOUT WHEN TO RETIRE

Daniel was a retired accountant. He wanted to spend the remaining years of his life traveling and exploring new activities. Krysten had spent many years as a full-time mother, and only in the last five years had returned to work that she found extremely fulfilling. Daniel wanted her to retire so that they would be free to travel more; Krysten felt committed to her work. They did not need her to work in order to sustain themselves financially, but she found the work highly meaningful.

I remarked, especially for Daniel's benefit, that Krysten's experience was quite common among women who had left the workforce to raise children and manage a home. Oftentimes once children are launched, they wish to return to paid or volunteer work as part of creating renewed, more diverse meaning in their lives. Hugo's psychiatric difficulties had left him dependent on Krysten for care and prolonged her sense of responsibility towards him, interfering somewhat with her plans to return to work. It seemed quite important that Krysten maintain her involvement with her work, and that Daniel understand and accept this as central to Krysten's wellbeing and happiness. Daniel acknowledged these points, and stated that he certainly wanted Krysten to feel happy.

The couple went on to plan some trips around Krysten's work commitments. Daniel also acknowledged that he was relying too much on fantasies about shared travel in figuring out how to make his retirement fulfilling. As I saw this couple during the coronavirus pandemic that began in 2020, he also acknowledged that it might be some time before they could safely travel, and that he needed to get on with pursuing some long-delayed dreams of engaging in new hobbies. Two weeks later, he reported that he had finally purchased a guitar and was taking lessons.

SUMMARY

Couples who otherwise are doing fairly well may reach an impasse around whether, and especially when, to attain certain life goals. Differences in their projected life chronologies can result in thoughts of dissolving the relationship. The Therapeutic Palette integrative approach can assist couples to reduce conflict in conversations around these issues and allow them to share and listen more compassionately to their respective sources of desire or reluctance to move to a new stage of life, and resolve these impasses.

CHAPTER 9

COUPLES WITH LOW OR NO PASSION AND PLEASURE

L AST CHANCE COUPLES WHO HAVE lost their desire for intimate passion and connection are often the most challenging couples to assist. In many cases, they come with a long history of high conflict, and one or both partners has responded to this conflict and the corresponding feelings of hurt, anger, resentment, and alienation with a loss of sexual desire and desire for any other sort of mutual pleasure. In others, the pleasure bond was never strong to begin with, and life's complexities and travails have dampened it to the point of extinction.

BASIC TECHNIQUES FOR RESTARTING PLEASURABLE CONNECTION

As described in Chapters 4 and 5 on working with high-conflict couples, it is important to introduce the theme of rebuilding pleasurable connection early on for all last chance couples, except those in which violence occurs. As was noted, helping couples communicate and more generally get along with less conflict does not automatically result in them reengaging in pleasurable activities (Fincham & Beach, 2010). Techniques like the 60-second pleasure point (Fraenkel, 1998b, 2011), which suggests small but regular bits of connection across the day; the "daily relational vitamin," statements of appreciation or admiration that can serve to soften the wall of alienation and resentment between partners; and a daily "how was your day, dear?" conversation, which provides opportunities for mutual soothing and decompression (Fraenkel, 1998a, 2011), are all useful with low- and no-passion couples—all can serve to restart pleasure and intimacy.

CREATING RHYTHMS OF RELATIONSHIP

As also described earlier, it is important that couples create regular rhythms of relationship—not only regular meetings to discuss and resolve problems, but regular times to meet for pleasure and intimacy. When I first suggest this to couples, frequently one partner or the other will roll their eyes and say despairingly, "So, now we have to schedule sex?" I respond by agreeing that the term *schedule* has the connotation of work and doesn't belong in the domain of pleasure. Yet other terms, such as *rhythms*, also refer to regularly occurring events but with more pleasant connotations—the rhythms of the seasons, of day and night, of our heartbeats, and of music and dance.

I note that one important myth about couple time that interferes with couples experiencing intimacy is the myth of spontaneity—the notion that despite our overscheduled lives, we hold out the hope that sex and other forms of intimacy will just happen and that both partners will be in the mood at the exact same moment (Fraenkel, 2011). Instead, I recommend couples create regular times for intimacy and, within those times, can be as spontaneous as they wish. I often use the analogy of a jazz group: There's plenty of improvisation going on, but if you don't show up for the gig on time, it won't happen. Even the act of musical improvisation depends on a solid rhythmic structure—the drummer and bass player set down the tempo and the groove, and the other musicians improvise around the set melodic and harmonic structure of the tune.

REVIVING AND EXPANDING THE COUPLE'S EARLY HISTORY OF PLEASURE

Hosting conversations about the history of the relationship, starting with how the partners met and what attracted each to the other, and what has transpired that led them to disengage, is also important, as partners may be afraid to reconnect lest they reinvigorate painful forms of interaction. If high-conflict communication was an issue, teaching couples the Speaker-Listener and Problem-Solving Techniques will provide them the tools to avoid such conflict and encourage them to reconnect without emotional risk.

SIMPLY BORED

Couples may also simply have become bored, having relied for too long on a few forms of pleasurable connection that no longer yield enjoyment (Aron et al., 2000; Coulter & Malouff, 2013; Graham, 2008; Strong & Aron, 2006). Or they may have relied on one another to provide stimulating conversation but, after years together, find there's not much new to share. A randomized-control study by Coulter and Malouff (2013) assigned one set of couples to a four-week intervention in which they were instructed to engage in exciting activities in a variety of suggested forms (adventurous, passionate, sexual, exciting, interesting, playful, romantic, and spontaneous) for 90 minutes per week, and compared them on self-rated romantic-relationship excitement to a matched wait list control group. They found that couples who engaged in these activities reported significantly higher relationship excitement, higher relationship satisfaction, and higher positive affect postintervention and four months later.

Therefore, couples should be encouraged to pick an activity that involves learning something new together, whether it be ballroom or other forms of dancing, yoga, Tai Chi, an artistic (e.g., pottery, painting) or musical activity (e.g., learning to play harmonica, recorder, or hand drums, or a music appreciation class for a form of music they're not so familiar with), a cooking class, or novel activities in nature (e.g., kayaking, rock climbing, birdwatching). They can also decide to read a novel, short stories, or poems together, or set out to watch the films of a particular director. As simple and commonsense as this suggestion would appear, couples often overlook obvious potential solutions to the passion problem, and sometimes spend too much time analyzing what relational issues have led them to this passionless state.

The main point to make to bored couples is that it's unrealistic to expect them to provide interesting stimulation to one another over many years—they need an outside stimulus or activity, and to explore the world together. This perspective is supported by the premises of the Creative Relational Movement approach to change: Couples often need to try new activities, even if they have doubts about whether these activities will change how they feel, and even if they are somewhat lacking in motivation and conviction, and see how the new activities may surprisingly change their feelings and thoughts, rather than hoping that repeated review of their story of a passionless marriage will automatically lead to change.

A corollary to the couple's work on escaping boredom by finding new activities is for each partner to look at whether they individually have become bored with how they spend leisure time. One source of attraction to a new partner is hearing about the activities that engage and enliven them. When people lose contact with nonwork sources of pleasure, excitement, and aliveness, they may lose that spark and energy that is part of what makes them attractive to others.

Vignette: Roberto and Lucia

After 25 years of marriage and raising two children to young adulthood, Roberto, 56, and Lucia, 51, an Argentinian American couple, rarely had sex or any other form of intimacy. Roberto's demanding albeit lucrative job in finance meant long hours at the office, and they rarely made time for one another. They got along fairly well and had no history of high conflict, but the passion and mutual attraction had gradually drained out of their relationship. They cared about each other but found their relationship boring. They were considering a separation, but wanted to try to improve the relationship to stay together, at least for the kids.

My encouragement to try some new activities had little effect. I then asked what each did for enjoyment on their own, and, aside from working out, neither had an active hobby. I asked whether each had ever entertained fantasies about trying something totally new. Lucia remarked that she had long wanted to take some courses in art history but kept putting it off. Likewise, Roberto said as a young man he was quite involved with photography but had never formally studied it, and dropped it once his career got busy. Each partner made a commitment to getting started on their individual leisure pursuits. This led each of them to feel more alive, and they suddenly found themselves attracted to one another once again. They began making love and together decided to visit museums and introduce each other to what they had learned in their respective courses.

INTIMACY WITHOUT WORDS

It is also important to emphasize that emotional intimacy and a sense of closeness can occur without words. Couple therapists have at times been caricatured for our overemphasis on verbal communication as the sole or most important conduit of intimacy. I often joke with couples that I may be one of the few therapists who believe that couples often talk too much! I explore with couples how they can create intimate time in nonverbal ways (other than sex, discussed below). Sitting on the couch reading different books together (or even scrolling through an online newspaper or social media—not checking emails) with legs entwined, going on a silent walk or hike, even eating a home-cooked meal silently and with full appreciation for the taste of the food can at times be more intimate than endless discussions and exchange of ideas, or regaling one's partner with tales of woe or triumph from the day.

INVITING ONE'S PARTNER INTO ONE'S PASSIONS

In addition, one or both partners may have foregone favored activities in an attempt to accommodate the other, and now longs to reengage in these activities. They may believe that their partner is still unwilling to try these activities, but faced with the possible end to the relationship, that partner may finally be willing.

Vignette: Cindy and Charles

This was the case for Cindy and Charles, the couple described in Chapter 5 in which Charles had tired of providing much daily soothing to Cindy. In his youth he had enjoyed more vigorous sports and outdoor activities, such as mountaineering and whitewater rafting, whereas Cindy preferred long walks on flat terrain that allowed for conversation. Now in his early 60s, having devoted most of his energy to soothing Cindy, and to work and time with the kids who were now well launched into adulthood, he strongly desired to return to those activities that he had put aside, anticipating that he might only have this decade of vigorous health remaining to experience these sorts of pleasures.

Although Cindy said it was fine by her if he pursued these activities without her, Charles wanted to share them with someone. Given Cindy's long-ago stated aversion to outdoorsy activities, Charles assumed he would need to leave the marriage and perhaps find someone else with whom he could share these forms of enjoyment. With the future of the relationship in the balance, and with her enhanced ability to self-soothe and not rely on Charles as much for emotional support,

Cindy agreed to push herself a bit and engage in some of these activities with Charles and found them quite invigorating. With Charles feeling "more alive" than he had in years, and enjoying Cindy joining him in a nonverbal, physical activity, his desire for sex with her returned.

IMPROVING SEXUAL INTIMACY

Some couples have more long-standing issues around sexual intimacy, either from the beginning of the relationship or that developed later—for instance, after the birth of children. Suzanne Iasenza (2020) has described in detail an approach she calls narrative relational sex therapy, which involves in-depth exploration of each partner's sexual history, beginning with their earliest memories of sexuality, through which conscious and unconscious themes around sexual contact, insecurities about one's body, trauma, and family- and culture-based proscriptions about sex are identified. She also presents a "sexual menu" to get a conversation started around undisclosed fantasies and desires that partners in sexually stuck couples have often not shared with one another, and with which they can begin to experiment in a nonjudgmental fashion.

Iasenza also coaches couples in "mindful narrative touch" (2020, p. 11), teaching them mindfulness practices and expanding on the pioneering technique of sensate focus, developed by Masters and Johnson (1966, 1975; Weiner & Avery-Clark, 2017). In sensate focus, each partner at first gives the other a sensual but not sexual massage (avoiding areas identified by each partner as erogenous), and the giver learns through verbal and nonverbal feedback what the receiver finds pleasurable and not pleasurable (depth of touch and strokes, rhythm, speed, and so on). Couples are then better acclimatized to each other's sources of physical pleasure and can go on to more direct sexual activity. Whereas Masters and Johnson encouraged partners to minimize the frequent tendency for "spectatoring"—watching how one is having sex during the act and judging one's effectiveness and adequacy in turning on one's partner (often anxiously), Iasenza asks partners to notice and discuss in therapy the content of the spectatoring, which is usually linked to problematic sexual-relational narratives.

Iasenza's integrative approach is quite comprehensive, and I recommend readers become familiar with it. In line with her approach and that of Perel (2007), I suggest working on the couple's sexual relationship before all their other issues are resolved, as soon as they are ready, and not to assume that decrease in conflict in other areas will automatically result in reemergence of partners' sexual desires. However, with last chance couples whose problems always include issues aside from sex and have led partners to hardened stances against and away from one another, it is always necessary to address these other issues somewhat before most partners are willing to reengage in physical connection.

SEX AS PLAY AND NONVERBAL COMMUNICATION

Although couples with long-standing issues around sex surely need to engage in the kind of in-depth therapeutic work Iasenza recommends, couples sometimes view sex as another form of relationship work. This can lead sex to become a rather goal-directed, humorless chore, followed by post-encounter evaluations (one or another form of, "Was it good for you? What can I do to improve?"). Introducing the notion that sex can be a play space filled with humor and spontaneity (see more details below) can lighten the mood and decrease performance anxiety. With a play space attitude, "mistakes" (being too forceful, not being forceful enough, moving too fast, too slow, kisses that are too dry or too wet, and so on) can be the source of spontaneous sexual comedy (corrected more easily) and giggled about, rather than being experienced and discussed as a moment of failure.

TAKING A CHANCE ON TOUCH: LET THE BODIES
DO THE TALKING

When partners have been in conflict for months or years, and there's been little to no physical affection or sex during that time, they may be hesitant to touch one another, never mind kiss or make love, even if in principle they wish to do so, and have discussed this desire in therapy. Even with conflict greatly reduced and a renewed commitment to remain together, partners may simply find it awkward to reconnect physically. In a way, they have returned to that moment many experience early in dating, when they've connected verbally and now the moment has come for the first kiss—inevitably a bit awkward to move from words to nonverbals, but if it works out and is well received, you're off and running!

To jumpstart the couple's physical connection, during a session in which partners report that things are generally going well and the conversation has been about how "we need to work on our sex life," I often tell the couple to make out right then, and, with a smile, I announce that I will be off-screen for a few minutes (if doing online therapy) or will leave the room and shut the door, if in person. This instruction inevitably evokes surprised laughter, but I insist they do it, and I leave, come back in a few minutes, and playfully ask how it went. Usually upon my return, I find the couple notably relaxed, sometimes a bit embarrassed, but beaming, and holding hands.

I follow up this kissing enactment with a transposition of a quote from the telephone industry—the slogan that alludes to searching the Yellow Pages with one's fingers. I remind the couple of this old slogan (some are too young to remember it, but many do), and say, "It's time to let your bodies do the talking." For couples that need a bit more convincing, I note that the parts of their brains that produce verbal language are not the parts they need to reconnect and communicate physically.

THE TEMPORAL SIDE OF SEX

One specific theme I frequently find interferes with sexual compatibility and pleasuring not emphasized much by Iasenza and other sexuality experts centers on the temporal side of sex. Partners often differ in their pace/tempo and rhythms in sexual behavior. In particular, cisgender heterosexual men often approach sex from the beginning with a fast pace, which does not allow women to become aroused and lubricated. They also may vary the pace/tempo and rhythm of their movements too much, shifting from fast to slow to fast, attending to one part of the woman's body and then moving quickly to another, rather than getting a "slow groove" going in one area (for instance, the clitoris during oral sex) and then seeing, feeling, listening for signs that the woman is getting increasingly aroused, and gradually increasing the pace.

I often meet with men individually to discuss this issue and use the analogy of being a jazz drummer whose role is to support the "arousal" of the soloists by laying down a steady groove while urging the soloist on with short, syncopated notes for emphasis and to build excitement. I reference the great Duke Ellington's song "It Don't Mean a Thing (If It Ain't Got That Swing)," and suggest that approaching lovemaking like a hard-hitting heavy metal drummer usually is not what a woman desires—rather, generally speaking, and in the words of a Pointer Sisters song, she wants him to approach sex (metaphorically and literally) with a "slow hand."

On the other hand, women and men vary tremendously in what they desire in terms of the tempo of lovemaking. Sometimes their desires are purely about what they find arousing, but sometimes may reveal underlying issues around sex.

Vignette: Daphne and Eric

Daphne was a 42-year-old concert pianist and Eric was a 44-year-old lawyer. They had two teenaged children, and sex had largely been absent for several years. When they did have sex, Daphne preferred it "hard"—fast and furious. Immediately after sex, she would get up and go back to other activities, especially practicing piano. Against gender stereotype, Eric longed for a slower, more sensual approach, and wanted cuddling before and after sex. He felt hurt and rejected by Daphne's sexual style.

Exploration of their approaches to sex revealed that Daphne had struggled since her teenage years with a serious eating disorder. Although she said she no longer binged and purged, she noted that she was highly attentive to her weight (she was quite slim and muscular, and worked out every day), and that she would panic and redouble her exercising if she gained more than two pounds. This concern about her body increased after having the two children. Her mother, who was quite slender, had been critical of Daphne's eating and her body, warning her not "to indulge" lest she gain weight. Daphne had studied piano since age five, and, although she never became well known, she was quite talented, worked hard on her performances, and tended to get anxious about playing in public due to her perfectionistic standards. Daphne explained that she preferred rapid sex because of continued self-criticism of her body, despite Eric's frequent statements that he found her beautiful.

For his part, Eric had been raised in a high-achieving family and had been successful in college and in his career. However, having attained a good deal of financial security, he now wanted to relax more and "enjoy life." He wanted more affection between himself and Daphne, as he had experienced little "free affection" in his family—his parents had doled out warm compliments only based on his academic and work achievements. He saw lovemaking as one area he wished to enhance, but found Daphne often noncommittal.

I suggested to Daphne that she might benefit from taking some more steps to accept her body and that this might shift her approach to sex toward the style desired by Eric, which she valued in principle but felt too anxious to relax into. I introduced her to David Epston's narrative therapy–based Anti-Anorexia/Anti-Bulimia League (http://www.narrativeapproaches.com/resources/anorexia-bulimia-archives-of-resistance/), an online resource where people, especially women, who have struggled with restrictive eating disorders share accounts of how they took a stand against these disorders and the many messages communicated through family and the larger media and cultures that encourage a problematic view of women's standards of beauty and bodies.

I encouraged Daphne to come up with an externalizing name for her concerns about her body, and she chose "The Gnawing." Daphne kept a record of times when she "took a stand" against The Gnawing and stopped checking her weight so frequently. She also experimented with a slower, more affectionate approach to sex with Eric, which would culminate in the kind of vigorousness she enjoyed. She also allowed herself to cuddle with him and allowed herself to enjoy his compliments about her physical beauty. Eric felt much more satisfied as a result.

REFRAMING SEX AS A PLAY SPACE

Weighted down by multiple work and other pressures, by their areas of conflict, and by their sense of disconnection, last chance couples often approach improving their sex life as another task or duty. The old adage "Marriage is hard work," which many couples sadly proclaim at the onset of therapy, infiltrates their attitudes toward sensuality and sexuality. I challenge this adage and note that with more effective forms of communication, sensitivity to one another's perspectives, needs, and desires, and a willingness to compromise, marriage or other long-term committed relationships do not have to be hard work at all. By learning effective communication and other ways of responding empathically to one another, couples often have their first experience in how much easier relationships can be.

Especially when partners approach sex with the instrumental goal of "making the partner come," this interferes with entering the sexual encounter freely and with the necessary parasympathetic activation that is associated with sexual arousal. With such couples, I note how their serious attitude about sex and their overfocus on goals impedes pleasurable connection. I introduce the frame of sex as a play space, where the pressures of life can be put aside. This simple reframe of the sexual encounter can be quite powerful in providing couples permission to enjoy themselves in the moment.

Vignette: Ted and Josephine

Ted and Josephine were a white couple in their mid-30s. Both had high-pressure jobs that left them exhausted at the end of the day. This contributed to their slow drift apart over the six years they been together. Adding to their stress were their unsuccessful attempts to get pregnant. Josephine had consulted with a fertility specialist, and the couple was trying to have more sex during her peak period of ovulation. These pressures and their sense of disconnection had led them to consider separation. At times, due to all the stress and pressure, Ted was unable to get an erection.

I validated their experiences of work stress, and the stress of dealing with fertility issues, and noted how they were now approaching sex as a chore. I encouraged them to do some mindful breathing and Qigong every day and especially before having sex, and to view sex as a play space, within which they could let go of stressors and simply focus on smell and touch, let go of the goal of getting pregnant, and immerse in the sensual moment.

Having seen that both had a sense of humor, I encouraged them to be silly with each other in bed. I also suggested that eroticism comes from the pleasurable tension between the "subjective and the objective"—knowing each other as individuals, their feelings and thoughts—and the pure enjoyment of each other's bodies. I modeled this sort of playing with the tension between appreciating each other's objective physical attributes and caring about each other's feelings by saying, in a low, Barry White–style lover voice, "Hey, babe, I'm gonna love ya just a little more—get over here and let me throw you around the bed!" And then switching to a higher-pitched, nerdy, emotionally-sensitive voice, "I mean, I *do* care about your *feelings* and all, I really, really do!"—and then back to Barry White-esque low voice, "now get over here, and let me looove you!" The couple laughed, and I noted Josephine's eyes flickered with a hint of excitement. The couple transformed their approach to sex, and within a month they were pregnant.

EXPLORING AND ENGAGING PARTNERS' FANTASIES AND SEXUAL PREFERENCES

Perel (2007) attributes the low desire and lack of sexual activity in many long-term relationships to partners not accepting their sexual fantasies or sharing those with their partners, for fear of rejection or shaming. She, along with Iasenza (2020), recommends exploring those fantasies as a matter of course. Iasenza recommends inviting these fantasies initially during individual sessions, whereas Perel often invites such discussions in conjoint sessions. Of course, in some instances, the couple raises the issue of fantasies and preferred activities themselves.

Vignette: Carl and Tim

Carl, a 41-year-old Irish American banker, and Tim, a 35-year-old Italian American florist, had been together for six years, but were on the cusp of ending the relationship. Among other issues, Tim, who described himself as "femme," enjoyed BDSM sex, especially involving dressing in leather. Carl, who had not disclosed his sexual orientation to his colleagues at the bank, had no interest in BDSM or leather, preferring more "straightforward" sex, in which he typically was the "top" and Tim was the "bottom." They had an arrangement in which Tim could visit BDSM dungeons as long as he was sure it was safe. Tim laughed and explained the rules for ensuring safety and ending encounters. Carl remained circumspect.

Despite this arrangement, their differences in sexual fantasies and preferences had led to a growing rift and loss of passion between them. On a recent visit to a large city in Germany, Tim ventured into a dungeon, with Carl upstairs waiting. At a certain point, Carl heard Tim crying out for help, went downstairs, and found Tim being beaten and choked by another man. Carl, who was quite tall and muscular, pulled the man off Tim, and the couple left. Carl found this incident extremely upsetting and was angry at Tim for being "so naive" about the risks of BDSM. Tim was also distressed about this event. He plaintively asked Carl if he would consider meeting him halfway, asking if Carl would consider wearing some leather during sex. Tim assured Carl that he would give up extradyadic BDSM adventures if Carl would do this for him. Two weeks later, Carl came to the session wearing a leather vest; Tim was ecstatic. The couple then began to explore more of Tim's fantasies, which Carl began to allow himself to enjoy.

Importantly, Tim's ability to influence Carl in this domain served to rebalance the broader power arrangement between them, as Carl had significantly greater financial power than Tim and was older. In addition, the couple lived in what had originally been Carl's apartment (although Tim had redecorated it), and Carl was physically larger than Tim. As a result of these power differences, Tim had often felt "less than" Carl, but this change in their sexual practices, based on Tim's desires, helped them feel more equal.

SUMMARY

Last chance couples that report low or no passion can be particularly challenging to assist, as they lack the energy of desire for connection. High-conflict couples, couples in which a partner has violated values or safety, and those mismatched in their desired life timelines may still hold some degree of disappointed desire, and partners still care about what the other thinks and feels about them. This energy, often expressed through conflict, can be transformed into enjoyable and emotionally safe connection. In couples in which none of these other issues pertain, but "the fire's out," partners can feel so disengaged that they cannot imagine continuing in a life together. Yet simple experiments in possibility with pleasure can revive their lust and love, and help the couple break out of the "ice sculpture" of apartness and discouragement.

PREPARATION FOR THE WORK
Self-Knowledge and Self-Care

Working with last chance couples can be invigorating and gratifying; it can also be overstimulating, disappointing, affronting, and exhausting. Even brief hostile and vituperative exchanges can get under our skin. Hearing emotional accounts of one partner's discovery that the other partner has engaged in an affair, or violence, or repeated overuse of substances, and hearing the other partner minimize or deny these behaviors can evoke moral outrage, disgust, or dismay based on our deepest-held values. Sitting with an economically privileged couple considering divorce because their passion has run dry, even though they have plenty of resources to engage in pleasure and have young children whose lives will be disrupted, can evoke the reaction that they are being selfish and spoiled. Working with a couple in which one partner is anxious about taking a next step in life like having children that his partner desperately wants when so many others do so without such distress can evoke irritation and mild contempt.

Additionally, the more one's reputation for helping couples has developed over time, the more one may receive referrals for last chance couples, who've tried couple therapy before without success. The pressure's on to make this therapy experience different and worthwhile.

I often think of this work as a kind of "open-hearted surgery"—it can get a bit urgent and messy as we delve into people's acquired hatred, loss of love, and their confusing communications. We need to be emotionally responsive to the people who put their hopes and trust in us, but the experience of diving into their conflicts can be at times unnerving and depleting. It is important that we therapists come to this challenging work with a good sense of our relational and moral triggers, and that we engage in regular self-care.

SELF-KNOWLEDGE

It is essential that we have a good grasp on our own family-of-origin histories, our own culturally transmitted beliefs about relationships and behaviors in them, and our own relationship histories so that we can distinguish between reactions that many therapists might have to what the couple presents—for instance, if partners insult each other in session, or one partner has engaged in violence or intimidation—and our own specific countertransference reactions. With my graduate students, I have each student create a genogram around two questions: (1) What aspects of your family and cultural background, including roles you played and challenging events, have contributed to one or more of your strengths as a therapist? (2) What aspects of your family and cultural background, including your social locations in terms of gender, gender identity, race, ethnicity, class, orientation to religious or spiritual values, challenges around physical ability, political and social beliefs, and others, may result in strong reactions to particular sorts of problems couples and families present? Some sample questions to consider (and this is by no means an exhaustive list!):

1. Were you raised in a family in which you often played the role of mediator between your parents, and at times were successful but often unsuccessful in decreasing their conflict—including that they ultimately divorced? How might that lead you to feel a bit overconfident about your powers to stop conflict (if they would just listen to you!), and also to feel the need to save the couples with whom you work (because you didn't save your parents' marriage despite your valiant efforts)?
2. Was there intimidation or violence in your family, with your father perpetrating the violence against your mother and possibly you and your siblings, leading you to side with your mother (irrespective of your gender identity) and now find it hard to connect with a male client who has done the same? Or was your mother highly critical of your father, of you and your siblings, who all felt unable to stand up to her? How might this trigger a high level of fear or disdain for a female client who acts similarly? Do your experiences

of upsetting high-volume conflict trigger you into intimidation or silence, or lead you to guide partners—who may both be okay with higher levels of emotion expression—into a rather emotionless form of communication which they find overly constraining?

3. Did a parent, grandparent, or other family member engage in substance overuse, and what impact did that have on you? How might this experience make it hard for you to tolerate a client who does the same, and to explore the underlying reasons for their overuse with them—or make you overly solicitous about their pain and ignore the effects their overuse is having on their partner?

4. How might you feel about people who inhabit locations that afford them greater privilege (especially unearned privileges of race, ethnicity, class) than you have experienced, and make you impatient or offended by their attitudes or behavior? For instance, I was raised middle class and, as some of the vignettes I've shared illustrate, in my practice I've worked with people of extraordinary wealth. At times I've found myself a bit unsympathetic to their complaints about their lives, given the enormous resources available to them. I've had to remember that everyone suffers in their own ways and monitor moments when I feel a bit of envy when a client talks about the difficulties managing their summer homes and their spacious apartments and their ranch in Montana, or the inconveniences they experienced at a five-star hotel.

5. How might your own struggles with anxiety, depression, or trauma, or your own relationship difficulties, make you sensitive to those issues in others, but also lead you to assume you know what they are feeling and going through without asking?

6. How might your cherished social and political values bump up against those of people who ascribe to quite different values?

For example, I am a left-leaning liberal, descended from socialist grandparents, and a few years ago worked with a gay male couple in which one partner described himself as Far Left, and the other as formerly centrist liberal but now Alt-Right (during the Trump era, no less). He also held a strong belief that "the Jews control all the world's wealth" and insisted on sharing the "facts" supporting this theory.

Initially alarmed at his beliefs (as was his partner of 16 years, who was considering ending their marriage due to their political differences), I found the best way to connect with him was first to describe my political and social orientation, and to apologize in advance if some of my questions or statements inadvertently had a judgmental tone (and invited him to point that out to me), and then to see this as a rare opportunity to get to know how someone whom I saw was quite bright came to adopt his Alt-Right stance. Indeed, there were moments in which I challenged him too vigorously, and he pulled back and wondered if the therapy could work, prompting me to apologize and work to repair our relationship. Ultimately, my modeling of genuine curiosity with him helped the other partner to soften his rejecting, outraged stance, and the two of them were able to find a consensus about areas of social justice work they could engage in together, and also to regain the base of pleasure and companionship that they'd enjoyed for years.

Likewise, in my work with Tamara and Terry (see Chapter 6), when Tamara spoke about how much her physical beauty meant to her and how she enjoyed appreciative comments from men in the street, I felt my feminist hackles raised, a strong desire to help her find greater value in her mind, and to "liberate" her from the sociocultural narratives that overemphasize women's looks over their minds and accomplishments. However, to do so directly would have felt insulting to her—as you'll recall, when I shared that some women might take offense at strange men commenting on their sexiness, she shrugged and said, "I guess I'm not much of a feminist that way." Likewise, when Terry spoke about Tamara and her looks in a proprietary manner, I found my feminist values evoked, and needed to settle down before addressing how this attitude might feel overly constraining for Tamara, to which he agreed. Critiquing him head-on would have ruptured our alliance.

Likewise, when the French American husband told his African American wife of many years (see Chapter 5) that he "didn't see [her] as Black, just as a human being," I felt a slight bit of contempt for my fellow white male, based on all my hard-earned and admittedly incomplete attempts to recognize my own white blindness and unearned privilege. I had to remember that I too was raised with the notion that the best way to deal with racial inequities was to accept everyone as "just human, and that we're all the same," when clearly, we are not so—culturally, and in terms of what our skin color affords us in terms of privilege or oppression on a day-to-day basis.

All these and many more questions should be considered as you engage in work with any client, and especially with last chance couples. It is useful to explore these issues with a therapist, a supervisor, or a colleague. The path to self-knowledge and examining one's sources of countertransference is unending. No matter how many different sorts of couples we've worked with and how long we've been in practice, it is critical to approach each new couple with what the

Zen Buddhists call beginner's mind—a deep openness to new experiences, to new learning, to failing to "get it right," and an attitude of deep humility in the face of this challenging work.

SELF-CARE

We therapists regularly recommend all manner of techniques for self-care: Mindfulness practices, time engaged in enjoyable nonwork activities, being less perfectionistic, daily statements of appreciation for the good things in our lives, exercise, good sleep hygiene, healthy eating and drinking. But in distributing this wisdom session after session, we may almost feel as though we don't need to engage in the same self-care practices, as we trudge on hour after hour with our clients—as if giving the advice is somehow equivalent to following it! To avoid burnout, a psychophysiological state of exhaustion and reactivity that can sneak up on us before we know it, it's crucial to engage in regular self-care. In one semester of my graduate courses, I have students present on a nonpsychology activity with which they've developed some skill and mastery, and that brings them pleasure.

I also have them reflect on how doing these activities can provide useful analogies for their work as therapists. Students have shared their engagement in sports, the arts, needlepoint, cooking and baking, watching films and manga cartoons, and much more. For me, self-care has centered on exercise, mindful breathing, Qigong and Tai Chi, time in nature, cooking, poetry, and, most importantly, on my life as a drummer and percussionist, which began long before I thought about becoming a psychologist and therapist. Playing music allows me a reprieve from the domain of words, an opportunity to express myself and connect with fellow musicians in ways that cannot be fully expressed in spoken language. Along the lines I've encouraged in my students, I've regularly drawn upon my life as a musician and drummer in particular to look at couples in unique ways, leading to my work on time and rhythm in couples (Fraenkel, 1994, 2001c, 2011) and the role of music and other arts in couple therapy (Fraenkel, 2020).

Whether or not you find ways to transfer some of your experiences and knowledge from these activities into your work as a therapist is much less important than making time to leave aside this difficult work of therapy for other forms of endeavor and experience. If we can't take our own advice, how can we expect our clients to do so?

Most of all, to hold the tensions last chance couples bring about whether to stay or to leave their relationship, we must enter the same liminal, not-yet-sure space we suggest to couples, and must see our efforts as experiments in possibility. Ideas and techniques that worked well with many prior couples may fall flat with the new one in front of us. We must bring our flexibility, creativity, and responsiveness to their unique situation, unique pain and desires, and unique selves. Although we're biased to help couples make it together, despite earnest (or perhaps half-hearted) attempts at change, they may improve, or not, and stay together, or not. We're there to give them their last best chance to figure it out. In the spirit of the Therapeutic Palette integrative approach, the therapist and the couple share the brush that gradually paints their picture, maps out their terrain of possibilities or impasses, and reveals the path that's best for them.

APPENDIX

TABLE OF THERAPEUTIC IDEAS AND TECHNIQUES

Ideas or Techniques	Chapter	Pages
Building the Therapeutic Alliance and Contract		
Creating a tentative therapeutic contract	Intro, 1	8, 39
Validating the ambivalent partner's desire to leave the relationship	Intro, 1	9, 38
Creating an initial focus on the present	Intro	10
Avoiding initial focus on strengths and positive narratives	Intro	12
Restarting pleasure while reducing pain	Intro	13
Role of courage and encouragement in therapy	1	23
Stating biases about improving relationship	1	39
Outlining plan of action	1	39
Inviting couples into a liminal space: suspending talk of future	1	40
Introduce idea that improvement is nonbinding	1	40
Showing interest in couple partners' areas of competence (work, etc.)	1	42
Discussing partners' doubts about therapy, challenges to expertise	1	44
Connecting with partners who've violated values or safety	1	45
Connecting across cultures and social locations: just ask	1	47–49

Teaching making statements of appreciation and admiration	2, 4	108, 184
Encouraging partners to respond to bids for attention	2, 4	108, 184
Teaching mutual soothing techniques	2, 4	108, 185, 214
Teach skills for repairing ruptures	4	211
Easy apologies	4	212
Neuroeducation about shame and guilt	4	213
Teaching mindfulness techniques for emotion regulation	2, 4	108
Teaching partners to take influence from one another	2, 4	108
Encouraging empathic discussion of differences	2, 4	109
Teaching Beginning Anew for Couples: mindfulness-based communication	4	206
Experiential/Emotionally focused therapy assessment questions	2	110
Emotionally focused therapy techniques	2	122
Softening (identifying vulnerability)	2	112
Evocative responding: drawing out and naming partners' feelings	2	112
Heightening: intensifying partners' emotions	2	112
Empathic conjecture: offering thoughts about what partners are feeling	2	112
Intergenerational couple therapy assessment questions	2	113
Intergenerational couple therapy techniques	2	116
Constructing problem-focused genograms	2	116
Examining effect of family-of-origin experiences on present relationship	2, 5	116
Encouraging partners to differentiate from family of origin	2, 5	116
Psychodynamic couple therapy assessment questions	2	117
Psychodynamic couple therapy techniques	2	117
Identifying intrapsychic conflicts	2	117
Naming and working with guilt and shame	2	117
Introducing idea/goal of mentalization and intersubjectivity	2	118
Examining patterns of transference and countertransference	2	119
Narrative therapy assessment questions	2	121
Narrative therapy techniques (practices)	2	122
Deconstructing the problem story	2	122

Creating self-genograms to examine therapist's strengths and challenges	Afterword	350
Therapist self-care	Afterword	353
Regular use of mindfulness practices	Afterword	353
Engaging regularly in pleasurable nonwork activities	Afterword	353

REFERENCES

ADAA. (2021). *Facts and statistics.* Anxiety and Depression Association of America. https://adaa.org/about-adaa/press-room/facts-statistics

Adair, K. C., Boulton, A. J., & Algoe, S. B. (2018). The effect of mindfulness on relationship satisfaction via perceived responsiveness: Findings from a dyadic study of heterosexual romantic partners. *Mindfulness, 9,* 597–609. https://doi.org/10.1007/s12671-017-0801-3

Albrecht, S. L., Bahr, H. M., & Goodman, K. L. (1983). *Divorce and remarriage: Problems, adaptations, and adjustments.* Westport, CT: Greenwood.

Alcoholics Anonymous (2001). *Alcoholics Anonymous: The story of how many thousands of men and women have recovered from alcoholism* (4th ed.). New York: Alcoholics Anonymous World Services, Inc.

Allen, E. S., & Atkins, D. C. (2012). The association of divorce and extramarital sex in a representative US sample. *Journal of Family Issues, 33,* 1477–1493.

Allen, E. S., & Rhoades, G. K. (2008). Not all affairs are created equal: Emotional involvement with an extradyadic partner. *Journal of Sex and Marital Therapy, 34,* 48–62.

Almeida, R. V., & Durkin, T. (1999). The cultural context model: Therapy for couples with domestic violence. *Journal of Marital and Family Therapy, 25,* 313–324. https://doi.org/10.1111/j.1752-0606.1999.tb00250.x

Amato, P. R. (2000). The consequences of divorce for adults and children. *Journal of Marriage and the Family, 62,* 1269–1287.

Amato, P. R., & Rogers, S. J. (1997). A longitudinal study of marital problems and subsequent divorce. *Journal of Marriage and the Family, 59,* 612–624.

Anderson, C. M., & Stuart, S. (1983). *Mastering resistance: A practical guide to family therapy.* New York: Guilford.

Aron, A., Norman, C., Aron, E., McKenna, C., & Heyman, R. (2000). Couples' shared participation in novel and arousing activities and experienced relationship quality. *Journal of Personality and Social Psychology, 78,* 273–284.

Asen, E., & Fonagy, P. (2012). Mentalization-based therapeutic interventions for families. *Journal of Family Therapy, 34,* 347–370.

Asen, E., & Fonagy, P. (2021). *Mentalization-based treatment with families.* New York: Guilford.

Atkins, D. C., Eldridge, K. A., Baucom, D. H., & Christensen, A. (2005). Infidelity and behavioral couple therapy: Optimism in the face of betrayal. *Journal of Clinical and Consulting Psychology, 73,* 144–150.

Atkinson, B. J. (2013). Mindfulness training and the cultivation of secure, satisfying couple relationships. *Couple and Family Psychology: Research and Practice, 2,* 73–94.

Back, M. D., Schmukle, S. C., & Egloff, B. (2006). Who is late and who is early? Big Five personality factors and punctuality in attending psychological experiments. *Journal of Research in Personality, 40,* 841–848.

Baer, R. A. (2003). Mindfulness training as a clinical intervention: A conceptual and empirical review. *Clinical Psychology: Science and Practice, 10,* 125–143.

Bateson, G. (1979). *Mind and nature: A necessary unity.* New York: E. P. Dutton.

Baucom, D. H., Epstein, N. B., Kirby, J. S., & LaTaillade, J. J. (2015). Cognitive-behavioral couple therapy. In A. S. Gurman, J. L. Lebow, & D. K. Snyder (Eds.), *Clinical handbook of couple therapy* (5th ed., pp. 23–60). New York: Guilford.

Baucom, B. R., McFarland, P. T., & Christensen, A. (2010). Gender, topic, and time in observed demand-wthdraw interaction in cross- and same-sex couples. *Journal of Family Psychology, 24,* 233–242.

Belsky, J., & Rovine, M. (1990). Patterns of marital change across the transition to parenthood. *Journal of Marriage and the Family, 52,* 109–123.

Benjamin, J. (1995). *Like subjects, love objects.* New Haven, CT: Yale University Press.

Benjamin, J. (2017). *Beyond doer and done to: Recognition theory, intersubjectivity and the third.* New York: Routledge.

Berg, E. C., Trost, M., Schneider, I. E., & Allison, M. T. (2001). Dyadic exploration of the relationship of leisure satisfaction, leisure time, and gender to relationship satisfaction. *Leisure Studies, 23*, 35–46.

Birchler, G. R., & Webb, L. J. (1977). Discriminating interaction behaviors in happy and unhappy marriages. *Journal of Consulting and Clinical Psychology, 45*, 494–495.

Birchler, G. R., Weiss, R. L., & Vincent, J. P. (1975). Multimethod analysis of social reinforcement exchange between maritally distressed and nondistressed spouse and stranger dyads. *Journal of Personality and Social Psychology, 31*, 349–360.

Blow, A. J., Sprenkle, D. H., & Davis, S. D. (2007). Is who delivers the treatment more important than the treatment itself? The role of the therapist in common factors. *Journal of Marital and Family Therapy, 33*, 298–317.

Bodenmann, G., & Randall, A. K. (2020). General and health-related stress and couples' coping. In K. S. Wampler & A. J. Blow (Eds.), *The handbook of systemic family therapy* (Vol. 3, pp. 253–268). London: John Wiley & Sons.

Bordin, E. S. (1979). The generalizability of the psychoanalytic concept of the working alliance. *Psychotherapy: Theory, Research, and Practice, 16*, 252–260.

Boyd-Franklin, N. (2003). *Black families in therapy: Understanding the African American experience* (2nd ed.). New York: Guilford.

Boyd-Franklin, N., & Karger, M. (2012). Intersections of race, class, and poverty: Challenges and resilience in African American families. In F. Walsh (Ed.), *Normal family processes: Growing diversity and complexity* (4th ed., pp. 273–296). New York: Guilford.

Bradbury, T. N., & Bodenmann, G. (2020). Interventions for couples. *Annual Review of Clinical Psychology, 16*, 99–123.

Bradbury, T. N., & Fincham, F. D. (1990). Attributions in marriage: Review and critique. *Journal of Personality and Social Psychology, 107*, 3–33.

Bradbury, T. N., Fincham, F. D., & Beach, S. R. H. (2000). Research on the nature and determinants of marital satisfaction: A decade in review. *Journal of Marriage and the Family, 62*, 964–980.

Brandt, J. E. (2005). Why she left: The psychological, relational, and contextual variables that contribute to a woman's decision to leave an abusive relationship. *Dissertation Abstracts International, 66*(08B), 4473.

Bruner, J. (1986). *Actual minds, possible worlds.* Cambridge, MA: Harvard University Press.

Buehlman, K. T., Gottman, J. M., & Fainsilber Katz, L. (1992). How a couple views their past predicts their future: Predicting divorce from an oral history interview. *Journal of Family Psychology, 5,* 295–318.

Bumburry, W. M., & Whitaker, C. A. (1988). *Dancing with the family: A symbolic-experiential approach.* New York: Routledge.

Burnside, J. (2020). *The music of time: Poetry in the twentieth century.* Princeton, N.J.: Princeton University Press.

Bynner, W. (1944). *The way of life according to Lao Tzu.* New York: Perigee.

Caetano, R., McGrath, C., Ramisetty-Mikler, S., & Field, C. A. (2005). Drinking, alcohol problems and the five-year recurrence and incidence of male to female and female to male partner violence. *Alcoholism: Clinical and Experimental Research, 29,* 98–106.

Caetano, R., Schafer, J., & Cunradi, C. B. (2001). Alcohol-related intimate partner violence among white, black, and Hispanic couples in the United States. *Alcohol Research and Health, 25,* 58–65.

Cano, A., & Leary, K. D. (2000). Infidelity and separations precipitate major depressive episodes and symptoms of nonspecific depression and anxiety. *Journal of Consulting and Clinical Psychology, 68,* 774–781.

Carpenter, C. J. (2012). Meta-analyses of sex differences in responses to sexual versus emotional infidelity: Men and women are more similar than different. *Psychology of Women Quarterly, 36,* 25–27.

Carvalho, A. F., Lewis, R. J., Derlega, V. J., Winstead, B. A., & Viggiano, C. (2011). Internalized sexual minority stressors and same-sex intimate partner violence. *Journal of Family Violence, 26,* 501–509. https://doi.org/10.1007/s10896-011-9384-2

Chambless, D. L., & Ollendick, T. H. (2001). Empirically supported psychological interventions: Controversies and evidence. *Annual Review of Psychology, 52,* 685–716.

Christensen, A., Dimidjian, S., & Martell, C. R. (2015). Integrative behavioral couple therapy. In A. S. Gurman, J. L. Lebow, & D. K. Snyder (Eds.), *Clinical handbook of couple therapy* (5th ed., pp. 61–94). New York: Guilford.

Christensen, A., & Heavey, C. L. (1990). Gender and social structure in the demand/withdraw pattern of marital conflict. *Journal of Personality and Social Psychology, 59,* 73–81.

Claxton, A., & Perry-Jenkins, M. (2008). No fun anymore: Leisure and marital quality across the transition to parenthood. *Journal of Marriage and Family, 70,* 28–43.

Cluff, R. B., Hicks, M. W., & Madseon, C. H. (1994). Beyond the circumplex model: I. A moratorium on curvilinearity. *Family Process, 33,* 455–470.

Colapinto, J. (1991). Structural family therapy. In A.S. Gurman & D.P. Kniskern (Eds.), *Handbook of family therapy,* Vol. 2, pp. 417–443. New York: Brunner/Mazel.

Coltrane, S. (2000). Research on household labor: Modeling and measuring the social embeddedness of routine family work. *Journal of Marriage and the Family, 62,* 1208–1233.

Constantino, M. J., Coyne, A. E., Boswell, J. F., Iles, B. R., & Visla, A. (2018). A meta-analysis of the association between patients' early perception of treatment credibility and their posttreatment outcomes. *Psychotherapy, 55,* 486–495.

Cooklin, A. (1982). Change in here-and-now systems vs systems over time. In A. Bentovim, G. G. Barnes, & A. Cooklin (Eds.), *Family therapy: Complementary frameworks of theory and practice* (Vol. 1, pp. 73–109). London: Academic Press.

Coulter, K., & Malouff, J. M. (2013). Effects of an intervention designed to enhance romantic relationship excitement: A randomized-control trial. *Couple and Family Psychology: Research and Practice, 2,* 34–44.

Cowan, P. A., & Cowan, C. P. (1988). Changes in marriage during the transition to parenthood: Must we blame the baby? In G. Y. Michaels & W. A. Goldberg (Eds.), *The transition to parenthood: Current theory and research* (pp. 114–154). Cambridge: Cambridge University Press.

Cowan, P. A., & Cowan, C. P. (2000). *When partners become parents: The big life change for couples.* Mahwah, NJ: Erlbaum.

Cowan, P. A., & Cowan, C. P. (2012). Normative family transitions, couple relationship quality, and healthy child development. In F. Walsh (Ed.), *Normal family processes: Growing diversity and complexity* (4th ed., pp. 428–451). New York: Guilford.

Cowan, P. A., Cowan, C. P., Pruett, M. K., Pruett, K., & Wong, J. (2009). Promoting fathers' engagement with children: Preventive interventions for low-income families. *Journal of Marriage and the Family, 71,* 663–679.

Crawford, D. W., Houts, R. M., Huston, T. L., & George, L. J. (2002). Compatibility, leisure, and satisfaction in marital relationships. *Journal of Marriage and Family, 64,* 433–449.

Crisp, P. (1987). Uncontained projective identification: The vicious circles of runaway feedback loops. *Psychoanalytic Psychology, 4,* 291–299.

Cummings, E. M., & Davies, P. (1994). *Children and marital conflict:*

The impact of family dispute and resolution. New York: Guilford Press.

Dalai Lama, & Goleman, D. (2003). *Destructive emotions: How can we overcome them?* New York: Bantam.

Dattilio, F. M. (2010). *Cognitive-behavioral therapy with couples and families: A comprehensive guide for clinicians.* New York: Guilford.

Davies, P. T., & Cummings, E. M. (2006). Interparental discord, family process, and developmental psychopathology. In D. Cicchetti & D. J. Cohen (Eds.), *Developmental psychopathology: Vol. 3 Risk, disorder, and adaptation* (2nd ed., pp. 86–128). Hoboken, N.J.: Wiley.

Davis, S. D., Lebow, J. L., & Sprenkle, D. H. (2012). Common factors of change in couple therapy. *Behavior Therapy, 43,* 36–48.

Devilly, G. J., & Borkovec, T. D. (2000). Psychometric properties of the credibility/expectancy questionnaire. *Journal of Behavior Therapy and Experimental Psychiatry, 31,* 73–86.

de Shazer, S. (1985). *Keys to solution in brief therapy.* New York: Norton.

Dictionary.com. (n.d.). Creativity. Retrieved February 14, 2022 from https://www.dictionary.com/browse/creativity

Doherty, W. J. (1995). *Soul searching: Why psychotherapy must promote moral responsibility.* New York: Basic Books.

Doherty, W. J. (2012, September/October). One brick at a time: Therapy is more craft than art or science. *Psychotherapy Networker,* 23–29.

Doherty, W. J. (2013). *Take back your marriage: Sticking together in a world that pulls us apart.* New York: Guilford.

Doherty, W. J., & Harris, S. M. (2017). *Helping couples on the brink of divorce: Discernment counseling for troubled relationships.* Washington, DC: American Psychological Association.

Doherty, W. J., Harris, S. M., & Wilde, J. L. (2015). Discernment counseling for "mixed-agenda" couples. *Journal of Marital and Family Therapy, 42,* 246–255. https://doi.org/10.1111/jmft.12132

Doss, B. D., Atkins, D. C., & Christensen, A. (2003). Who's dragging their feet? Husbands and wives seeking marital therapy. *Journal of Marital and Family Therapy, 29,* 165–177.

Doss, B. D., Simpson, L. E., & Christensen, A. (2004). Why do couples seek marital therapy? *Professional Psychology: Research and Practice, 6,* 608–614.

Drapkin, M. L., McCrady, B. S., Swingle, J., Epstein, E. E., & Cook, S. M. (2005). Exploring bidirectional couple violence in a clinical sample of female alcoholics. *Journal of Studies on Alcohol, 66,* 213–219.

Driver, J., Tabares, A., Shapiro, A. F., & Gottman, J. M. (2012). Couple interaction in happy and unhappy marriages: Gottman laboratory studies. In F. Walsh (Ed.), *Normal family processes: Growing diversity and complexity* (4th ed., pp. 57–77). New York: Guilford.

Dyck, V. & Daly, K. (2006). Rising to the challenge: Fathers' role in the negotiation of couple time. *Leisure Studies, 25*, 201–217.

Epstein, N. B., Werlinich, C. A., & LaTaillade, J. J. (2015). Couple therapy for partner aggression. In A. S. Gurman, J. L. Lebow, & D. K. Snyder (Eds.), *Clinical handbook of couple therapy* (5th ed., pp. 389–411). New York: Guilford.

Esterling, B. A., L'Abate, L., Murray, E. J., & Pennebaker, J. W. (1999). Empirical foundations for writing in prevention and psychotherapy: Mental and physical health outcomes. *Clinical Psychology Review, 19*, 79–96.

Eubanks, C. F., Muran, J. C., & Safran, J. D. (2018). Alliance rupture repair: A meta-analysis. *Psychotherapy, 55*, 508–519.

Falconier, M. K., Nussbeck, F., Bodenmann, G., Schneider, H., & Bradbury, T. N. (2015). Stress from daily hassles in couples: Its effects on intradyadic stress, relationship satisfaction, and physical and psychological well-being. *Journal of Marital and Family Therapy, 41*, 221–235. https://doi.org/10.1111/jmft.12073

Falicov, C. J. (1998). *Latino families in therapy*. New York: Guilford.

Falicov, C. J. (2016). The multiculturalism and diversity of families. In T. Sexton & J. L. Lebow (Eds.) *Handbook of family therapy* (pp. 66–85). New York: Routledge.

Falicov, C. J. (2017). Multidimensional Ecosystemic Comparative Approach (MECA). In J. L. Lebow, A. Chambers, & D. C. Breunlin (Eds.), *Encyclopedia of couple and family therapy* (pp. 1955–1960). New York: Springer. https://doi.org/10.1007/978-3-319-15877-8_848-1

Fiese, B. H. (2006). *Family routines and rituals*. New Haven, CT: Yale University Press.

Fiese, B. H., Tomcho, T. J., Douglas, M., Josephs, K., Poltrock, S., & Baker, T. (2002). A review of 50 years of research on naturally occurring family routines and rituals: Cause for celebration? *Journal of Family Psychology, 16*, 381–390. https://doi.org/10.1037//0893-3200.16.4.381

Fincham, F. D., & Beach, S. R. H. (2010). Of memes and marriage: Toward a positive relationship science. *Journal of Family Theory and Review, 2*, 4–24. https://doi.org/10.1111/j.1756-2589.2010.00033.x

Fishbane, M. D. (2013). *Loving with the brain in mind: Neurobiology and couple therapy*. New York: Norton.

Fishbane, M. D. (2015). Couple therapy and interpersonal neurobiology. In A. S. Gurman, J. L. Lebow, & D. K. Snyder (Eds.), *The clinical handbook of couple therapy* (5th ed., pp. 681–701). New York: Guilford.

Fishbane, M. D. (2019). Healing intergenerational wounds: An integrative relational-neurobiological approach. *Family Process, 58,* 796–818.

Fonagy, P., Gergely, G., Jurist, E. L., & Target, M. (2002). *Affect regulation, mentalization, and the development of the self.* New York: Other Press.

Fraenkel, P. (1994). Time and rhythm in couples. *Family Process, 33,* 37–51.

Fraenkel, P. (1995). The nomothetic-idiographic debate in family therapy. *Family Process, 34,* 113–121.

Fraenkel, P. (1996). Zeit und Rhythmus in Paarbeziehungen. *Familiendynamik, 21,* 160–182.

Fraenkel, P. (1997). Systems approaches to couple therapy. In W. K. Halford & H. Markman (Eds.), *Clinical handbook of marriage and couples interventions* (pp. 379–413). London: John Wiley.

Fraenkel, P. (1998a). Time and couples, part I: The decompression chamber. In T. Nelson & T. Trepper (Eds.), *101 interventions in family therapy* (Vol. 2, pp. 140–144). Binghamton, NY: Haworth.

Fraenkel, P. (1998b). Time and couples, part II: The sixty second pleasure point. In T. Nelson & T. Trepper (Eds.), *101 interventions in family therapy* (Vol. 2, pp. 145–149). Binghamton, NY: Haworth.

Fraenkel, P. (1999). All about fathers. *NYU Child Study Center Newsletter, 4,* 1–4.

Fraenkel, P. (2001a). The beeper in the bedroom: Technology has become a therapeutic issue. *Psychotherapy Networker, 25,* 22–29, 64–65.

Fraenkel, P. (2001b). Getting a kick out of you: The jazz Taoist key to love. In J. Levine & H. Markman (Eds.), *Why do fools fall in love?* (pp. 61–66). San Francisco: Jossey-Bass.

Fraenkel, P. (2001c). The place of time in couple and family therapy. In K. J. Daly (Ed.), *Minding the time in family experience: Emerging perspectives and issues* (pp. 283--310). London: JAI.

Fraenkel, P. (2005). Whatever happened to family therapy? *Psychotherapy Networker, 29,* 30–39, 70.

Fraenkel, P. (2009). The therapeutic palette: A guide to choice points in integrative couple therapy. *Clinical Social Work Journal, 37,* 234–247.

Fraenkel, P. (2011). *Sync your relationship, save your marriage: Four steps to getting back on track.* New York: Palgrave Macmillan.

Fraenkel, P. (2017). Integration in couple and family therapy. In J. Lebow, A. Chambers, & D Breunlin (Eds.), *Encyclopedia of couple and family therapy*, Vol. 3, pp. 1501–1506. New York: Springer International Publishing. doi: 10.1007/978-3-319-15877-8_534-1

Fraenkel, P. (2018). Time in family and couple therapy. J.L. Lebow et al. (Eds.), *Encyclopedia of couple and family therapy*, Vol. 4, pp. 2938–2943. New York: Springer International Publishing, https://doi.org/10.1007/978-3-319-15877-8_954-1

Fraenkel, P. (2019a). Incest and relational trauma: The systemic narrative feminist model. In P. Pitta & C. Datchi (Eds.), *Integrative couple and family therapies: Treatment models for complex clinical issues* (pp. 47–70). Washington, DC: American Psychological Association. https://dx.doi.org/10.1037/0000151-003

Fraenkel, P. (2019b). Love in action: An integrative approach to last chance couple therapy. *Family Process, 58*, 569–594.

Fraenkel, P. (2020). Integrating music into couple therapy theory and practice. *Clinical Social Work Journal, 48*, 319–333. https://doi.org/10.1007/s10615-020-00755-y

Fraenkel, P. (2022). Therapeutic palette integrative couple therapy. In J. L. Lebow & D. K. Snyder (Eds.). *Clinical handbook of couple therapy* (6th ed., pp. 339–361). New York: Guilford.

Fraenkel, P., Benson, K., St. James, C., & Bowen, M. (2022). Intimate partner violence: A focus on queer families, families and substance use, and military couples: Clinical applications. In S. Browning & B. van Eeden-Moorefield (Eds.), *Treating contemporary families: Toward a more inclusive clinical practice* (pp. 93–126). Washington, DC: American Psychological Association.

Fraenkel, P., & Capstick, C. (2012). Contemporary two-parent families: Navigating work and family challenges. In F. Walsh (Ed.), *Normal family processes: Growing diversity and complexity* (4th ed., pp. 78–101). New York: Guilford.

Fraenkel, P., & Markman, H. J. (2002). Prevention of marital disorders. In D. S. Glenwick & L. A. Jason (Eds.), *Innovative strategies for promoting health and mental health across the life span* (pp. 245–271). New York: Springer.

Fraenkel, P., & Pinsof, W. M. (2001). Teaching family therapy-centered integration: Assimilation and beyond. *Journal of Psychotherapy Integration, 11*, 59–85.

Fraenkel, P., & Wilson, S. (2000). Clocks, calendars, and couples: Time and the rhythms of relationships. In P. Papp (Ed.), *Couples on the fault line: New directions for therapists* (pp. 63–103). New York: Guilford.

Fraley, R. C., Hudson, N. W., Hefferman, M. E., & Segal, N. (2015). Are adult attachment styles categorial or dimensional? A taxometric analysis of general and relationship-specific attachment orientations. *Journal of Personality and Social Psychology, 109*, 354–368.

Fraley, R. C., Roisman, G. I., Booth-LaForce, C., & Owen, M. T. (2013). Interpersonal and genetic origins of adult attachment styles: A longitudinal study from infancy to early adulthood. *Journal of Personality and Social Psychology, 104*, 817–838.

Frank, J. D., & Frank, J. B. (1993). *Persuasion and healing: A comparative study of psychotherapy* (3rd ed.). Baltimore, M.D.: The John Hopkins University Press.

Frankl, V. E. (2019). *The doctor and the soul: From psychotherapy to logotherapy*. New York: Vintage.

Freedman, J., & Combs, G. (1996). *Narrative therapy: The social construction of preferred realities*. New York: Norton.

Fruzetti, A. E. (2006). *The high-conflict couple: A dialectical behavior therapy guide to finding peace, intimacy, and validation*. Oakland, CA: New Harbinger.

Garfield, R. (2016). *Breaking the male code: Unlocking the power of friendship*. New York: Avery.

Gerson, R., Hoffman, S., Sauls, M., & Ulrici, D. (1993). Family-of-origin frames in couples therapy. *Journal of Marital and Family Therapy, 19*, 341–354.

Gibson, J. J. (1979). *The ecological approach to visual perception*. Boston, MA: Houghton Mifflin Harcourt.

Gilligan, C. (1982). *In a different voice: Psychological theory and women's development*. Cambridge, MA: Harvard University Press.

Gladwell, M. (2008). *Outliers: The story of success*. New York: Little, Brown.

Glass, S. P. (2002). Couple therapy after the trauma of infidelity. In A. S. Gurman & N. S. Jacobson (Eds.), *Clinical handbook of couple therapy* (3rd ed., pp. 488–507). New York: Guilford.

Glass, S. P. (2003). *Not "just friends": Protect your relationship from infidelity and heal the trauma of betrayal*. New York: Free Press.

Glass, S. P., & Wright, T. M. (1985). Sex differences in type of extramarital involvement and marital satisfaction. *Sex Roles, 12*, 1101–1120.

Glass, S. P., & Wright, T. M. (1992). Justifications for extramarital relationships: The association between attitudes, behaviors and gender. *Journal of Sex Research, 29*, 361–387.

Glebova, T., Bartle-Haring, S., Gangamma, R., Knerr, M., Ostrom Delaney, R., Meyer, K., McDowell, T., Adkins, K., & Grafsky, E. (2011). Therapeutic alliance and progress in couple therapy: Multiple per-

spectives. *Journal of Family Therapy, 33,* 42–65. https://doi.org/10
.1111/j.1467-6427.2010.00503.x

Goldner, V. (1985). Feminism and family therapy. *Family Process, 24,*
31–47.

Goldner, V. (1998). The treatment of violence and victimization in intimate relationships. *Family Process, 37,* 263–286.

Goldner, V. (2004). When love hurts: Treating abusive relationships. *Psychoanalytic Inquiry, 24,* 346–372. https://doi.org/10
.1080/07351692409349088

Goldner, V. (2014). Romantic bonds, binds, and ruptures: Couples
on the brink. *Psychoanalytic Dialogues, 24,* 402–418. https://doi
.org/10.1080/10481885.2014.932209

Goldner, V., Penn, P., Sheinberg, M., & Walker, G. (1990). Love and
violence: Gender paradoxes in volatile attachments. *Family Process,
29,* 343–364.

Goldsmith, M. (2007). *What got you here won't get you there.* New
York: Hachette.

Goleman, D. (1995). *Emotional intelligence: Why it can matter more
than IQ.* New York: Bantam.

Good, J. M. M. (2007). The affordances for social psychology of the
ecological approach to social knowing. *Theory & Psychology, 17,*
265–295. https://doi.org/10.1177/0959354307075046

Goolishian, H. A., & Anderson, H. (1992). Strategy and intervention
versus nonintervention: A matter of theory? *Journal of Marital and
Family Therapy, 18,* 5–15.

Gordon, K. C., Baucom, D. H., & Snyder, D. K. (2005). Treating couples
recovering from infidelity: An integrative approach. *Journal of Clinical Psychology, 61,* 1393–1405.

Gordon, K., Kaddouma, A., Baucom, D. H., & Snyder, D. K. (2015).
Couple therapy and the treatment of affairs. In A. S. Gurman, J. L.
Lebow, & D. K. Snyder (Eds.), *Clinical handbook of couple therapy*
(5th ed., pp. 412–444). New York: Guilford.

Gottman, J. M. (1994). *What predicts divorce?* Hillsdale, NJ: Erlbaum.

Gottman, J. M. (2011). *The science of trust: Emotional attunement for
couples.* New York: Norton.

Gottman, J. M., Coan, J., Carrere, S., & Swanson, C. (1998). Predicting
marital happiness and stability from newlywed interactions. *Journal of Marriage and the Family, 60,* 5–22.

Gottman, J. M., Driver, J., & Tabares, A. (2015). Repair during marital
conflict in newlyweds: How couples move from attack-defend to
collaboration. *Journal of Family Psychology, 26,* 85–108.

Gottman, J. M., & Gottman, J. S. (2015a). Gottman couple therapy. In

A. S. Gurman, J. L. Lebow, & D. S. Snyder (Eds.), *Clinical handbook of couple therapy* (5th ed., pp. 129–157). New York: Guilford.

Gottman, J. M., & Gottman, J. S. (2015b). *10 principles for doing effective couples therapy*. New York: Norton.

Gottman, J. M., & Gottman, J. S. (2018). *The science of couples and family therapy: Behind the scenes at the Love Lab*. New York: Norton.

Gottman, J. M., Notarius, C., Gonzo, J., & Markman, H. J. (1979). *A couple's guide to communication*. Champaign, IL: Research Press.

Graham, J. M. (2008). Self-expansion and flow in couples' momentary experiences: An experience sampling study. *Journal of Personality and Social Psychology, 95*, 679–694.

Gratwick Baker, K. (2015). Bowen family systems couple coaching. In A. S. Gurman, J. L. Lebow, & D. K. Snyder (Eds.), *The clinical handbook of couple therapy* (5th ed., pp. 246–267). New York: Guilford.

Grayson, J. (2014). *Freedom from obsessive-compulsive disorder: A personalized recovery program for living with uncertainty*. New York: Penguin.

Greenan, D. E., & Tunnel, G. (2002). *Couple therapy with gay men*. New York: Guilford.

Greenberg, L. S. (2011). *Emotion-focused therapy*. Washington, D.C.: American Psychological Association.

Gross, J. J. (Ed.). (2015). *Handbook of emotion regulation* (2nd ed.). New York: Guilford.

Gurman, A. S. (2011). Couple therapy research and the practice of couple therapy: Can we talk? *Family Process, 50*, 280–292.

Gurman, A. S. (2015). Functional analytic couple therapy. In A. S. Gurman, J. L. Lebow, & D. S. Snyder (Eds.), *Clinical handbook of couple therapy* (5th ed., pp. 192–223). New York: Guilford.

Gurman, A., & Fraenkel, P. (2002). The history of couple therapy: A millennial review. *Family Process, 41*, 199–260.

Gurman, A. S., Lebow, J. L., & Snyder, D. K. (Eds.). (2015). *Clinical handbook of couple therapy* (5th ed.). New York: Guilford.

Haley, J. (1993). *Uncommon therapy: The psychiatric techniques of Milton H. Erickson, M.D.* New York: Norton.

Haley, J. (1987). *Problem-solving therapy* (2nd ed.). Hoboken, N.J.: Jossey-Bass.

Halford, W. K. (2011). *Marriage and relationship education: What works and how to provide it*. New York: Guilford

Halford, W. K., Hayes, S., Christensen, A., Lambert, M., Baucom, D. H., & Atkins, D. (2012). Towards making progress feedback an effective common factor in couple therapy. *Behavior Therapy, 43*, 49–60.

Hardy, K. V., & Bobes, T. (2016). *Culturally sensitive supervision and training: Diverse perspectives and practical applications.* New York: Routledge.

Hare-Mustin, R. T. (1978). A feminist approach to family therapy. *Family Process, 17,* 181–194.

Hazan, C., & Shaver, P. R. (1987). Romantic love conceptualized as an attachment process. *Journal of Personality and Social Psychology, 52,* 511–524.

Hazan, C., & Shaver, P. R. (1994). Deeper into attachment theory. *Psychological Inquiry, 5,* 68–79.

Heidegger, M. (1962). *Being and time.* New York: Harper & Row.

Hendrick, C., & Hendrick, S. S. (1994). Attachment theory and close relationships. *Psychological Inquiry, 5,* 38–41.

Henline, B. H., Lamke, L. K., & Howard, M. D. (2007). Exploring perceptions of online infidelity. *Personal Relationships, 14,* 113–128.

Herman, J. L. (1992). *Trauma and recovery: The aftermath of violence—from domestic abuse to political terror.* New York: Basic Books.

Hertlein, K. M., & Piercy, F. P. (2005). A theoretical framework for defining, understanding, and treating internet infidelity. *Journal of Couple and Relationship Therapy, 4,* 79–91.

Hertlein, K. M., & Piercy, F. P. (2006). Internet infidelity: A critical review of the literature. *Family Journal, 14,* 366–371.

Hill, M. S. (1988). Marital stability and spouses' shared time. *Journal of Family Issues, 9,* 427–451.

Holman, T. B. & Epperson, A. (1984). Family and leisure: A review of the literature with research recommendations. *Journal of Leisure Research, 16,* 277–294.

Holtzworth-Munroe, A., Marshall, M. A., Meehan, J. C., & Rehman, U. (2003). Physical aggression. In D. K. Snyder & M. A. Whisman (Eds.), *Treating difficult couples: Helping clients with coexisting mental and relationship disorders* (pp. 201–230). New York: Guilford.

Horvath, A. O., & Bedi, R. P. (2002). The alliance. In J. C. Norcross (Ed.), *Psychotherapy relationships that work: Therapist contributions and responsiveness to patients* (pp. 37–69). New York: Oxford University Press.

Hoyt, M. F. (2015). Solution-focused couple therapy. In A. S. Gurman, J. L. Lebow, & D. K. Snyder (Eds.), *Clinical handbook of couple therapy* (5th ed., pp. 300–332). New York: Guilford.

Hughes, S. M., Farley, S. D., & Rhodes, B. C. (2010). Vocal and physiological changes in response to the physical attractiveness of conversational partners. *Journal of Nonverbal Behavior, 34,* 155–167. https://doi.org/10.1007/s10919-010-0087-9

Iasenza, S. (2020). *Transforming sexual narratives: A relational approach to sex therapy.* New York: Routledge.

Imber-Black, E. (1999). *The secret life of families: Making decisions about secrets: When keeping secrets can harm you, when keeping secrets can heal you—and how to know the difference.* New York: Bantam.

Imber-Black, E. (2011). The evolution of Family Process: Contexts and transformations. *Family Process, 50,* 267–279.

Imber-Black, E., Roberts, J., & Whiting, R. A. (2003). *Rituals in families and family therapy* (2nd ed.). New York: Norton.

Jackson, D. (1965). Family rules: Marital quid pro quo. *Archives of General Psychiatry, 12,* 585–594.

Jacobson, N. S., & Christensen, A. (1998). *Acceptance and change in couple therapy: A therapist's guide to transforming relationships.* New York: Norton.

Jahnke, R., Larkey, L., Rogers, C., Etnier, J., & Lin, F. (2010). A comprehensive review of health benefits of Qigong and Tai Chi. *American Journal of Health Promotion, 24,* 1–25.

Janoff-Bulman, R. (1992). *Shattered assumptions: Towards a new psychology of trauma.* New York: Free Press.

Johnson, C. A., Stanley, S. M., Glenn, N. D., Amato, P. R., Nock, S. L., Markman, H. J., & Dion, M. R. (2001). *Marriage in Oklahoma: 2001 baseline statewide survey on marriage and divorce.* Stillwater: Oklahoma State University Bureau for Social Research.

Johnson, S. M. (2015). Emotionally focused couple therapy. In A. S. Gurman, J. L. Lebow, & D. K. Snyder (Eds.), *Clinical handbook of couple therapy* (5th ed., pp. 97–128). New York: Guilford.

Johnson, S. M. (2019). *Attachment theory in practice: Emotionally focused therapy (EFT) with individuals, couples, and families.* New York: Guilford.

Johnson, S. M. (2020). *The practice of emotionally focused couple therapy* (3rd ed.). New York: Routledge.

Jordan, P. L., Markman, H. J., & Stanley, S. M. (2001). *Becoming parents: How to strengthen your marriage as your family grows.* San Francisco: Jossey-Bass.

Jurist, E. (2018). *Minding emotions: Cultivating mentalization in psychotherapy.* New York: Guilford.

Kabat-Zinn, J. (2003). Mindfulness-based interventions in context: Past, present, and future. *Clinical Psychology: Science and Practice, 10,* 144–156.

Kabat-Zinn, J. (2005). *Wherever you go there you are: Mindfulness meditation in everyday life* (10th anniv. ed.). New York: Hyperion.

Kagan, J. (2010). *The temperamental thread: How genes, culture, time, and luck make us who we are.* New York: Dana Press.

Kagan, J., & Snidman, N. (2009). *The long shadow of temperament.* Cambridge, MA: Belknap.

Kahneman, D. (2011). *Thinking, fast and slow.* New York: Farrar, Straus & Giroux.

Keeney, B. P., & Cromwell, R. E. (1979). Temporal cycles and sequences in family systems. *Journal of Comparative Family Studies, 10*, 19–33.

Keith, D. (2015). *Continuing the experiential approach of Carl Whitaker: Process, practice and magic.* Phoenix: Zeig, Tucker & Theisen.

Kelly, S., Wesley, K. C., Maynigo, T. P., Omar, Y., Clark, S. M., & Humphrey, S. C. (2019). Principle-based integrative therapy with couples: Theory and a case example. *Family Process, 58*, 532–549. https://doi.org/10.1111/famp.12442

Kerr, M. E., & Bowen, M. (1988). *Family evaluation: An approach based on Bowen theory.* New York: Norton.

Khaddouma, A., Gordon, K. C., & Strand, E. B. (2017). Mindful mates: A pilot study of the relational effects of mindfulness-based stress reduction on participants and their partners. *Family Process, 56*, 636–661.

Khong, C. (2014). *Beginning anew: Four steps to restoring communication.* Berkeley, CA: Parallax.

Killian, K. D. (2013). *Interracial couples, intimacy, and therapy: Crossing racial borders.* New York: Columbia University Press.

Knobloch-Fedders, L. M., Pinsof, W. M., & Mann, B. J. (2007). Therapeutic alliance and treatment progress in couple psychotherapy. *Journal of Marital and Family Therapy, 33*, 245–257.

Knudson-Martin, C. (1997). The politics of gender in family therapy. *Journal of Marital and Family Therapy, 23*, 431–447.

Knudson-Martin, C. (2012). Changing gender norms in families and society: Toward equality amid complexities. In F. Walsh (Ed.), *Normal family processes: Growing diversity and complexity* (4th ed., pp. 324–346). New York: Guilford.

Knudson-Martin, C. (2013). Why power matters: Creating a foundation of mutual support in couple relationships. *Family Process, 52*, 5–18. https://doi.org/10.1111/famp.12011

Knudson-Martin, C. (2015). When therapy challenges patriarchy: Undoing gendered power in heterosexual couple relationships. In C. Knudson-Martin, M. Wells, & S. K. Samman (Eds.), *Socio-emotional relationship therapy: Bridging emotion, societal context, and couple interaction* (pp. 15–26). New York: Springer.

Knudson-Martin, C., & Huenergardt, D. (2010). A socio-emotional approach to couple therapy: Linking social context and couple interaction. *Family Process, 49,* 369–386.

Knudson-Martin, C., & Mahoney, A. (Eds.). (2009). *Couples, gender, and power: Creating change in intimate relationships.* New York: Springer.

Koerner, E. F. K. (1992). The Sapir-Whorf hypothesis: A preliminary history and a bibliographical essay. *Journal of Linguistic Anthropology, 2,* 173–198.

Köhler, W. (1947). *Gestalt psychology: The definitive statement of the Gestalt theory.* New York: Liveright.

Kramer, U., & Stiles, W. B. (2015). The responsiveness problem in psychotherapy: A review of proposed solutions. *Clinical Psychology Science and Practice, 22,* 277–295.

Kuhn, T. (1986). *The structure of scientific revolutions* (2nd ed.). Chicago: University of Chicago Press.

La Guardia, J. G., Ryan, R. M., Couchman, C. E., & Deci, E. L. (2000). Within-person variation in security of attachment: A self-determination theory perspective on attachment, need fulfillment, and well-being. *Journal of Personality and Social Psychology, 79,* 367–384.

Lammers, J., Stoker, J. I., Jordan, J., Pollman, M., & Stapel, D. A. (2011). Power increases infidelity among men and women. *Psychological Science, 22,* 1191–1197.

Larson, J. H., Crane, D. R., & Smith, C. W. (1991). Morning and night couples: The effect of wake and sleep patterns on marital adjustment. *Journal of Marital and Family Therapy, 17,* 53–65.

Larson, R. W., & Almeida, D. M. (1999). Emotional transmission in the daily lives of families: A new paradigm for studying family process. *Journal of Marriage and the Family, 61,* 5–20.

LaSala, M. C. (2005). Extradyadic sex and gay male couples: Comparing monogamous and nonmonogamous relationships. *Families in Society, 85,* 405–412.

Lebow, J. L. (2014). *Couple and family therapy: An integrative map of the territory.* Washington, DC: American Psychological Association.

Lebow, J. L. (2015). Separation and divorce issues in couple therapy. In A. S. Gurman, J. L. Lebow, & D. K. Snyder (Eds.), *Clinical handbook of couple therapy* (5th ed., pp. 445–463). New York: Guilford.

Lee, D. N., & Schögler, B. (2009). Tau in musical expression. In S. Malloch & C. Trevarthen (Eds.), *Communicative musicality: Exploring the basis of human companionship* (pp. 83–104). Oxford: Oxford University Press.

Leigh, R. C. (1989). Reasons for having and avoiding sex: Gender, sexual orientation and relationship to sexual behavior. *Journal of Sex Research, 35*, 199–200.

Leuchtmann, L., Horn, A. B., Randall, A. K., Kuhn, R., & Bodenmann, G. (2018). A process-oriented analysis of the three-phase method: A therapeutic couple intervention strengthening dyadic coping. *Journal of Couple and Relationship Therapy, 17*, 251–275.

Levenson, R. W., & Gottman, J. M. (1983). Marital interaction: Physiological linkage and affective exchange. *Journal of Personality and Social Psychology, 45*, 587–597.

Levenson, R. W., & Gottman, J. M. (1985). Physiological and affective predictors of change in relationship satisfaction. *Journal of Personality and Social Psychology, 49*, 85–94.

Levine, R. (1997). *A geography of time.* New York: Basic Books.

Lewandowski, G. W., & Ackerman, R. A. (2006). Something's missing: Need fulfillment and self-expansion as predictors of susceptibility to infidelity. *Journal of Social Psychology, 146*, 389–403.

Liddle, H. A. (2014). Adapting and implementing an evidence-based treatment with justice-involved adolescents: The example of multidimensional family therapy. *Family Process, 53*, 516–528.

Linville, D., Chronister, K., Marsiglio, M., & Brown, T. B. (2012). Treatment of partner violence in gay and lesbian relationships. In J. J. Bigner & J. L. Wetchler (Eds.), *Handbook of LGBT-affirmative couple and family therapy* (pp. 327–342). New York: Brunner-Routledge.

Madanes, C. (1981). *Strategic family therapy.* Hoboken, N.J.: Jossey-Bass.

Madden, C. (2014). *After a good man cheats: How to rebuild trust and intimacy with your wife.* New York: Train of Thought Press.

Mark, K. P., Janssen, E., & Milhausen, R. R. (2011). Infidelity in heterosexual couples: Demographic, interpersonal, and personality-related predictors of extradyadic sex. *Archives of Sexual Behavior, 40*, 971–982.

Markman, H. J., & Rhoades, G. K. (2012). Relationship education research: Current status and future directions. *Journal of Marital and Family Therapy, 38*, 169–200. https://doi.org/10.1111/j.1752-0606.2011.00247.x

Markman, H. J., Rhoades, G. K., Stanley, S. M., Ragan, E. P., & Whitton, S. W. (2010). The premarital communication roots of marital distress and divorce: The first five years of marriage. *Journal of Family Psychology, 24*, 289–298.

Markman, H. J., Stanley, S., & Blumberg, S. L. (2010). *Fighting for your marriage* (Deluxe 3rd ed.). San Francisco: Jossey-Bass.

Marks, S. R., Huston, T. L., Johnson, E. M., & MacDermid, S. M. (2001).

Role balance among white married couples. *Journal of Marriage and Family, 63,* 1083–1098.

Martin, D. J., Garske, J. P., & Davis, K. M. (2000). Relation of the therapeutic alliance with outcome and other variables: A meta-analytic review. *Journal of Consulting and Clinical Psychology, 68,* 438–350.

Masters, W. H., & Johnson, V. E. (1966). *Human sexual response.* Boston: Little, Brown.

Masters, W. H., & Johnson, V. E. (1975). *The pleasure bond: A new look at sexuality and commitment.* Boston: Little, Brown.

May, R. (1975). *The courage to create.* New York: Norton.

McCrady, B. S., & Epstein, E. E. (2015). Couple therapy and alcohol problems. In A. S. Gurman, J. L. Lebow, & D. K. Snyder (Eds.), *Clinical handbook of couple therapy* (5th ed., pp. 555–584). New York: Guilford.

McDowell, T., Knudson-Martin, C., & Bermudez, J. M. (2017). *Socioculturally attuned family therapy: Guidelines for equitable theory and practice.* New York: Routledge.

McGoldrick, M., Carter, B., & Garcia-Preto, N. (2011). *The expanded family life cycle: Individual, family, and social perspectives* (4th ed.). Boston: Pearson.

McGoldrick, M., Gerson, R., & Petry, S. (2008). *Genograms: Assessment and intervention* (3rd ed.). New York: Norton.

McGoldrick, M., & Hardy, K. V. (2019). *Re-visioning family therapy: Addressing diversity in clinical practice* (3rd ed.). New York: Guilford.

McGoldrick, M., & Shibusawa, T. (2012). The family life cycle. In F. Walsh (Ed.), *Normal family processes: Growing diversity and complexity* (4th ed., pp. 375–398). New York: Guilford.

Merriam-Webster. (n.d.a). Create. In *Merriam-Webster.com dictionary.* Retrieved February 16, 2022, from https://www.merriam-webster .com/dictionary/create

Merriam-Webster. (n.d.b). Encourage. In *Merriam-Webster.com dictionary.* Retrieved February 15, 2022, from https://www .merriam-webster.com/dictionary/encourage

Miller, S. L., & Maner, J. K. (2008). Coping with romantic betrayal: Sex differences in responses to partner infidelity. *Evolutionary Psychology, 6,* 413–426.

Minuchin, S. (1974). *Families and family therapy.* Cambridge, MA: Harvard University Press.

Minuchin, S., Reiter, M. D., & Borda, C. (2014). *The craft of family therapy: Challenging uncertainties.* New York: Routledge.

Monson, C. M., & Fredman, S. J. (2015). Couple therapy and posttraumatic stress disorder. In A. S. Gurman, J. L. Lebow, & D. K. Snyder (Eds.), *Clinical handbook of couple therapy* (5th ed., pp. 531–554). New York: Guilford.

Moore, L. E., Tambling, R. B., & Anderson, S. R. (2013). The intersection of therapy constructs: The relationship between motivation to change, distress, referral source, and pressure to attend. *The American Journal of Family Therapy, 41,* 245–258.

Moore-Ede, M. C., Sulzman, F. M., & Fuller, C. A. (1982). *The clocks that time us.* Cambridge, MA: Harvard University Press.

Newman, B., Reeve, K. F., Reeve, S. A., & Ryan, C. S. (2003). *Behaviorspeak: A glossary of terms in applied behavior analysis.* Monee, IL: Dove and Orca.

Nhat Hanh, T. (1990). *Present moment wonderful moment.* Berkeley, C.A.: Parallax.

Nhat Hanh, T. (2001). *Anger: Wisdom for cooling the flames.* New York: Riverhead.

Nhat Hanh, T. (2006). *Understanding our mind.* Berkeley, C.A.: Parallax.

Nhat Hanh, T. (2015). *Inside the now: Meditations on time.* Berkeley, C.A.: Parallax.

Nielsen, A. C. (2016a). Projective identification in couples. *JAMA, 67,* 593–624.

Nielsen, A. C. (2016b). *A roadmap for couple therapy: Integrating systemic, psychodynamic, and behavioral approaches.* New York: Routledge.

Notarius, C., & Buongiorno, I. (1992). *Waiting time until seeking couples' therapy or any other couples intervention* [Unpublished study]. Catholic University of America.

Olson, D. H. (1986). Circumplex model VII: Validation studies and FACES III. *Family Process, 25,* 337–351.

Osgood, C. E., Suci, G. J., & Tannenbaum, P. H. (1957). *The measurement of meaning.* Urbana: University of Illinois Press.

Osypiuk, K., Thompson, E., & Wayne, P. M. (2018). Can Tai Chi and Qigong postures shape our mood? Toward an embodied cognition framework for mind-body research. *Frontiers in Human Neuroscience, 12,* 1–12. https://doi.org/10.3389/fnhum.2018.00174

Owen, J., Duncan, B., Anker, M., & Sparks, J. (2012). Initial relationship goal and couple therapy outcomes at post and six-month follow-up. *Journal of Family Psychology, 26,* 179–186. DOI: 10.1037/a0026998

Panksepp, J., & Trevarthen, C. (2009). The neuroscience of emotion in music. In S. Malloch & C. Trevarthen (Eds.), *Communicative musi-*

cality: Exploring the basis of human companionship (pp. 105–146). Oxford: Oxford University Press.

Papp, P., & Imber-Black, E. (1996). Family themes: Transmission and transformation. *Family Process, 35,* 5–20.

Papp, P., Scheinkman, M., & Malpas, J. (2013). Breaking the mold: Sculpting impasses in couples' therapy. *Family Process, 52,* 33–45. https://doi.org/10.1111/famp.12022

Parker, A. E., Hablerstadt, A. G., Dunsmore, J. C., Townley, G., Bryant, A., Jr., Thompson, J. A., & Beale, K. S. (2012). "Emotions are a window into one's heart": A qualitative analysis of parental beliefs about children's emotions across three ethnic groups. *Monographs of the Society for Research in Child Development, 77,* 1–136.

Pennebaker, J. W. (1997). Writing about emotional experiences as a therapeutic process. *Psychological Science, 8,* 162–166.

Pennebaker, J. W. (2004). *Writing to heal: A guided journal for recovering from trauma and emotional upheaval.* New York: New Harbinger.

Perel, E. (2007). *Mating in captivity: Unlocking erotic intelligence.* New York: HarperCollins.

Perel, E. (2017). *The state of affairs: Rethinking infidelity.* New York: HarperCollins.

Pierce, T., & Lydon, J. (2001). Global and specific relational models in the experience of social interactions. *Journal of Personality and Social Psychology, 80,* 613–631.

Piña, D. L., & Bengtson, V. L. (1993). The division of household labor and wives' happiness: Ideology, employment, and perceptions of support. *Journal of Marriage and the Family, 55,* 901–912.

Pinderhughes, E. (1989). *Understanding race, ethnicity, and power: The key to efficacy in clinical practice.* New York: Free Press.

Pinsof, W. M. (1994). An integrative systems perspective on the therapeutic alliance: Theoretical, clinical, and research implications. In A. O. Horvath & L. S. Greenberg (Eds.), *The working alliance: Theory, research, and practice* (pp. 173–195). New York: John Wiley & Sons.

Pinsof, W.M. (1995). *Integrative problem-centered therapy.* New York: Basic Books.

Pinsof, W. M., Breunlin, D., Russell, W., Lebow, J. L., Chambers, A. L., & Rampage, C. (2018). *Integrative systemic therapy: Metaframeworks for problem solving with individuals, couples, and families.* Washington, DC: American Psychological Association.

Pittendrigh, C. S. (1972). On temporal organization in living systems.

In H. Yaker, H. Osmond, & F. Cheek (Eds.), *The future of time* (pp. 179–218). New York: Anchor.

Pittman, F. (1989). *Private lies: Infidelity and the betrayal of intimacy.* New York: Norton.

Powers, M. B., Vedel, E., & Emmelkamp, P. M. G. (2008) Behavioral couples therapy (BCT) for alcohol and drug use disorders: A meta-analysis. *Clinical Psychology Review, 28*, 952–962.

Prochaska, J. O., & DiClemente, C. C. (1992). Stages of change in the modification of problem behaviors. In M. Hersen, R. M. Eisler, & P. M. Miller (Eds.), *Progress in behavior modification* (pp. 184–214). Sycamore, I.L.: Sycamore Press.

Reitmeijer, C. A., Bull, S. S., & McFarlane, M. (2001). Sex and the internet. *AIDS, 15*, 1433–1434.

Repetti, R. L., Taylor, S.E., & Seeman, T. E. (2002). Risky families: Family social environments and the mental and physical health of offspring. *Psychological Bulletin, 128*, 330–366.

Resick, P. A., Monson, C. M., & Rizvi, S. (2007). Posttraumatic stress disorder. In D. H. Barlow (Ed.), *Clinical handbook of psychological disorders: A step-by-step treatment manual* (4th ed., pp. 65–122). New York: Guilford.

Richards, J. C., Jonathan, N., & Kim, L. (2015). Building a circle of care in same-sex couple relationships: A socio-emotional relational approach. In C. Knudson-Martin, M. A. Wells, & S. K. Samman (Eds.), *Socio-emotional relationship therapy: Bridging emotion, societal context, and couple interaction* (pp. 93–105). Cham, Switzerland: AFTA SpringerBriefs in Family Therapy.

Robinson, J., & Spitze, G. (1992). Whistle while you work? The effect of household task performance on women's and men's well-being. *Social Science Quarterly, 73*, 844–861.

Rosenthal, R. N. (2013). Treatment of persons with substance use disorder and co-occurring other mental disorders. In B. S. McCrady & E. E. Epstein (Eds.), *Addictions: A comprehensive guidebook* (2nd ed., pp. 659–707). New York: Oxford University Press.

Santisteban, D. A., Suarez-Morales, L., Robbins, M. S., & Szapocznik, J. (2006). Brief strategic family therapy: Lessons learned in efficacy research and challenges to blending research and practice. *Family Process, 45*, 259–271.

Satir, V. (1983). *Conjoint family therapy* (3rd ed.). Paolo Alto, CA: Science & Behavior.

Scheff, L., & Edmiston, S. (2010). *The cow in the parking lot: A Zen approach to overcoming anger.* New York: Workman.

Scheinkman, M. (2005). Beyond the trauma of betrayal: Reconsidering affairs in couples therapy. *Family Process, 44*, 227–244.

Scheinkman, M. (2008). The multi-level approach: A road map for couple therapy. *Family Process, 47*, 197–213.

Scheinkman, M., & Fishbane, M. (2004). The vulnerability cycle: Working with impasses in couple therapy. *Family Process, 43*, 279–299.

Schneider, K. J., & Krug, O. T. (2017). *Existential-humanistic therapy* (2nd ed.). Washington, DC: American Psychological Association.

Schneider, J. P. (2002). The new "elephant in the living room": Effects of compulsive cybersex behaviors on the spouse. In A. Cooper (Ed.), *Sex and the internet: A guidebook for clinicians* (pp. 169–186). New York: Brunner-Routledge.

Schwartz, P. (1994). *Peer marriage: How love between equals really works*. New York: Free Press.

Schwartz, R. C., & Sweezy, M. (2020). *Internal family systems therapy* (2nd ed.). New York: Guilford.

Selvini Palazzoli, M., Boscolo, L., Cecchin, G., & Prata, G. (1985). *Paradox and counterparadox: A new model in the therapy of the family in schizophrenic transaction*. Lanham, M.D. Jason Aronson.

Seybold, K. S., Hill, P. C., Neumann, J. K., & Chi, D. (2001). Physiological and psychological correlates of forgiveness. *Journal of Psychology and Christianity, 20*, 250–259.

Sexton, T., Gordon, K. C., Gurman, A., Lebow, J. L., Holtzworth-Munroe, A., & Johnson, S. (2011). Guidelines for classifying evidence-based treatments in couple and family therapy. *Family Process, 50*, 377–392.

Sheinberg, M., & Fraenkel, P. (2001). *The relational trauma of incest: A family-based approach to treatment*. New York: Guilford.

Siegel, D. J. (2012). *The developing mind: How relationships and the brain interact to shape who we are* (2nd ed.). New York: Guilford.

Siegel, D. J. (2015). Foreword. In J. M. Gottman & J. S. Gottman., *10 principles for doing effective couples therapy* (pp. xi–xii). New York: Norton.

Siegel, J. P. (2015). Object relations couple therapy. In A. S. Gurman, J. L. Lebow, & D. K. Snyder (Eds.), *Clinical handbook of couple therapy* (5th ed., pp. 224–245). New York: Guilford.

Sifneos, P. (1991). Affect, emotional conflict, and deficit: An overview. *Psychotherapy and Psychosomatics, 56*, 116–122.

Simon, G. M. (2015). Structural couple therapy. In A. S. Gurman, J. L. Lebow, & D. K. Snyder (Eds.), *Clinical handbook of couple therapy* (5th ed., pp. 358–384). New York: Guilford.

Smith Benjamin, L. (2002). *Interpersonal diagnosis and treatment of personality disorders* (2nd ed.). New York: Guilford.

Smyth, J. M., Nazarian, D., & Arigo, D. (2008). Expressive writing in the clinical context. In A. J. J. M. Vingerhoets, I. Nykíček, & J. Denollet (Eds.), *Emotion regulation: Conceptual and clinical issues* (pp. 215–233). New York: Springer.

Snyder, D. K., & Mitchell, A. E. (2008). Affective reconstructive couple therapy: A pluralistic, developmental approach. In A. S. Gurman (Ed.), *Clinical handbook of couple therapy* (4th ed., pp. 353–382). New York: Guilford.

Solomon, A. H. (2017). *Loving bravely: 20 lessons of self-discovery to help you get the love you want.* Oakland, CA: New Harbinger.

Solomon, M., & Tatkin, S. (2011). *Love and war in intimate relationships: Connection, disconnection, and mutual regulation in couple therapy.* New York: Norton.

Sprenkle, D. H., Davis, S. D., & Lebow, J. L. (2009). *Common factors in couple and family therapy: The overlooked foundation for effective practice.* New York: Guilford.

Spring, J. A. (2020). *After the affair: Healing the pain and rebuilding trust when a partner has been unfaithful* (3rd ed.). New York: Harper.

Stanley, S. M., Whitton, S. W., Clements, M. L., & Markman, H. J. (2006). Sacrifice as a predictor of marital outcomes. *Family Process, 45,* 289–303.

Steinglass, P. (1987). A systems view of family interaction and psychopathology. In: T. Jacob (Ed.), *Family interaction and psychopathology: Theories, methods and findings* (pp. 25–65). New York: Plenum Press.

Stiles, W. B., Honos-Webb, L., & Surko, M. (1998). Responsiveness in psychotherapy. *Clinical Psychology: Science and Practice, 5,* 439–458.

Stith, S. M., McCollum, E. E., & Rosen, K. H. (2011). *Couples treatment for domestic violence: Finding safe solutions.* Washington, DC: American Psychological Association.

Stith, S. M., Rosen, K. H., McCollum, E. E., & Thomsen, C. J. (2004). Treating intimate partner violence within intact couple relationships: Outcomes of multi-couple versus individual couple therapy. *Journal of Marital and Family Therapy, 30,* 305–318. https://doi.org/10.1111/j.1752-0606.2004.tb01242.x

Stricker, G., & Trierweiler, S. J. (1995). The local clinical scientist: A bridge between science and practice. *American Psychologist, 50,* 995–1002. https://doi.org/10.1037/0003-066X.50.12.995

Strong, G., & Aron, A. (2006). The effect of shared participation in novel and challenging activities on experienced relationship quality: Is it mediated by high positive affect? In K. Vohs & E. Finkel (Eds.), *Self and relationships: Connecting intrapersonal and interpersonal processes* (pp. 342–259). New York: Guilford.

Subirana-Malaret, M., Gahagan, J., & Parker, R. (2019). Intersectionality and sex and gender-based analyses as promising approaches in addressing intimate partner violence treatment programs among LGBT couples: A scoping review. *Cogent Social Sciences, 5*(1), 1644982. https://doi.org/10.1080/23311886.2019.1644982

Such, E. (2006). Leisure and fatherhood in dual-earner families. *Leisure Studies, 25*, 185–199.

Tambling, R. B. (2012). A literature review of therapeutic expectancy effects. *Contemporary Family Therapy, 34*, 402–415. https://doi.org/10.1007/s10591-012-9201-y

Tedeschi, R. G., & Calhoun, L. G. (2004). Posttraumatic growth: Conceptual foundations and empirical evidence. *Psychological Inquiry, 15*, 1–18.

Thibaut, J. W., & Kelly, H. H. (1959). *The social psychology of groups.* New York: Wiley.

Thomassin, K., Bucsea, O., Chan, K. J., & Carter, E. (2019). A thematic analysis of parents' gendered beliefs about emotion in middle childhood boys and girls. *Journal of Family Issues, 40*, 2944–2973.

Tolin, B. (2006). *101 common clichés of Alcoholics Anonymous: The sayings the newcomers hate and the oldtimers love.* Self-published.

Tolle, E. (2004). *The power of now: A guide to spiritual enlightenment.* New York: New World Library.

Tracey, T. J., & Kokotovic, A. M. (1989). Factor structure of the Working Alliance Inventory. *Psychological Assessment: A Journal of Consulting and Clinical Psychology, 1*, 207–210.

Trillingsgaard, T., Baucom, K. J. W., & Heyman, R. E. (2014). Predictors of change in relationship satisfaction during the transition to parenthood. *Family Relations, 63*, 667–679.

Tuber, S. (2008). *Attachment, play, and authenticity: A Winnicott primer.* New York: Jason Aronson.

van der Kolk, B. A. (2014). *The body keeps the score: Brain, mind, and body in the healing of trauma.* New York: Penguin.

Viereck, G. S. (1929, October 26). What life means to Einstein: An interview by George Sylvester Viereck. *Saturday Evening Post,* pp. 17, 110–113, 114, 117. https://www.saturdayeveningpost.com/wp-content/uploads/satevepost/what_life_means_to_einstein.pdf

Wachs, K., & Cordova, J. V. (2007). Mindful relating: Exploring mindfulness and emotion repertoires in intimate relationships. *Journal of Marital and Family Therapy, 3*, 464–481.

Wachtel, E. (2019). *The heart of couple therapy: Knowing what to do and how to do it.* New York: Guilford.

Wachtel, P. L. (2010). Beyond "ESTs": Problematic assumptions in the pursuit of evidence-based practice. *Psychoanalytic Psychology, 27*, 251–272. https://doi.org/10.1037/a0020532

Walsh, F. (Ed.). (2009). *Spiritual resources in family therapy* (2nd ed.). New York: Guilford.

Walsh, F. (Ed.). (2012). *Normal family processes: Growing diversity and complexity* (4th ed.). New York: Guilford.

Walsh, F. (2019). Social class, rising inequality, and the American Dream. In M. McGoldrick & K. V. Hardy (Eds.), *Re-visioning family therapy: Addressing diversity in clinical practice* (3rd ed., pp. 73–90). New York: Guilford.

Walters, M., Carter, B., Papp, P., & Silverstein, O. (1988). *The invisible web: Gender patterns in family relationships.* New York: Guilford.

Watson, M. F. (2013). *Facing the black shadow.* Self-published.

Watzlawick, P., Beavin-Bavelas, J. T., & Jackson, D. D. (1967). *The pragmatics of human communication: A study of interactional patterns, paradoxes, and pathologies.* New York: Norton.

Watzlawick, P., Weakland, P. H., & Fisch, R. (1974). *Change: Principles of problem formation and problem resolution.* New York: Norton.

Weiner, L., & Avery-Clark, C. (2017). *Sensate focus in sex therapy.* New York: Routledge.

Welter-Enderlin, R. (1993). Secrets of couples and couples therapy. In E. Imber-Black (Ed.), *Secrets in families and family therapy* (pp. 48–65). New York: Norton.

Whisman, M. A., & Beach, S. R. H. (2015). Couple therapy and depression. In A. S. Gurman, J. L. Lebow, & D. K. Snyder (Eds.), *Clinical handbook of couple therapy* (5th ed., pp. 585–605). New York: Guilford.

Whisman, M. A., Dixon, A. E., & Johnson, B. (1997). Therapists' perspectives of couple problems and treatment issues in couple therapy. *Journal of Family Psychology, 11*, 361–366.

Whisman, M. A., & Snyder, D. K. (2007). Sexual infidelity in a national survey of American women: Differences in prevalence and correlates as a function of method of assessment. *Journal of Family Psychology, 21*, 147–154.

White, M. (1988, Summer). The externalizing of the problem and the re-authoring of lives and relationships. *Dulwich Centre Newsletter*, 3–21.

White, M. (1991a). Deconstruction and therapy. *Dulwich Centre Newsletter, 3*, 21–40.

White, M. (1991b). Outside expert knowledge. *Australian and New Zealand Journal of Family Therapy, 12*, 207–214.

White, M. (1992). Deconstruction and therapy. In D. Epston & M. White (Eds.), *Experience contradiction, narrative, and imagination: Selected papers of David Epston and Michael White 1989–1991*. Adelaide: Dulwich Centre.

White, M. (1995). Behaviour and its determinants or action and its sense: Systems and narrative metaphors. In M. White (Ed.), *Reauthoring lives: Interviews and essays* (pp. 214–221). Adelaide: Dulwich Centre.

Williams, K. (2011). A socio-emotional relational framework for infidelity: The relational justice approach. *Family Process, 50*, 516–528.

Williams, K., & Knudson-Martin, C. (2013). Do therapists address gender and power in infidelity? A feminist analysis of the treatment literature. *Journal of Marital and Family Therapy, 39*, 271–384. https://doi.org/10.1111/j.1752-0606.2012.00303.x

Wilson, E. O. (1998). *Consilience: The unity of knowledge*. New York: Vintage.

Winfrey, O. (2016, January 4). *Interview with Thich Nhat Hanh* [Video]. YouTube. https://www.youtube.com/watch?v=dG2mMU1loGk

Winnicott, D. W. (1971). *Playing and reality*. London: Routledge.

Wolcott, I. H. (1986). Seeking help for marital problems before separation. *Australian Journal of Sex, Marriage and Family, 7*, 154–164.

Wood, B. (1985). Proximity and hierarchy: Orthogonal dimensions of family interconnectedness. *Family Process, 24*, 487–507.

Wright, J., Sabourin, S., Mondor, J., McDuff, P., & Mamodhoussen, S. (2006). The clinical representativeness of couple therapy outcome research. *Family Process, 46*, 301–316.

INDEX

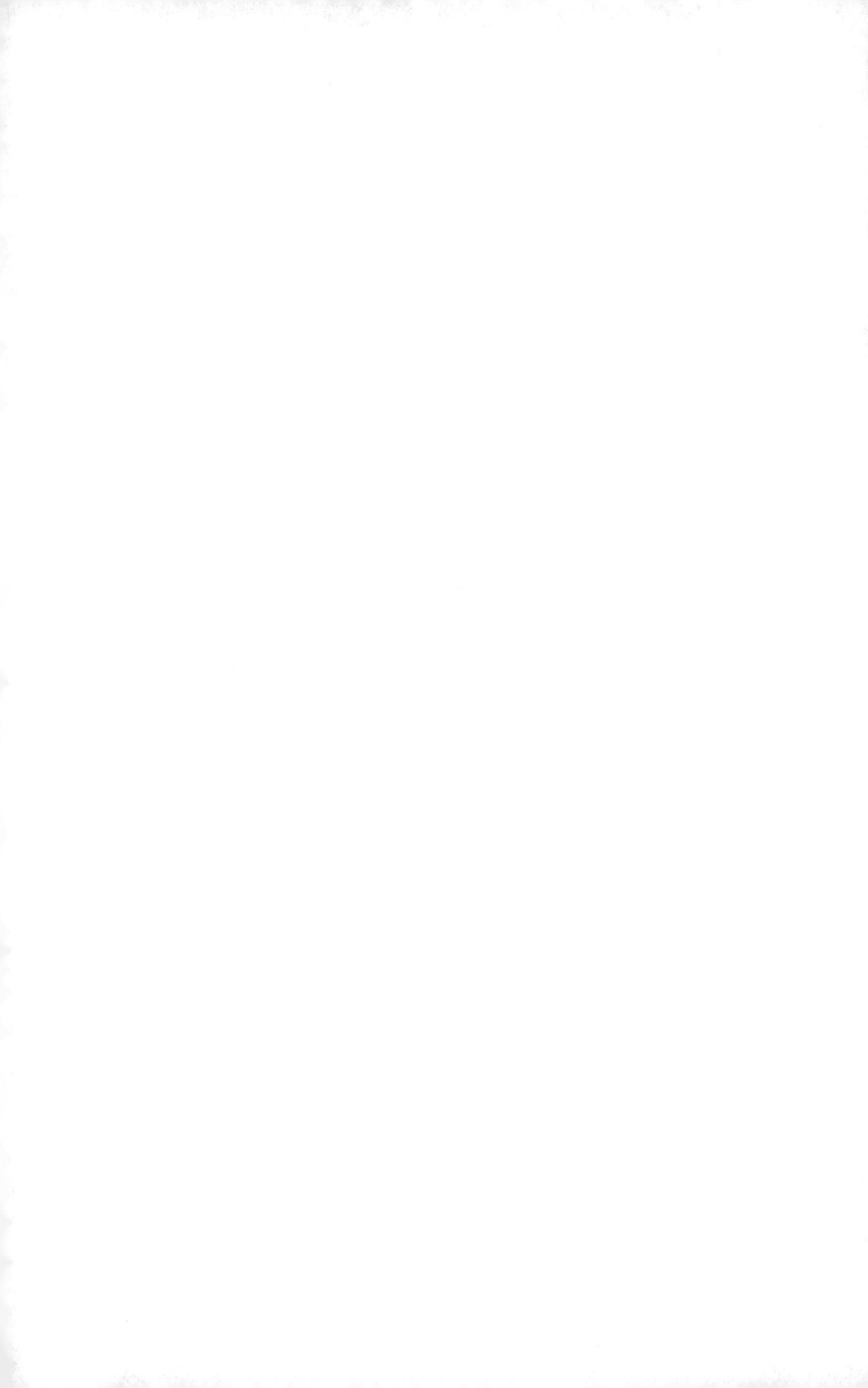

ABOUT THE AUTHOR

Peter Fraenkel, PhD, is associate professor of psychology at City College of New York; former faculty at the Ackerman Institute for the Family and NYU Medical Center; and is in private practice in New York City. He has published on a wide range of topics including integrative approaches to couple and family therapy, distress and divorce prevention, time issues in couples and families, collaborative family program development for minoritized groups, and family-based trauma. He is the author of *Sync Your Relationship, Save Your Marriage: Four Steps to Getting Back on Track* (2011, Palgrave-Macmillan), and coauthor of *The Relational Trauma of Incest: A Family-Based Approach to Treatment* (2001, Guilford). Dr. Fraenkel lectures and conducts therapist trainings internationally. He received the American Family Therapy Academy's 2012 award for Innovative Contribution to Family Therapy. He is a former vice president and current board member of AFTA, and a reviewer for several family therapy journals.